Evaluation
and
Management
of Gait
Disorders

NEUROLOGICAL DISEASE AND THERAPY

Series Editor

WILLIAM C. KOLLER

Department of Neurology
University of Kansas Medical Center
Kansas City, Kansas

Evaluation and Management of Gait Disorders

edited by
Barney S. Spivack

Norwalk Hospital
Norwalk, Connecticut
Yale University School of Medicine
New Haven, Connecticut

Marcel Dekker, Inc.   New York • Basel • Hong Kong

To Robin Oshman and to Josh Spivack,
who have encouraged me to remain mobile

Library of Congress Cataloging-in-Publication Data

Evaluation and management of gait disorders / edited by Barney S.
Spivack.
    p.   cm. -- (Neurological disease and therapy ; 35)
    Includes bibliographical references and index.
    ISBN 0-8247-9586-5 (hardcover : alk. paper)
    1. Gait disorders in old age. I. Spivack, Barney S.
II. Series: Neurological disease and therapy ; v. 35.
    [DNLM: 1. Gait. 2. Movement Disorders--etiology. 3. Movement
Disorders--diagnosis. 4. Movement Disorders--therapy. W1 NE33LD
v. 35 1995]
RC376.5.E94   1995
616.8'3--dc20
DNLM/DLC
for Library of Congress   94-24238
                                               CIP

The publisher offers discounts on this book when ordered in bulk quantities.
For more information, write to Special Sales/Professional Marketing at the
address below.

This book is printed on acid-free paper.

Marcel Dekker, Inc.
270 Madison Avenue, New York, New York 10016

Current printing (last digit):

10 9 8 7 6 5 4 3 2 1

PRINTED IN THE UNITED STATES OF AMERICA

Series Introduction

The goal of the *Neurological Disease and Therapy* series is to publish comprehensive books on topics of importance to the clinical neurologist, and which cover aspects of basic science as well as provide practical clinical information. The series covers a broad spectrum of neurological disorders, and has included topics such as Parkinson's disease, stroke, Alzheimer's disease, sleep disorders, many aspects of epilepsy, multiple sclerosis, tics and Tourette's syndrome, cerebellar diseases, trauma of the head and spine, brain tumors, and myasthenia gravis. The series has also focused on many therapeutic issues including the use of monamine oxidase inhibitors and botulinum toxin, and has addressed such general areas as neurotoxicology, neurovirology, and tremor disorders. Specific books have dealt with neuroepidemiology and neurology. It is hoped that these important reference texts will aid the clinician in managing their patients. Future books in the series will concentrate on applying our emerging knowledge in neurology to the care of patients in the clinic.

Evaluation and Management of Gait Disorders by Dr. Barney S. Spivack is an important contribution to the neurological series. Disturbances of mobility and gait are common problems seen in neurological practice, particularly in older individuals. Gait disorders can be due to lesions almost anywhere in the nervous system and represent a challenge to the treating physician. Aspects of treatment, including drugs, surgery, and rehabilitation, are discussed. This book provides anatomical, biomechanical, and physiological information on how all humans walk. Chapters 1 and 2 discuss clinical gait analysis and neural control of locomotion. Chapter 3 provides an excellent overview of neurological diseases causing gait disturbances. Gait dysfunction due to vestibular disease, cerebellar disease, and extrapyramidal disease is the subject of Chapters 4–6. Gait apraxia and gait abnormalities in elderly patients are addressed in Chapters 7 and 8. Chapters 9 and 10 deal with orthopedic disorders that can interfere with ambulation as well as the effects of medication. Chapter 11 is devoted to the important topic of falls in the elderly. The subjects of neuromuscular disease, rehabilitation, and the impact of physical activity on functional capability are addressed in Chapters 12–14. Patients presenting in the clinic with abnormal gaits can represent a significant diagnostic and management problem for the clinician. *Evaluation and Management of Gait Disorders* will be of value to all health-care professionals who are involved in the evaluation and management of individuals who have difficulty with balance and ambulation.

William C. Koller

Foreword

Understanding and treating disorders of mobility require a multidisciplinary perspective. Thus orthopedics, neurology, otolaryngology, physical therapy, and, more recently, geriatric medicine are all involved in treating these disorders. Much is already known about the biomechanics of mobility, and technology promises to add substantially to this database in the foreseeable future. By contrast, much less is known about the neural control of mobility and progress, while ongoing, has been slow.

Much has been written about the effects of neurological dysfunction on gait and balance, but no major breakthroughs have occurred. Early studies described the effects of basal ganglia and other degenerative diseases on gait. Much additional interest was generated following the description of normal pressure hydrocephalus (NPH) in the mid-1960s. Although interest in NPH was short-lived, it was replaced by an increasing emphasis on mobility in Parkinson's disease. In recent years, the increasing importance of vascular disease in the genesis of mobility dysfunction has been recognized. The neurologist's perspective, how-ever, is limited by his or her ability to describe the pathophysiology in only a small number of patients.

Second to cognitive impairment, problems of mobility, including falls, are the most pressing problems that older persons face. In recogniz-ing the magnitude and importance of this problem, funding agencies, most notably the National Institute on Aging, have provided financial support to help define the multiplicity of factors that conspire to produce mobility disorders and to move toward effective treatment. The focus is not directed toward treating specific disease pathophysiology but rather toward understanding the general mechanisms underlying mobility disor-ders and effecting improved general treatment strategies (e.g., physical therapy). This is currently an active area of research.

Also of importance is the increasing awareness of biomechanical dysfunction that may limit mobility. Joint replacement and increased understanding of the role of the foot and ankle, as well as strength, have made many of these disorders potentially treatable. Vestibular disorders can now be assessed due to the availability of sophisticated vestibular testing (e.g., computerized posturography and vestibular oculography). Treatment strategies are also evolving in this area. These technological advances have made it possible to study the mechanics of balance and mobility with both less costly equipment and greater precision. Thus, gait and balance analysis has become a reality outside of well-established centers.

This book presents a significant body of new information. Further-more, its multidisciplinary approach allows the reader to view mobility disorders in a broader context than in the past, thus providing an effec-tive contemporary perspective for diagnosis and treatment of patients with these conditions.

Leslie Wolfson, M.D.
Professor and Chair
Department of Neurology
University of Connecticut School of Medicine
Farmington, Connecticut

Preface

Disturbances of mobility and gait are common problems in current medical practice as physicians encounter an increasing number of older persons and others with chronic diseases limiting physical function. Mobility impairments contribute significantly to disability, activity limitation, and poor quality of life, and represent a major public health issue. The inability to transfer or ambulate independently is an important determinant of the need to provide home or institutional long-term care.

The increasing appreciation of the impact of mobility and gait impairments has been accompanied by a demand for medical educational materials at the undergraduate and graduate levels. Individuals with gait disorders present to physicians within varied medical disciplines. This volume is offered in the hope that it will be of value to neurologists, physiatrists, geriatricians, internists, family practitioners, medical students, physicians-in-training, and other medical specialists and researchers who evaluate and manage individuals with these impairments. Other health professionals, including therapists, nurse specialists, and physician extenders, may also find this book valuable, as may bioengineers and scientists engaged in balance and gait research.

There are several characteristics about the content and organization of this book that make it useful. Our approach and orientation has been to aid the clinician in the evaluation and management of individuals who have difficulty in ambulation. We review biomechanical, anatomical, and physiological factors in normal gait and gait patterns in healthy older persons, providing a basis for clinical gait analysis. Neurological diseases causing gait abnormalities, with reviews of extrapyramidal disease, gait apraxia, vestibular and cerebellar dysfunction, are emphasized. Other medical illnesses contributing to motor impairment and the adverse effects of medications on mobility and gait in older persons are highlighted. The appropriate evaluation of individuals who fall and recommended methods to minimize fall risk are presented. The adverse effects of immobilization, a common final pathway for many acute and chronic illnesses, are reviewed. Contributions from the gait laboratory are presented. The evaluation of walking devices and other adaptive aids and appropriate rehabilitation medicine modalities are reviewed, as most clinicians will be working with health professionals within this discipline in the management of individuals with gait problems. The importance of ongoing physical activity in later life and its impact on fitness and independent function is presented in the final chapter.

Our aim has been to bring together clinically relevant data from a number of different specialties which may supplement a more discipline-specific text. Much of what is included in this text is not found in neurology, general medicine, geriatric medicine, or subspecialty texts.

This volume will provide clinicians with a sound foundation in the assessment and management of gait disorders. It should enable physicians to better care for the disproportionate burden of illness borne by our increasingly large population of older individuals and others with mobility impairment.

I am grateful to Mr. Paul Dolgert, Executive Editor of Marcel Dekker, Inc., Medical Division, for providing this opportunity and to Ms. Elyce Misher, Production Editor, for her editorial assistance. I also appreciate the direction and encouragement provided by Dr. Steven Gambert and Dr. William Koller, and am grateful to Ms. Louisa Zajac of the Hospital for Special Care in New Britain, Connecticut and to Ms. Gloria Seymour of Norwalk Hospital, Norwalk, Connecticut for their assistance in the preparation of this monograph.

Barney S. Spivack

Contents

Contributors

Dennis J. Chapron, R.Ph., M.S.   Associate Professor, School of Pharmacy, University of Connecticut, Storrs, and University of Connecticut Health Center, Farmington, Connecticut

Sander L. Glatt, M.D.   Associate Professor, Department of Neurology, University of Kansas Medical Center, Kansas City, Kansas

Ming-Hsia Hu, P.T., Ph.D.   Associate Professor, School of Physical Therapy, College of Medicine, National Taiwan University, Taipei, Taiwan, Republic of China

Melvin H. Jahss, M.D.   Clinical Professor, Orthopedic Surgery, Mount Sinai School of Medicine; Chief, Orthopedic Foot Service, Hospital for Joint Diseases, New York, New York

James Oat Judge, M.D. Assistant Professor, Division of Geriatrics, Department of Medicine, University of Connecticut Health Center, Farmington, Connecticut

Wendy S. Kellner, M.D. Chief, Inpatient Rehabilitation, Department of Physiatry Medicine, Hospital for Special Care, New Britain, Connecticut

William C. Koller, M.D., Ph.D. Professor and Chairman, Department of Neurology, University of Kansas Medical Center, Kansas City, Kansas

David E. Krebs, Ph.D., P.T. Professor and Director, MGH Institute of Health Professions, Massachusetts General Hospital; Department of Orthopaedics, Harvard Medical School; and Department of Mechanical Engineering, Massachusetts Institute of Technology, Boston, Massachusetts

Joyce Lockert, M.S., P.T. MGH Institute of Health Professions, Massachusetts General Hospital, Boston, Massachusetts

Kevin C. O'Connor, M.D. University of Medicine and Dentistry of New Jersey, Newark, New Jersey

Lisa Oestreich, M.D. Department of Neurology, University of Rochester, Rochester, New York

Sylvia Ōunpuu, M.Sc. Gait Analysis Laboratory, Department of Orthopedics, Newington Children's Hospital, Newington, Connecticut

Aftab E. Patla, Ph.D. Professor, Neural Control Lab, Department of Kinesiology, University of Waterloo, Waterloo, Ontario, Canada

Linda S. Pescatello, Ph.D., F.A.C.S.M. Director, Health Promotion, New Britain General Hospital, New Britain, Connecticut

Kathleen M. Shannon, M.D. Department of Neurology, Rush-Presbyterian-St.Luke's Medical Center, Chicago, Illinois

Lewis Sudarsky, M.D. Assistant Chief, Neurology Service, Veterans Affairs Medical Center, West Roxbury; Assistant Professor, Department of Neurology, Harvard Medical School, Boston, Massachusetts

Rein Tideiksaar, Ph.D. Assistant Professor and Director, Falls and Immobility Program, Department of Geriatrics, Mount Sinai Medical Center, New York, New York

B. Todd Troost, M.D. Chairman and Professor, Department of Neurology, Bowman Gray School of Medicine, Wake Forest University, Winston-Salem, North Carolina

Robert E. White, M.D. Medical Director, Rehabilitation Hospital of Lafayette, Lafayette, Louisiana

Marjorie Woollacott, Ph.D. Department of Exercise and Movement Science, University of Oregon, Eugene, Oregon

1

Clinical Gait Analysis

SYLVIA ÕUNPUU

Newington Children's Hospital, Newington, Connecticut

I. INTRODUCTION

Gait analysis is defined as the objective documentation of gait. This is a broad definition for a large assortment of techniques ranging from observational gait analysis to computer-assisted three-dimensional (3-D) analysis of movement, all of which are referred to as "gait analysis." Computerized gait analysis, if defined as consisting of 3-D motion analysis, dynamic electromyography, and force plate data acquisition, more accurately defines the state of the art in terms of the technology that is available for clinical decision making. By providing objective documentation, including a description of how a patient walks (joint kinematics and temporal and stride variables) and information about the potential causes of movement abnormalities (joint kinetics and electromyographic data), clinicians are better equipped to make treatment decisions intended to improve a patient's ambulatory ability. This is very important in complex gait abnormalities where it is often difficult to observe and absorb all the problems at all joints. Computerized gait analysis does not replace the more traditional tools used in clinical decision making, such as assessments of joint range of motion and muscle strength and radiography. It should be used in conjunction with these tools to provide a more complete description of the patient. This is because gait analysis provides information about the movement (gait) which may differ from the information obtained when the patient is at rest. Gait analysis, however, does not dictate a specific treatment philosophy, such as multiple-level surgeries, but rather facilitates the decision-making process for the treatment of gait abnormalities. It does, however, allow for more complex treatment decisions by providing more complete information about a patient and allowing the clinician to evaluate more effectively the results of treatment.

Formal measurement of biomechanical parameters alone may not reveal how well individuals ambulate in their own environment. The functional approach to the assessment of mobility (Performance-Oriented Mobility Screen), which incorporates gait assessment and evaluates gait initiation, step height, length, symmetry and continuity, path deviation, trunk stability, walk stance, and turning while walking, is reviewed in Chapter 11. This functional approach to the assessment of mobility is especially valuable in the evaluation of frail older adults in whom there is a high prevalence of gait disorders due to the combined effects of neuromuscular and orthopedic diseases, sensory impairments, and side effects of commonly prescribed medications.

The purpose of this chapter is to introduce the reader to computer-aided gait analysis as a method of documentation and evaluation of gait abnormalities. Gait analysis provided by one laboratory does not necessarily provide the same amount of quality of information as that provided by another. Even more importantly, information that appears similar at the surface, for example, hip joint angle, may not be measured in the same manner from one laboratory to the next. The following pages will describe a method of computerized gait analysis specific to the system used at the Newington Children's Hospital Gait Analysis Laboratory. It is important for any clinician who is using gait analysis as a part of the treatment decision-making process to have basic knowledge about methods of data collection and correlation with the anatomy as well as appreciation for the methods of calculation of the various gait parameters. This chapter will focus on variables used to describe gait such as joint kinematics (joint motion), joint kinetics, temporal parameters, and muscle activation (electromyography).

II. CLINICAL GAIT ANALYSIS

A. Definition and Purpose

Clinical gait analysis may be defined as the systematic assessment of human locomotion through objective documentation of gait patterns. The purposes of gait analysis are to: (1) document an individual's gait function; (2) aid in treatment decision making for the correction of gait abnormalities; and (3) aid in treatment evaluation. The most common use of routine clinical gait analysis is in the surgical decision-making process for ambulatory children with neuromuscular disorders such as cerebral palsy (1–9). A valuable contribution to this process is the evaluation of the orthopedic intervention after a patient regains strength. This is probably the next most common use of clinical gait analysis. The information gained in treatment evaluation allows for change and progress in treatment protocol development. Gait analysis used as documentation of patient function over time or for evaluation of less invasive treatment such as drug therapy has been generally limited to research applications. When a better understanding of specific pathologies such as Parkinson's disease is available, it is possible that, for example, gait analysis will become a routine tool for evaluating a patient's status to determine prognosis. Also, computerized gait analysis lends itself well to research because of utilization of computerized data storage.

B. The Appropriate Patient Referral

Computerized gait analysis may be appropriate for any adult or child who has a gait problem that requires treatment. It is most commonly used on patients with neuromuscular disorders because of the complexity of the associated gait abnormalities and subsequent difficulty in making clinical decisions that may be invasive and irreversible. This includes disorders such as cerebral palsy, stroke, traumatic brain injury, and myelomeningocele, to name a few. For these patient populations, gait analysis is primarily used to help make decisions for orthopedic surgeries rather than for more conservative treatment methods such as physical therapy and orthotics. Gait analysis is also very useful as a research tool in applications such as the long-term evaluation of progressive disorders or evaluation of the effect of different types of orthotic and prosthetic devices on gait.

Gait analysis techniques may not be appropriate for all people with gait abnormalities. There are a few restrictions that are measurement system specific. These issues are discussed in the Section V.C.

C. Gait Analysis Methods

The necessary components for a complete gait analysis include: (1) videotaping, before the application of external measurement devices applied during the motion data collection; (2) joint range of motion and strength; (3) bony abnormalities (determined clinically and radiographically); (4) temporal and stride parameters; (5) joint kinematics (motion) in three dimensions; (6) joint kinetics (if force plate information can be obtained); and (7) muscle activation patterns during gait. The integration of all this information will provide the most complete picture of an individual's ambulation. The following sections provide brief descriptions of these seven components.

1. Videotaping

Videotaping provides qualitative documentation about the way a person walks. It is very difficult to evaluate the "smoothness" or "fluidity" of a gait pattern without a video record. The ability to obtain simultaneous coronal and sagittal plane views with a split screen increases the clinician's appreciation of the degree of "out-of-plane" motion seen in many gait disorders. Furthermore, slow motion and stop-framing enhanced video techniques and zooming capabilities, which can provide close-up views of the feet, may be the only means of evaluating the motion and position of the hind foot. Video records taken during the motion data collection also provide a good check for potential problems that may not be noticed during actual data collection, such as a partially detached marker or an atypical stride.

2. Clinical Assessment

The clinical assessment provides information about the joint range of motion, joint contractures, and muscle strength that can be correlated with joint kinematics and kinetics to help determine the potential causes of gait abnormalities (Table 1). The specific measures required will depend somewhat on the patient's underlying condition. When evaluating patients with gait disorders, the following measures have been found useful: hip flexion/extension, abduction/adduction, and internal/external rotation; knee flexion/extension and distal hamstring tightness; ankle plantarflexion/dorsiflexion; forefoot and hindfoot inversion/eversion. These measures are limited because of their subjective nature and, therefore, should be used in conjunction with objective measures. Also, strength measures obtained from children need to be interpreted with caution because of potential difficulties in cooperation, understanding, and producing "maximal" resistive effort. Clinical assessment also includes evaluation of the predominant type of muscle tone if applicable.

3. Bony Abnormalities

Assessment of bony abnormalities such as tibial torsion and femoral anteversion also assist in determining the cause of gait abnormalities. Computerized axial tomographic and Magilligan radiographic methods are commonly used to measure femoral anteversion. Femoral anteversion may also be estimated by a palpation method as described by Ruwe et al. (10). The patient is placed in a prone position with the knee flexed to 90 degrees (Fig. 1). The shank is then rotated externally while palpating the position of the femoral neck. When the femoral neck is parallel to the table (or the greater trochanter is in its most lateral position) the angle between the shank and the vertical is measured (11). Noninvasive techniques, such as measuring the foot–thigh angle or bimalleolar axis (11), are most commonly used in the estimation of tibial torsion. In both these techniques, the patient lies prone with the knee flexed to 90 degrees. The orientation of the foot is measured in relation to the knee axis or the long axis of the thigh (Fig. 1). Unfortunately, the intraobserver variability for the estimation of tibial torsion is quite high.

4. Temporal and Stride Variables

This component of gait analysis includes measures such as velocity, cadence, stride length, step length, and percentage of stance to swing. These measures can provide an indication of the level of function when compared to normal values. They can also be compared to previous values from the same patient to evaluate treatment effects. A potential problem in using these measures in the evaluation of treatment arises in children who typically undergo stature changes in the time between treatment evaluations. Temporal and stride variables are stature dependent. For example, step and stride lengths and walking velocity will typically increase with an increase in stature. Therefore, these measurements must be corrected in some manner to account for changes in

Table 1 Preoperative and Postoperative Clinical Examination Results

| | Preop | | | | Postop | | | |
| | Motion | | Strength | | Motion | | Strength | |
	right	left	right	left	right	left	right	left
Hips								
flexion	F	F	5	4	F	F	4+	4+
extension (knee @ 0°)	−5	−5	5	4	−10	−5	5	4+
extension (knee @ 90°)			5	4			5	4
abduction (hip @ 0°)	45	20	4+	4	35	30	5	4
abduction (hip @ 90°)	45	25			−	−		
adduction	F	F			F	F		
internal rotation	30	75			35	45		
external rotation	50	10			45	40		
femoral anteversion	5	60			5	5		
Knees								
extension (hip @ 0°)	5	0			0	0		
extension (hip @ 90°)	−35	−55	5	4+	−45	−50	5	4
hamstring tightness	M>L	M			M>L	M		
flexion	F	F	5	4−	F	F	5	4
Ankles								
dorsiflexion (knee @ 0°)	15	−5			10	−15		
dorsiflexion (knee @ 90°)	20	0	5	1	15	0	4+	1
plantarflexion	F	F	5	2−	F	F	4	1
Forefoot								
inversion	F	F	5	1+	F	F	4+	2−
eversion	F	F	5	U	F	F	5	U

Table 1 Continued

	Preop				Postop			
	Motion		Strength		Motion		Strength	
	right	left	right	left	right	left	right	left
Hindfoot								
inversion	F	F			F	F		
eversion	F	0			F	F		
foot–thigh angle	10+	10+			15+	5+		
Reflexes								
Duncan Ely	−	2			−	−		
ankle clonus	−	+			−	−		
confusion	−	+			−	+		
Leg lengths	87.5	88.0			95.0	94.0		

F, full range; U, unable to isolate; M, medial; L, lateral

height. Also, these measurements are very "mood" dependent with large variations possible. When comparing with normal temporal and stride values, the values should be matched by height, not age. In children with stature below normal for age, age-matched comparison may result in overestimation of the "expected" values. Conversely, in older patients, these measurements decrease according to age. Therefore, temporal and stride variables should be matched by age in these patients.

Temporal and stride measurements are also referred to as "outcome" measures because they cannot be applied directly to the cause of gait abnormalities or used in treatment decision making. As a result, their utility as a stand-alone tool is somewhat limited for clinical decision making.

Temporal and stride measurements are typically calculated using the motion measurement system along with foot switches. Foot switches are small devices that are applied to the base of the foot in specific locations to indicate when a specific portion of the foot is not in contact with the ground. Many simpler methods of obtaining this information have been developed for use when a motion system is not available. These include foot prints and instrumented walkways.

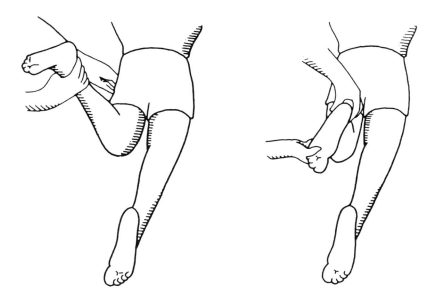

Figure 1   Techniques for estimating femoral anteversion (left) and foot–thigh angle (right) during the clinical examination.

5. Joint Kinematics

Joint kinematics include variables used to describe the spatial movement of the body without considering the forces that cause the movement. These include linear and angular displacements, linear and angular velocities, and linear and angular accelerations. Angular displacements that describe the motion of the joints during the gait cycle are the most commonly reported. The actual angle definitions for these variables, which may vary depending on the laboratory, are given in the next section. Currently, one of the most successful techniques for obtaining joint motion data for clinical use is the use of reflective marker systems. Reflective joint markers are aligned with respect to specific bony landmarks on the pelvis and both lower extremities (Fig. 2). Through the recording of reflected infrared light, the three-dimensional location of each marker is determined. Joint angle motion is then determined using Euler angles (12, 13).

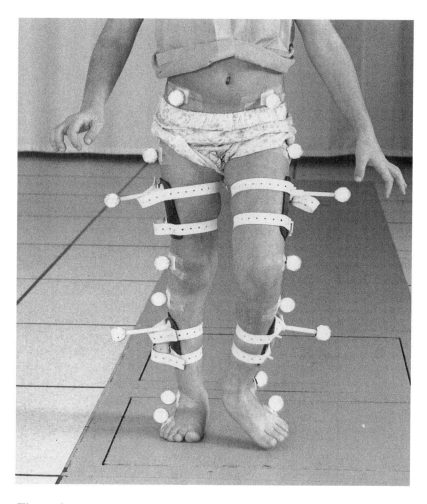

Figure 2 Patient walking with joint markers. Joint markers are used to define segments and joint locations; right and left ASIS, PSIS wand (not seen in figure), proximal marker along long axis of thigh, wand on midthigh, lateral femoral epicondyle, wand on midshank, lateral malleolus, and lateral fifth metatarsal head markers.

6. Joint Kinetics

Relative to the descriptive joint kinematics, joint kinetics provide more information about the cause of motion abnormalities (14,15). Calculations can be made only when force plate and joint kinematic information are obtained simultaneously. Force plate data are valid only if one foot falls within the boundaries of the force plate. As a result, in patients with very small step lengths, valid force plate data will not be possible and joint kinetics cannot be calculated.

For clinical gait applications, the joint kinetic data most typically used are joint moments and joint powers. Joint moments refer to a body's response to an external load and indicate the dominant muscle group. For example, a net knee extensor moment means the knee extensors are dominant. Joint powers refer to the net rate of generating or absorbing energy and are the product of the joint moment and the joint angular velocity. Joint powers are related to the type of muscle contraction. A net power generation is associated with concentric contraction and net power absorption is associated with eccentric muscle contraction.

Joint kinetics, which are determined mathematically, cannot be observed like joint kinematics. Therefore, they are less intuitive and require some knowledge about the method of calculation. Two methods used to calculate joint kinetics are the resultant ground reaction force method and the inverse dynamic method; both are reported routinely in the literature (13). The resultant ground reaction force (GRF) method, which is based on the position of body segments in relation to the resultant ground reaction force, is calculated by multiplying the resultant GRF (obtained from the force plate) by the perpendicular distance from the estimated joint center of rotation. The errors associated with this method are discussed in detail in a paper by Wells (16). In brief, the error increases as the joint is proximal and it is not possible to calculate the joint moments and powers that occur in the swing phase. The second method, which involves a process commonly referred to as inverse dynamics, uses Newton's Laws of Motion and includes the effect of body segment masses and moments of inertia in the final moment calculations. Although both methods make assumptions, the second and more complex method is recommended (for detailed discussions of methods used to calculate joint moments and powers, see Refs. 13 and 17).

Another complicating factor in the interpretation of joint kinetic data is the inconsistency in the conventions used. For data presented in this chapter, plots indicate the net muscle moment. Therefore, the data represent the body's response to an external load and correspond to the electromyographic (EMG) data collected. Another approach plots the "external" moments applied to the body. This method does not corroborate with other data collected and thus requires the interpreter to take a second step to determine the body's response.

7. Muscle Activity

The muscle activity during locomotion may be measured using dynamic EMG. The EMG techniques used in clinical gait analysis typically provide the clinician with on/off information of a particular muscle during the gait cycle. Electromyographic signal amplitude information is limited if normalization techniques are not used. Unfortunately, normalization techniques are not practical for routine clinical application. Normalization to maximum levels of voluntary contraction is difficult in clinical populations when pain is involved and when the patient is young, and impossible in these populations where voluntary isolated motion is not possible. Normalization to the maximum or average level of activity over the gait cycle is another common method of EMG amplitude normalization (18). Unfortunately, absolute amplitude information is lost when any of these normalization methods are performed (19). The amplitude of an EMG signal is also affected by other factors such as interelectrode distance and distance between electrode and muscle tissue of interest (17). Therefore, it is not valid to compare the EMG amplitude across muscles or in the same muscle on different limbs. Dynamic EMG does not provide information related to the strength or force generated by a muscle during contraction unless the signal recorded during gait is normalized (or represented in relation) to a known force or a maximum voluntary contraction (19).

Muscle activation is measured by placing electrodes on (surface) or in (fine wire) the particular muscle of interest. Surface electrodes are used for individual muscles or muscle groups just under the skin surface. Fine wire electrodes are typically used for deep muscles such as the posterior tibialis and toe flexors. The advantages of each electrode type have been discussed in detail (17, 20). Generally, fine wire electrodes should be used when necessary, that is, when the muscle of interest is deep (under other surface muscles) or when the surface muscle of interest is very small. Using surface electrodes on "small" muscles poses the risk of "cross-talk"—when activity of an adjacent muscle is recorded along with activity from the muscle of interest. The use of fine wire electrodes for large surface muscles provides no advantage over the surface electrode in the quality of EMG signal (21). Fine wire electrodes may also cause cramping and increase the level of spasticity in children with spastic disorders. This may ultimately modify a patient's "typical" walking pattern.

For quality control, the raw (or original) EMG signal must be examined initially to evaluate the signal for potential artifacts that may not be evident after the signal is processed. Then, different techniques such as full-wave rectification, linear enveloping, and integration can be used to process the raw EMG signal (17). Each has advantages depending on the application of the EMG data. Some type of processing is necessary if EMG data are to be averaged across strides or patients.

D. Test Protocol

The actual time required for a gait analysis assessment varies depending on the number of tests performed and the level of cooperation of the patient. As a result, the time taken to perform a gait analysis varies from laboratory to laboratory, despite the common title of gait analysis. A full gait analysis that includes all the above parameters will require approximately 3–3.5 h. The analysis is usually performed in the following order: videotaping, clinical assessment, motion analysis, and EMG. Fine wire EMG is collected last if required. Motion and EMG data are not collected simultaneously to avoid overencumbering the patient with hardware. Evaluation of barefoot as well as brace conditions can extend the length of a test. Multiple gait strides of each condition are also collected to determine if a patient is walking consistently from stride to stride. Testing can be completed with walking aids such as walkers or crutches if these aids do not interfere with the markers or consistently block their view from the cameras. If walking aids cannot be used, hand-held assistance (whereby two people help the patient walk through the test space) may be required.

III. NORMAL GAIT

Normal gait can be described by tracking the motion of a specific joint throughout the gait cycle or by looking at each phase of the gait cycle and defining the motion/position of all joints. First, however, it is necessary to understand the joint angle definitions before attempting to interpret joint kinematic data on plots. The reader is referred to the Appendix for terminology related to Section III.A.

A. Joint Kinematics

This section will describe normal joint kinematics for the pelvis, hip, knee, and ankle in the coronal, sagittal, and transverse planes of motion. Each angle's anatomical definition is included along with a description of the joint motion and a plot of the motion with respect to the gait cycle. Joint angle definitions are dependent on the marker set used to collect the data and thus are laboratory dependent. Although this does not make much difference at the knee which is intuitively the relationship between the thigh and shank, the hip angle is less clear and may be a representation of the thigh segment to the vertical (used when pelvis position is not monitored) or the thigh in relation to the pelvis. Unfortunately, in the literature both angle definitions are used under the same title: hip flexion/extension. Differences in marker set placement and thus joint angle definitions, however, limit the ability of data to be compared directly from laboratory to laboratory.

Like most gait variables, joint kinematics are best communicated through the use of plots (Fig. 3). Plots are the most efficient way to communicate "time series" data because they relate the degrees of motion to the timing of events in the gait cycle. Unfortunately, the format of joint kinematic plots varies depending on the laboratory, a situation which has contributed to the confusion new clinicians experience when interpreting gait data. The following is a description of the format used at the Newington Gait Laboratory, which is one of the more common formats seen in the literature (Fig. 3). The vertical axis represents the degrees of motion at a specific joint. Usually, the neutral position of the joint is at zero degrees, which is represented by a horizontal line in the middle or at the bottom of the graph. The vertical axis is also labeled according to the position of the joint on either side of neutral (for example, flexion and extension). The horizontal axis represents time and usually is given in units of percent of gait cycle. The stance phase begins at initial contact or 0% of the gait cycle. The vertical line at 60% of the gait cycle indicates toe-off, which marks the beginning of the swing phase or the last 40% of the gait cycle. All joint kinematic plots in this chapter are graphed in this format. Some variations in plotting formats are seen in the literature such as the beginning the gait cycle with the swing phase or expressing time intervals in seconds rather than percent of the gait cycle. Unfortunately, this inconsistency results in confusion.

During normal gait, the majority of motion occurs in the sagittal plane. In pathological gait, there is typically reduced motion in the

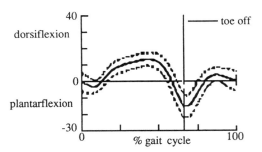

Figure 3 Typical plot format used for the presentation of kinematic and kinetic data. The following is an example of normal ankle motion in the sagittal plane.

sagittal plane and much greater motion in the coronal and transverse planes. Motion in these two planes is a function of compensations needed as coping responses for limited motion and deviations in the sagittal plane or a direct result of the underlying condition. Therefore, clinicians must compare motion in each plane with normal motion. The following is a description of normal gait kinematics for children after gait maturation, which occurs at about age 5 (22). After a child matures, gait patterns are similar to those found in young adults. Gait kinematics and kinetics begin to show consistent changes in older adults (23). These include reductions in range of motion and changes in temporal and stride parameters that are not consistent in relation to stature as found in younger adults.

Before the joint motion is described, the precise angle definition is given. The exact angle is determined by the joint and segment marker locations that should ultimately relate in some logical way to the anatomy. Unfortunately, joint marker positions vary from laboratory to laboratory because of different alignment protocols. Joint angles, that is, hip, knee, and ankle, are relative angles and describe the relationship between adjacent segments. The joint angles define the motion of the distal segment in relation to the proximal segment. As such, observers should be oriented so that they view the motion of the second segment from the appropriate position on the first segment. The only exceptions to this are pelvic motion and foot progression. Pelvic motion is the motion of the pelvis in relation to the laboratory coordinate system and foot progression is the orientation of the foot to the line of progression.

Motion will also be described with respect to the phases of the gait cycle (Figs. 4 and 5).

1. Sagittal Plane

Pelvis   Pelvic motion is defined as the absolute position of the pelvis in relation to the laboratory. It is the angle between the line connecting the anterior superior iliac spine (ASIS) and the posterior superior iliac spine (PSIS) to the horizontal [Fig. 6(a)]. The normal pelvis is usually tilted anteriorly between 4 to 10 degrees. A mild oscillating pattern causes an increasing anterior tilt during midstance and initial swing; the overall range of motion of about 4 degrees [Fig. 6(a)]. If the line joining the ASIS to PSIS were parallel to the floor, there would be zero tilt (as indicated by the horizontal axis of the plot).

Hip   The hip joint is defined as the relative angle between a line perpendicular to the pelvic transverse plane and the long axis of the thigh after both lines are projected onto the pelvic sagittal plane [Fig. 6(b)]. As a result, information about the absolute position of the thigh (i.e., whether the thigh reaches a vertical position) is not given by this variable. The hip extends throughout stance phase from maximum flexion (37 degrees), which is attained in terminal swing, to maximum extension in terminal stance (6 degrees); flexion begins in preswing and continues throughout the swing phase [Fig. 6(b)]. In normal gait, the overall range of motion is about 43 degrees.

Knee   The knee joint is defined as the angle between the long axis of the thigh and the long axis of the shank. Knee motion is characterized by two waves of flexion/extension, one in stance and one in swing [Fig. 6(c)]. The knee flexes in loading response (20 degrees) and then extends; it begins flexing again in terminal stance, reaching about 45 degrees of flexion at toe-off. The second peak knee flexion (64 degrees) occurs at approximately 33% of the swing phase. This is critical for foot clearance of the swing limb, which is in the range of a few millimeters in normal gait. The knee normally does not extend fully at an initial contact or in terminal stance. Normal range of knee motion is about 60 degrees.

Ankle   The ankle joint is defined as the angle between the long axis of the shank and the plantar aspect of the foot. The overall range of motion is about 30 degrees with two waves of plantarflexion followed by dorsiflexion [Fig. 6(d)]. Peak dorsiflexion (12 degrees) is reached in terminal stance followed by peak plantarflexion (18 degrees) in initial swing.

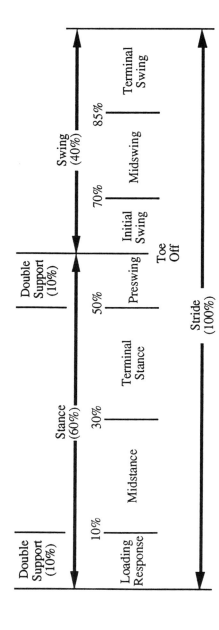

Figure 4   Graphic depicting the phases of the gait cycle and their proportions as percentages of the gait cycle.

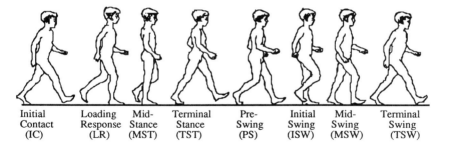

Initial Contact (IC)	Loading Response (LR)	Mid-Stance (MST)	Terminal Stance (TST)	Pre-Swing (PS)	Initial Swing (ISW)	Mid-Swing (MSW)	Terminal Swing (TSW)

Figure 5 The phases of the gait cycle shown with the corresponding body position for sagittal plane motion.

Ankle motion in stance is also frequently defined by the ankle rockers as illustrated in Figure 7. First rocker takes place from initial contact to foot flat, or the loading response portion of the gait cycle. During this phase, there is controlled lowering of the foot to the ground with a relative plantarflexion motion at the joint. This motion is controlled by the eccentric contraction of the ankle dorsiflexors and thus is consistent with a net power absorption. Second rocker takes place from midstance through terminal stance when the tibia is rotating forward over the plantigrade foot. This motion is controlled by the eccentric contraction of the ankle plantarflexors (power absorption). Finally, third rocker takes place in preswing when the heel is lifting from the ground and the ankle is actively plantarflexing. This motion is produced by the concentric contraction of the ankle plantarflexors (power generation).

2. Coronal Plane

Pelvis Pelvic motion refers to the absolute position of the pelvis in relation to the laboratory and is measured as the angle between the line connecting the ASISs and the horizontal [Fig. 8(a)]. The pelvis rises from midswing and loading response and drops from midstance to initial swing. The overall range of motion of the pelvis is about 8 degrees with the neutral position (pelvis parallel to the floor) occurring in midstance and midswing [Fig. 8(a)].

Hip The hip joint is defined as the relative angle between a line perpendicular to the pelvic transverse plane and the long axis of the thigh after both lines are projected onto the pelvic coronal plane [Fig. 8(b)]. As a result, absolute position of the thigh (i.e., whether the thigh

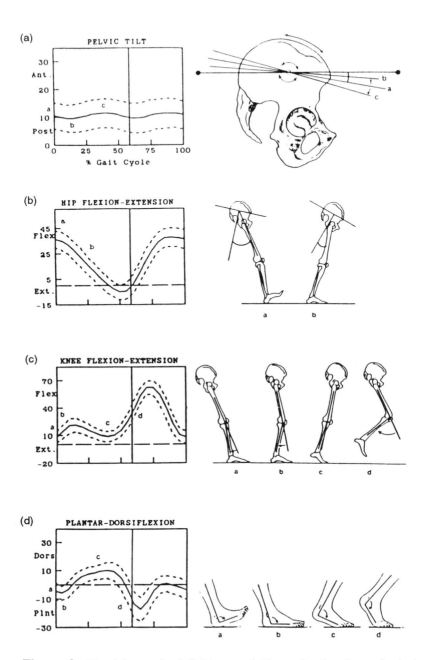

Figure 6 The joint angle definitions and kinematics for the sagittal plane motion of the (a) pelvis; (b) hip; (c) knee; and (d) ankle.

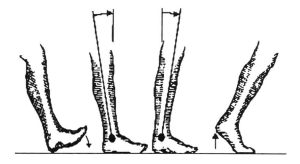

first rocker   second rocker   third rocker

Figure 7   A drawing of the ankle joint rockers.

reaches a vertical position) is not given. Hip motion in the coronal plane mimics the motion of the pelvis in the coronal plane [Fig. 8(b)]. The hip generally reaches peak adduction during loading response and progressively abducts throughout the remainder of stance, reaching peak abduction in initial swing. The overall range of motion of 13 degrees.

3. Transverse Plane

Pelvis   Pelvic motion is defined as the absolute position of the pelvis in relation to the laboratory. It is defined by the angle between the line connecting the ASIS's to a line perpendicular to the line of progression. The overall range of motion of the pelvis is about 8 degrees, consisting of a few degrees of internal rotation at initial contact, external rotation during stance, slight external rotation at toe-off, and internal rotation in swing [Fig. 9(a)]].

Hip   The hip joint is defined as the relative angle between a line joining the ASISs and a line connecting the medial and lateral epicondyles after the latter have been projected onto the pelvic transverse plane (note that the line joining the ASISs already exists in this plane) [Fig. 9(b)]. As a result, absolute position of the thigh is not given. The thigh in relation to the pelvis is slightly internally rotated throughout the majority of the stance phase and externally rotates in initial swing with an overall range of motion of about 8 degrees [Fig. 8(b)].

Foot Progression   The foot progression angle is the angle between the long axis of the foot (as represented by the second metatarsal

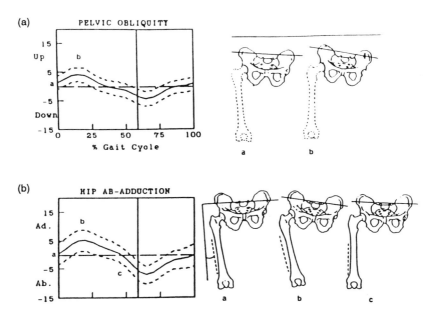

Figure 8   The joint angle definitions and kinematics for the coronal plane motion of the (a) pelvis and (b) hip.

projected onto the floor) and the line of progression [Fig. 9(c)]. In normal gait, the foot is rotated slightly external to the direction of progression; however, there is large intrasubject variability [Fig. 9(c)]. The foot externally rotates in initial swing with an overall range of motion of approximately 6 degrees.

The plots described above have been arranged in a format illustrated in Figure 10 which provides a summary of the motion of the lower extremities and pelvis in three planes on one page. This is a useful format that allows for easy comparison across joints and planes. The data on the plots represent the mean [1 standard deviation (s.d.)] of normal children ranging in age from 5 to 14 years. These data are representative of normal adult patterns (22).

B. Temporal and Stride Variables

Temporal and stride variables are stature dependent and show many changes during the development of gait and during growth. As a result, a

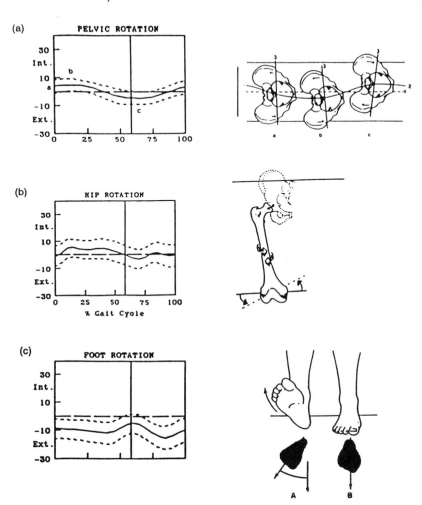

Figure 9 The joint angle definitions and kinematics for the transverse plane motion of the (a) pelvis; (b) hip; (c) foot progression.

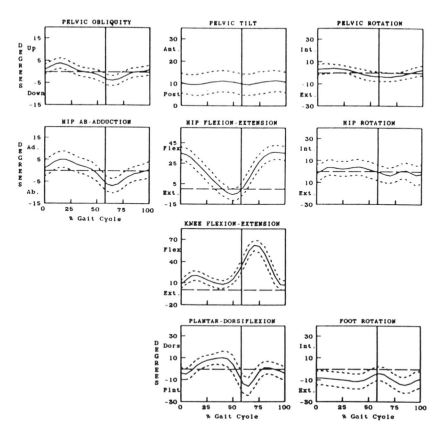

Figure 10   Joint kinematics in the coronal (first column), sagittal (second column), and transverse (third column) planes (mean ± 1 s.d.). Data are normalized to 100% of the stride; stance phase is followed by swing and toe-off is indicated by the vertical line.

normal database for these variables must include information across various statures. The most comprehensive work evaluating the changes in these parameters through the maturation of gait has been completed by Sutherland and coworkers (24). These measures generally vary greatly in normal adult gait because of differences in stature as well as other variables that affect these measurements. The normal values we use for comparison of children ranging in age from 5–20 are included in Table 2.

Table 2 Summary of the Temporal and Stride Variables for Groups of Children with Normal Gait. The groups are divided according to leg length. The expected temporal and stride parameter ranges may be determined by selecting the group with the appropriate leg length and then referring to the reported ranges for other selected parameters.

	Leg length (cm)	Height (in.)	Step (cm)	Stride (cm)	Cadence (steps/min)	Velocity (cm/s)
Group 1 (*n*=12)						
mean	58	47	47	94	139	109
s.d.	2.2	1.4	2.6	5.9	10.5	9.7
maximum	61	49	52	104	160	127
minimum	54	45	43	80	122	94
Group 2 (*n*=10)						
mean	65	51	56	109	131	119
s.d.	1.7	1.9	5.5	7.1	7.5	7.9
maximum	67	53	68	120	141	134
minimum	61	48	48	97	114	107
Group 3 (*n*=12)						
mean	70	53	56	114	133	127
s.d.	2.1	1.1	3.7	8.2	12.3	13.8
maximum	73	55	63	130	160	144
minimum	68	51	51	106	111	99
Group 4 (*n*=10)						
mean	78	58	62	123	126	130
s.d.	2.8	2.1	3.7	6.8	8.8	8.6
maximum	82	63	68	139	139	143
minimum	74	55	56	110	111	114
Group 5 (*n*=12)						
mean	87	64	65	128	114	122
s.d.	2.8	2.1	4.3	8.5	8.5	12.0
maximum	92	69	73	142	133	146
minimum	83	61	59	116	103	100

C. Muscle Activity

Normal muscle activity has been documented by many groups (20, 25–27). The work of Sutherland and associates on the development of gait (24) includes the changes in muscle activation patterns that occur up until 7 years of age when they approximate normal adult patterns. The presentation of these normative data comes in two formats, the bar plot (25) and

Table 3   Normal Muscle Activity During Gait

1. Hip abductors
    active during stance for pelvic stability
    during loading response
        controls pelvic drop on swing side by limiting stance side hip adduction
        eccentric contraction
    during midstance
        produces pelvis rise on swing side by producing stance side hip abduction
        concentric contraction
2. Gluteus maximus
    active terminal swing and loading response
        produces hip extension
        concentric contraction
    muscle elongated before contraction during hip flexion in swing
3. Iliacus
    active in terminal preswing and initial swing
        initiates hip flexion
        concentric contraction
    elongation before contraction during hip extension in first half of stance
4. Quadriceps
    activity varies with walking velocity
    active during initial contact and loading response
        initially restricts/controls knee flexion
        eccentric contraction
        secondly active knee extension
        concentric contraction
    at higher velocities activity is seen at toe-off
        slow knee flexion
        eccentric contraction
5. Hamstrings
    active during terminal swing
        decelerate swinging leg
        eccentric contraction
    active during loading response
        hip extension
        concentric contraction
    elongation before shortening during hip flexion in swing
6. Adductors
    individual variation is high
    active during toe-off and initial swing
        aid in hip flexion
        concentric contraction

Table 3   Continued

---

active during terminal swing
   internally rotate femur
7. Triceps surae
   active during midstance and terminal stance
   controls forward progression of the tibia during ankle dorsiflexion
      initially elongation/eccentric
   ankle plantarflexion
      concentric contraction
   peroneal action is similar
8. Tibialis anterior and toe extensors
   active during loading response
      control lowering of the forefoot to the floor
      eccentric contraction
   active at toe-off and in-swing
      dorsiflex the ankle for clearance
      concentric contraction

---

the ensemble-averaged linear envelope (26). When interpreting the raw EMG signal, it becomes apparent that muscles do not generally show precise on and off patterns but show a gradual onset and cessation of activity. This information is not available in the bar plot and may result in misinterpretation of the EMG signal. Also, variability of the EMG signal is high with respect to the other gait variables (28). These points should be kept in mind when interpreting the pathological EMG signal.

Types of Muscle Contraction   The principal function of muscles is to accelerate (concentric contraction) and decelerate (eccentric contraction) angular motions of the limbs and stabilize (isometric contraction) position. During gait, muscles contract in one of three ways depending on the point in the gait cycle: concentric contraction occurs when a muscle is shortening under tension; eccentric contraction occurs when a muscle is lengthening under tension; and isometric contraction occurs when a muscle develops tension without a change in length. Table 3 provides descriptions of normal muscle activity of some of the major muscle groups during gait (29).

Most muscles are active at the beginning and end of the swing and the stance phases with minimal muscle activity in midstance and midswing. Generally, elongation of the muscle occurs through passive stretch or eccentric contraction before shortening contractions take place. The normal activity of the major muscle groups that are active during gait are presented in the bar graph in Figure 11. This can be used as an easy and quick reference when interpreting EMG data, as long as one keeps in mind that the onset and termination of muscle activity and the individual variation in muscle activity are not well illustrated in each graph.

D. Joint Kinetics

Once mature gait patterns have been developed, the joint kinetics assume very specific patterns. These patterns generally remain similar

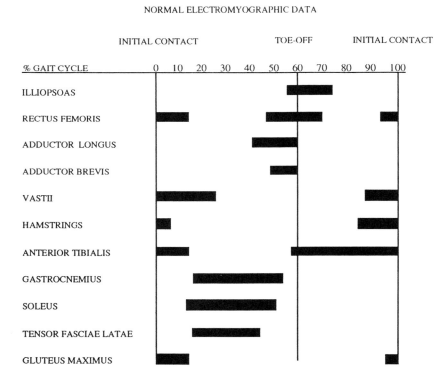

Figure 11   Bar graph representing the timing of muscle activity with respect to the gait cycle. Stance phase is separated from swing phase by the vertical solid line at 60% of the gait cycle.

across people with changes noted only in the peak amplitudes, primarily as a result of changing velocities (17) and body mass. The peak joint moments and powers increase as walking velocity increases. The normal sagittal plane joint kinematics and kinetics for the hip, knee, and ankle are plotted in Figure 12, and were calculated as described by Davis et al. (12) and Kadaba et al. (30). This format was selected so that the motion followed by the moment and then the power could be examined sequentially for a specific phase in the gait cycle. This helps to synthesize all of the components collected in gait analysis. For example, during midstance, the motion of the ankle can be determined on the motion plot, that is, ankle dorsiflexion. Looking at the moment plot over the same portion of the gait cycle, there is a net ankle plantarflexor moment that indicates the ankle plantarflexors are active. Finally, looking again at the same portion of the gait cycle in the power plot, there is a net power absorption that is associated with an eccentric muscular contraction. This is what would be expected as the ankle is dorsiflexing under the control of the ankle plantarflexors; thus the muscle is lengthening under tension. The step-by-step process can be used to evaluate all the joints at each phase in the gait cycle. A detailed description of the joint kinetics with respect to the phases of the gait cycle is given in the next section.

As with the joint kinematic data, joint moments and powers are best presented in a plot format. Both the joint moments and joint powers are normalized with respect to the body weight (measured in kilograms) to reduce the variability that is related to an individual's body mass. The net muscle moment is generally referred to as extensor (negative) or flexor (positive). The joint powers are labeled as generation (positive) and absorption (negative).

E. Gait with Respect to the Phases of the Gait Cycle

The following is a description of normal gait variables in the sagittal plane with respect to the events and phases of the gait cycle (Figs. 4 and 5). This coordinates the various components of gait to help create a better understanding of the mechanics of normal gait. In this section, the resultant GRF will be mentioned during the stance phase. The body's response to this force will be described in terms of the net muscle moment and power generated at the joint. This provides a better basis for understanding the sequence of muscle firing and subsequent movement that occurs during normal gait. The resultant ground

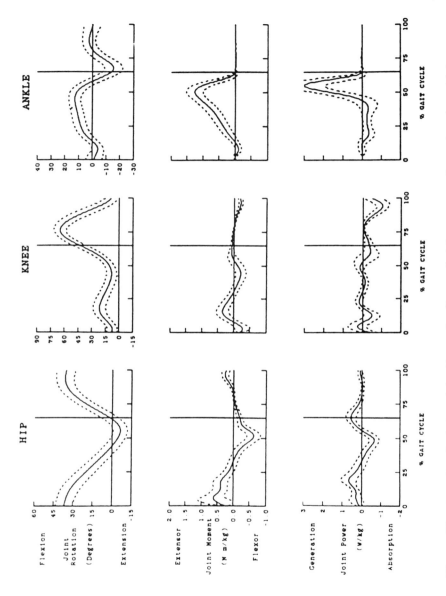

Figure 12 Normal sagittal plane joint kinematics (first row), joint moments (second row), and joint powers (third row) for the hip, knee, and ankle.

reaction force is a vector of which the position and magnitude can be obtained with the use of a force plate. It is the force acting on the body when it is in contact with the ground. Its point of action is at the center of pressure which is also calculated by the force plate. This information is also summarized in Table 4.

1. Stance Phase

Initial Contact(IC) (0% of the gait cycle)   This event is the moment when the foot makes contact with the floor. The hip is flexed, the knee is almost fully extended, and the ankle is in neutral position. In normal gait, ground contact is made with the heel contacting the floor.

Loading Response (LR) (0–10% of the gait cycle)   This is the initial double support that continues until the opposite limb leaves the floor. The purpose of this phase is to provide shock absorption while maintaining forward progression and stance stability. During LR, the ankle plantarflexes until the foot is flat on the floor (first rocker). This motion is driven by the resultant ground GRF which passes posterior to the ankle joint center causing the ankle to plantarflex. This movement is controlled by the ankle dorsiflexors (net dorsiflexor muscle moment) as they contract eccentrically (power absorption). The knee flexes during this phase and is controlled by a net knee extensor moment through eccentric contraction (power absorption) of the knee extensors. The hip extends from initial contact throughout this phase. This motion is produced by a net hip extensor moment through concentric contraction of the hip extensors.

Midstance (MST) (10–30% of the gait cycle)   This is the initial single support phase and is equivalent to the swing phase of the opposite limb (i.e., extends from toe-off to initial contact of the opposite limb). The purpose of this phase is to advance the body over the stance phase limb while maintaining stability. During MST, the ankle dorsiflexes as the tibia moves over the plantigrade foot (second rocker). The resultant GRF is passing anterior to the ankle joint tending to produce ankle dorsiflexion. This motion is controlled by the net ankle plantarflexor moment through eccentric contraction of the ankle plantarflexors. The knee is extending during this portion of the gait cycle. The resultant GRF is passing posterior to the knee joint center and is resisted by the a net knee extensor moment through concentric contraction of the knee extensors. Toward the end of this phase, the ankle plantarflexors may also contribute to knee extension by controlling the forward motion of the tibia. The hip continues to extend during this phase. The resultant

Table 4   Summary of the Major Components of Gait with Respect to the Phases of the Gait Cycle

Phases		Ankle	Knee	Hip
LR	external load[a]	plantarflex	flex	flex
	joint movement[b]	plantarflexing	flexing	extending
	dominant moment[c]	dorsiflexors	extensors	extensors
	associated power[d]	absorption	absorption	generation
MST	external load	dorsiflex	flex	flex
	joint movement	dorsiflexing	extending	extending
	dominant moment	plantarflexors	extensors	extensors
	associated power	absorption	generation	generation
TST	external load	dorsiflex	extend	flex
	joint movement	plantarflexing	extending/flexing	extending
	dominant moment	plantarflexors	plantarflexors	ligamentous
	associated power	generation	negligible	absorption
PSW	external load	dorsiflex	flex	extend
	joint movement	plantarflexing	flexing	flexing
	dominant moment	plantarflexor	extensor (small)	flexors
	associated power	generation	absorption	generation
ISW	external load	plantarflex (small)	flex	none
	joint movement	plantar/dorsiflexing	flexing	flexing
	dominant moment	dorsiflexor (small)	extensor (small)	flexor
	associated power	negligible	absorption	generation
MSW	external load	plantarflex (small)	extend	extend
	joint movement	dorsiflexing	extending	flexing
	dominant moment	dorsiflexor (small)	negligible	negligible
	associated power	negligible	negligible	negligible
TSW	external load	plantarflex (small)	extend	extend
	joint movement	minimal plantarflexing	extending	minimal extending
	dominant moment	dorsiflexors (small)	flexors	extensors
	associated power	negligible	absorption	generation

[a]Motion at the joint produced by the resultant GRF (when the foot is in contact with the ground), inertial forces and gravity.
[b]Joint's motion during the specific phase.
[c]The body's response to the external loads and indicates the dominant muscle group.
[d]The type of muscular contraction of the associated muscle; absorption and generation refer to eccentric and concentric muscular contraction, respectively.
LR, loading response; MST, midstance; TST, terminal stance; PSW, preswing; ISW, initial swing; MSW, midswing; TSW, terminal swing

GRF passes anterior to the hip joint center tending to flex the hip. This motion is resisted by a net hip extensor moment through the continued concentric contraction of the hip extensors.

Terminal Stance (TST) (30–50% of the gait cycle)   Single support continues through the end of this phase when the swing limb comes in contact with the ground. The purpose of this phase is the continued advancement beyond the stance foot through the forward fall of the trunk. During TST, the ankle actively plantarflexes (third rocker). The resultant GRF is passing anterior to the ankle joint center tending to produce ankle dorsiflexion. This is resisted by a net ankle plantarflexor moment as the ankle plantarflexors contract concentrically. This results in a large power generation burst. The knee continues to extend during the initial portion of this phase until it reaches maximum extension and begins to flex. The resultant GRF passes very close to the knee joint center tending initially to extend and then flex the knee. When the GRF is anterior to the knee it helps maintain the knee in extension and produce stance phase stability with minimal activity of the knee musculature required. In the end of this phase, as the knee starts to flex, the GRF passes posterior to the knee tending to flex the knee and thus contributing to the force necessary to propel the stance limb into swing. Concentric contraction of the gastrocnemius contributes to the net knee flexor moment. The hip extends to the maximum extension during TST. The resultant GRF has now passed posterior to the hip joint center tending to cause hip extension. This is resisted by a net hip flexor moment. Examination of dynamic EMG reveals that the hip flexors are not active, suggesting that the movement is produced by ligamentous structures. As the hip continues to extend, there is lengthening of these structures and associated power absorption.

Preswing (PSW) (50–60% of the gait cycle)   This phase represents the second double support phase and begins with the contact of the opposite swing limb and ends with toe-off of the stance limb. The purpose of this phase is to propel the limb into swing primarily through the contribution of the hip flexors and diminishing but continued contribution of the ankle plantarflexors. During PSW the ankle continues to plantarflex as the lower extremity unweights. The point of action of the resultant GRF, the center of pressure, continues to the distal aspect of the foot tending to dorsiflex the ankle as in the previous two phases. This force is initially resisted by a net ankle plantarflexor moment through concentric contraction of the ankle plantarflexors. The resultant

GRF rapidly reduces in amplitude as the body weight shifts to the opposite limb and there is a rapid reduction of the ankle plantarflexor moment and associated power absorption. This coincides with the termination of ankle plantarflexor activity. The knee continues to flex rapidly to about 40 degrees of flexion at toe-off. The resultant GRF is much more posterior to the knee center. From peak hip extension at the beginning of this phase the hip begins to flex. The resultant GRF passes posterior to the hip joint center tending to extend the hip. This is resisted by a net hip flexor moment through concentric contraction of the hip flexors. The peak power generation of the hip flexors occurs at toe-off as they help propel the limb into swing.

Toe-off (TO) (60% of the gait cycle)   This event marks the transition between the stance and swing phase and typically occurs at about 60% of the gait cycle in normal gait. The hip is slightly flexed, the knee is flexed to approximately 40 degrees, and the ankle is plantarflexed but not yet at peak plantarflexion. In normal gait, the great toe is the last part of the stance limb to leave the ground.

2. Swing Phase

Initial Swing (ISW) (60–73% of the gait cycle)   This phase is the beginning of the second single support phase and begins when the foot leaves the ground until it passes opposite the stance limb. This phase occupies about one-third of the swing phase. The purpose of this phase is to continue to advance the swing limb while providing sufficient clearance of the foot from the ground. In normal gait, clearance of the foot is approximately 2 mm, illustrating the control necessary for normal walking (17). During ISW, the ankle continues to plantarflex and then begins to dorsiflex rapidly to aid in clearance. Ankle dorsiflexion is produced by the concentric contraction of the anterior tibial muscles. The moment and powers at the ankle joint during the swing phase are not large as there is no resultant GRF in swing and the inertial contributions of the foot segment below the ankle joint are small. The knee continues to flex rapidly to peak knee flexion of approximately 64 degrees at the transition between ISW and midswing. Knee flexion occurs primarily passively from a combination of simultaneous active hip flexion and the momentum gained during third rocker. As with the ankle, minimal joint moments and powers are recorded during this phase. The knee continues to flex during ISW. A net hip flexor moment through the concentric contraction of the hip flexors produced this movement. The net hip flexor moments also flex the hip joint during this phase.

Midswing (MSW) (73–87% of the gait cycle)   This phase represents the middle third of the swing phase and corresponds with single limb stance of the opposite limb. The purpose of MSW is to continue to advance the swing limb while providing sufficient clearance of the foot from the ground. The ankle reaches its peak dorsiflexion for the swing phase during MSW. This is produced through concentric contraction of the anterior tibial muscles. The level of contraction of these muscles quickly reduces in this phase, allowing the ankle to begin to plantarflex slightly. After reaching peak flexion at the beginning of MSW, the knee begins to extend rapidly, primarily through momentum as minimal EMG activity is recorded during this portion of the gait cycle. This is one mechanism of reducing energy consumption by minimizing muscle activity.

Terminal Swing (TSW) (87–100% of the gait cycle)   This phase represents the last third of the swing phase and terminates with initial contact of the swing limb. The purpose of this phase is to continue forward advancement of the swing limb and maintain clearance as well as prepare for initial contact. The ankle plantarflexes slightly. However, the ankle dorsiflexors begin to contract at a higher level to prepare for initial contact. Tension development in the anterior tibialis is necessary before it is required to resist the resultant GRF in LR. The knee rapidly extends during this phase, initially through momentum, and toward the end through contraction of the quadriceps. The extension ends before initial contact as a net knee flexor moment through eccentric contraction of the knee flexors (hamstrings) decelerates the forward rotation of the shank segment with respect to the thigh segment. Coactivation of the knee flexors and extensors before initial contact provides stability for the knee at weight acceptance. Finally, the hip reaches maximum flexion at the beginning of this phase and tends to extend slightly just before initial contact. Gravity as well as activity of the hip extensors produces hip extension. The muscle activity results in a net hip extensor moment through a corresponding concentric contraction.

F. Coronal Plane

The previous discussion focused on the sagittal plane where the majority of motion occurs during normal gait. An understanding of normal gait in the coronal plane is also necessary because abnormalities are seen in this plane as well. In normal gait, the motion, moments, and powers are minimal at the knee and ankle. The motions are actually so small that the signal-to-noise ratio is high, limiting the clinical utility of these specific measures. At the hip, however, more motion occurs which has very specific patterns. At initial contact the hip is in about neutral position (0 degrees of abduction/adduction in relation to the pelvis). During LR, the shock absorption phase, the hip adducts under the control of the hip abductors. The resultant GRF passes medial to the hip joint center tending to adduct the hip. This is resisted by net hip abductor muscle moment through eccentric contraction of the hip abductors as they absorb the initial impact. During MST and TST, the hip abducts through concentric contraction of the hip abductors as the resultant GRF is maintained medial to the hip joint center. In PSW there is a rapid drop-off in the net hip abductor moment as body weight is transferred to the opposite limb.

IV. CASE STUDY

The following case study has been selected to illustrate how computerized gait analysis can be used in the treatment decision making and evaluation of individuals with gait abnormalities. In our gait laboratory, data from a gait test are evaluated by both an orthopedist affiliated with the laboratory and the kinesiologist or physical therapist who performed the test. It will become evident in this case study that interpretation of the results is based not only on the information presented at the time of the gait analysis but also is a function of the amount of experience of the people involved in the review. This experience is attained by evaluating numerous cases both before and after surgery is performed. The evaluation of postoperative gait analyses is a routine procedure in our laboratory. All patients are called in for a repeat gait analysis approximately 1 year after treatment. At that time, a postoperative test is performed in the same manner as the preoperative test so that a similar data set is available for comparison.

A. Preoperative Assessment

1. Patient History

Patient WW has a diagnosis of cerebral palsy, left spastic hemiplegia. He was the product of a full-term birth with no known complications. At the age of 2, he underwent cardiac surgery and suffered a cardiovascular accident. WW had a left tendo-Achilles lengthening (TAL) in January 1978 followed by a repeat TAL in January 1981; he was 3 and 6 years of age, respectively. WWs preoperative gait analysis was performed in September 1989 at 15 years of age.

2. Clinical Assessment

The clinical assessment highlights the asymmetry of involvement in this boy; he has limited strength and range of motion on the left side (Table 4), especially tight hip adductors, medial hamstrings and heel cord as well as excessive femoral anteversion and spasticity of the rectus femoris (Duncan Ely test) and triceps surae (positive clonus). The left side also shows greater weakness than the right.

3. Muscle Activity

Electromyographic data confirm the greater involvement of the left side (Fig. 13). Specifically, there is inappropriate activity of the rectus femoris in midswing, inappropriate activity of the hamstrings in mid- and terminal stance, premature firing of the gastroc-soleus beginning in terminal swing, underactivity of the anterior tibialis in loading response, and premature shut-off in terminal swing.

4. Preoperative Joint Kinematics and Kinetics

Multiple strides of data (a minimum of three) are initially assessed to determine if the gait abnormalities are consistent from stride to stride. An analysis of the joint kinematic and kinetic plots reveals very high stride-to-stride consistency in the sagittal and transverse planes. Therefore, for each condition, only one plot in each plane of the right and left sides will be used to illustrate the joint kinematics and kinetics (Figs. 14 and 15).

Coronal Plane   Pelvic motion is slightly variable from stride to stride and amodular. At the hip, there is asymmetry with excessive abduction at initial contact, progressive adduction in stance, and abduction in swing on the right side. The left hip shows the opposite pattern with excessive adduction at initial contact, progressive abduction in stance, and adduction in swing. The hip motion is a result of the asymmetry seen in the pelvic motion in the transverse plane (see discussion below).

Sagittal Plane   At the pelvis there is a slightly posterior baseline pelvic tilt with increasing lordosis during left lower extremity stance. Greater dynamic involvement of the left hip flexors may contribute to

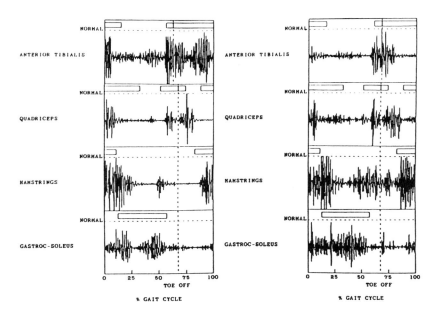

Figure 13   Raw EMG tracings of the left (first column) and right (second column) for the rectus femoris, hamstrings, gastrocnemius/soleus, and anterior tibialis muscles. The normal expected activity is indicated on the bars above each raw signal.

this problem. At the hips, there is asymmetry with reduced range of motion (ROM) on the left side. The reduced relative hip flexion during the initial part of stance would be expected, considering the increased posterior pelvic tilt at this point in the gait cycle. Left hip joint kinetics are within normal limits. Right knee motion is within normal limits. On the left side, during loading response, there is progressive extension of the knee to a hyperextended position in midstance. Spasticity of the triceps surae and poor quadriceps control are the mechanisms contributing to this problem. This is confirmed by the knee moment which is flexor throughout the majority of stance with associated power absorption. In swing, the left knee shows delayed and less-than-normal peak flexion in swing. Inappropriate quadriceps activity and quadriceps spasticity contribute to this problem. At the ankle, there is normal modulation and range of motion in the sagittal plane. On the left side drop

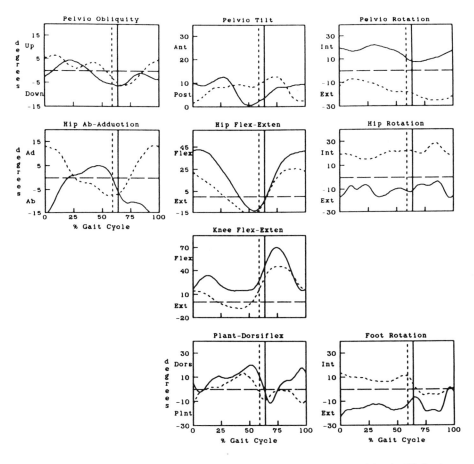

Figure 14 A comparison of the joint kinematic data on the right (solid line) versus the left (dashed line); data were collected during barefoot walking prior to surgical intervention.

foot in terminal swing is exhibited. Shut-off of the left anterior tibialis may contribute to this problem. The associated joint kinetics shows a plantarflexor moment throughout the stance phase secondary to the poor prepositioning of the foot at initial contact. The associated power pattern shows an inappropriate generation in midstance and less-than-normal generation in terminal stance.

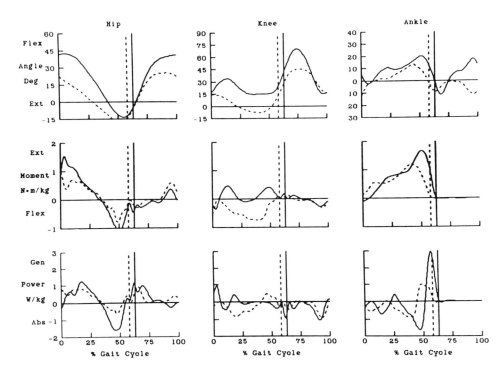

Figure 15 A comparison of the joint kinetic data on the right (solid line) versus the left (dashed line); data were collected during barefoot walking prior to surgical intervention.

Transverse Plane   The pelvis is asymmetrical with the left hemipelvis held external to the right throughout the gait cycle. This is a result of excessive femoral anteversion (internal hip rotation) of the left hip as seen on the hip rotation plot. The right hip has compensatory external rotation during gait (available hip ROM can be confirmed on the clinical exam). Visual gait analysis of this child suggests bilateral internal hip rotation. The asymmetry of the pelvis and the position of the hip are difficult to appreciate in the transverse plane without the gait analysis motion data. Left foot progression is internal with respect to the direction of progression. This is a result of the excessive internal hip rotation, which is not corrected fully by the external left hemipelvis rotation. Comparing this with the normal foot–thigh angle measurement and noting the lack of any forefoot adduction confirm this result.

5. Surgical Decisions

Based on the gait analysis and clinical findings, the following procedures were performed on the left side during one operative session: medial hamstrings lengthening, rectus femoris transfer to the sartorius, and a femoral (intertrochanteric) derotation osteotomy. Medial hamstrings lengthening was performed because of the reduced knee extension at initial contact and excessive knee flexion in stance. Only the medial aspect of the hamstrings was lengthened because on palpation of the popliteal fossa during the clinical evaluation of hamstrings length (popliteal angle), the medial component was taut, not the lateral. It is also postulated that when a proximal femoral derotation osteotomy is performed there is a tendency to tighten the medial aspect of the hamstrings and lengthen the lateral. Transfer of the left rectus femoris to the sartorius is a procedure used to maintain knee flexion in swing in the presence of simultaneous hamstrings surgery. This decision is based partly on previous experience and research (31) which show that rectus femoris transfer surgery is necessary when preoperative knee range of motion (during gait) is less than 80% of normal and hamstrings lengthening is being performed. If no rectus femoris transfer is completed, the peak knee flexion in swing will decrease. Other criteria for the performance of this surgery is inappropriate activity of the rectus femoris in midswing, a positive Duncan Ely test, reduced knee range of motion (less than 80%), and reduced time to and degree of peak knee flexion in swing. Finally, an intertrochanteric femoral derotation osteotomy is recommended because of the excessive internal rotation of the left hip in relation to the pelvis. It is also known through the evaluation of similar children with this type of involvement (hemiplegia with minimal upper extremity involvement) that correction of the femoral anteversion will help correct the compensatory rotation of the pelvis. Previous experience also indicates that when asymmetrical pelvic rotation is corrected, asymmetry at the hips in the coronal plane is reduced. It was decided not to perform heel cord surgery because this patient had already had two tendo-Achilles lengthenings. This decision was made despite the limited dorsiflexion noted on clinical assessment and the limited sagittal plane motion during gait.

The proposed procedures were performed when the patient was 15 years old.

B. Postoperative Assessment

1. Joint Kinematic and Kinetic Changes

Plots showing right and left joint kinematics that were obtained 1 year after the surgery (Fig. 16) should be compared with preoperative motion plots (Fig. 14) to observe the changes seen in all three planes of motion. These changes are also described below.

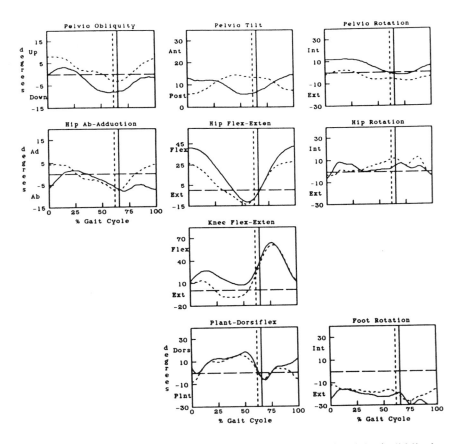

Figure 16   A comparison of the joint kinematic data on the right (solid line) versus the left (dashed line); data were collected during barefoot walking 1 year after surgical intervention.

Coronal Plane Postoperatively, the pelvis and hip show normal modulation. Elimination of the asymmetry in the transverse plane at the hip and subsequently the pelvis resulted in this change.

Sagittal Plane Postoperatively, there is a reduction in the excessive range of motion of the pelvis with associated increased symmetry at the hip. Joint kinetic patterns at the hip are more normal. Knee flexion modulation in swing is improved with normal time to and amount of peak knee flexion. Ankle motion and kinetics are unchanged.

Transverse Plane Postoperatively, motion at the pelvis, hips, and feet is within normal limits except for a small asymmetry at the pelvis, with the left hemipelvis rotated posteriorly and right hemipelvis rotated internally, as a result of the left femoral derotation osteotomy. With increased rotation of the left hip, the patient is able to assume a normal position and thus adjust the pelvis to a more normal position.

The patient was tested while wearing a left posterior leaf spring (PLS) orthosis; the following changes are noted on the left side: (1) the drop foot in swing is eliminated through the forefoot support provided by the orthosis; (2) the spasticity of the ankle, as demonstrated by power generation in midstance, is reduced with the PLS; (3) the patient is still capable of power generation in terminal stance with the PLS; and (4) the knee hyperextension and corresponding excessive flexor moment and power absorption in stance are reduced. The changes in kinematics noted at the ankle are compared in the barefoot condition versus the PLS condition (Fig. 17).

Conclusions One year postoperatively, WW exhibits changes in his gait pattern that are associated with a more functional gait. The only remaining problem is excessive knee extension during stance on the left side, an effect of the tightness and spasticity in the ankle plantarflexors despite the two previous interventions on this muscle. The problem, however, is somewhat relieved when the patient wears the PLS. Stretching of the heel cord and possibly intramuscular lengthening of the gastrocnemius for the future are recommended.

V. OTHER CONSIDERATIONS

Clinicians need to consider the following additional points when interpreting gait analysis data: the importance of detecting stride-to-stride variations in gait, the potential of error when using two-dimensional

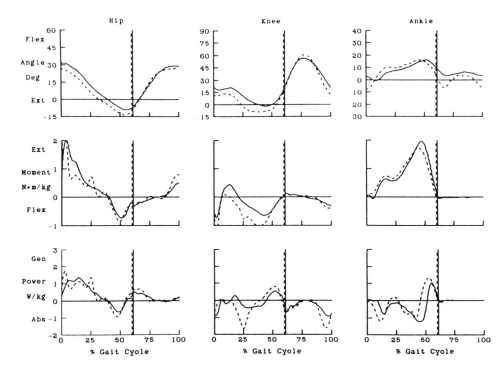

Figure 17 A comparison of the left ankle and the left knee kinematic and kinetic data collected on the barefoot (dashed line) and the PLS (solid line) walk; data were collected during barefoot walking 1 year after surgical intervention.

techniques to document three-dimensional motion, and limitations of gait analysis. Also included in this section will be a brief discussion of the use of gait analysis as a research tool.

A. Stride-to-Stride Variability

The stride-to-stride variations in gait patterns are difficult to determine from visual analysis of gait alone. Because of their important implications, they merit careful, objective assessment alone. For example, if a patient has adequate dorsiflexion on one stride and less than normal dorsiflexion on the next, the treatment decision will generally be more conservative.

A knowledge of the variability in normal gait patterns is essential when interpreting abnormal gait. The stride-to-stride and day-to-day variability of normal gait has been studied previously in adults (32, 33). The findings indicate that within-day variability is generally low but becomes higher the longer the period of time studied. A study using similar tools of assessment showed that the within-day variability of gait patterns in children was similar to adults (34). In patients with cerebral palsy who had either bilateral or unilateral involvement, within-day repeatability was similar and in some cases better than in normal children.

B. Two-Dimensional Versus Three-Dimensional Gait Analysis Techniques

Two-dimensional (2-D) gait analysis, which assumes motion is planar, was the most commonly employed technique in the initial attempts at clinical gait analysis (5, 35). Two-dimensional gait data are easier to collect and process and the equipment used to attain the data is less expensive. Motion during pathological (36) and even normal gait (22), however, is not 2-D. In a recent study, Davis et al. (37) compared the error associated by applying 2-D techniques to 3-D motion. Mean root-mean-square differences of 5 degrees in plantarflexion/dorsiflexion angles were found in normal gait and mean root-mean-square differences of 30 degrees in plantar flexion/dorsiflexion were noted in abnormal gait. To add to this problem, these errors were highly variable in abnormal gait, which eliminates the possibility of predicting and correcting for such errors.

The errors incurred when comparing data collected in 3-D to the same data reduced to a 2-D representation for the ankle joint kinematics, moment, and power are illustrated in Figure 18. Although the differences in ankle kinematics would not change a clinical decision, the differences in the ankle moment and power suggest differences in the underlying condition which may affect a treatment decision and the evaluation of changes in gait postoperatively.

Error in sagittal plane motion collected in 2-D will occur if motion is also taking place in the transverse and/or the coronal plane. Transverse plane motion is very common in patients with cerebral palsy who have femoral anteversion and corresponding internal hip rotation. Coronal plane motion is very common when patients have limited sagittal plane motion and circumduct the hip to aid in clearance of the swing limb. These two problems often occur simultaneously. The effect of

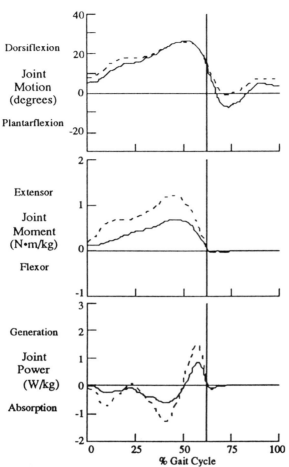

Figure 18 A comparison of kinematic, moment, and power data for the ankle joint in the sagittal plane when computed in three dimensions (dashed line) and two dimensions (solid line).

"out-of-plane" motion on the sagittal plane knee angle is illustrated in Figure 19. As more external or internal rotation of the hip occurs, the larger the apparent knee joint angle becomes from the sagittal view [Fig. 19(a)]. Similarly, as more hip abduction occurs, the smaller the apparent knee joint angle becomes in the sagittal view [Fig. 19(b)]. A similar

(a) sagittal plane

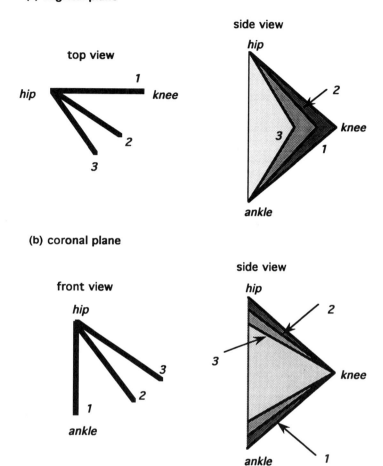

(b) coronal plane

Figure 19 Illustration showing the errors in a 2-D representation of the knee joint angle in the sagittal plane when motion occurs in (a) the transverse plane and (b) the coronal plane. The degree of out-of-plane motion is illustrated on the left with the corresponding effect on the knee joint angle in the sagittal plane illustrated on the right. Position 1 indicates no out-of-plane motion and position 3 indicates the largest degree of out-of-plane motion.

problem occurs when measuring joint angles directly from a video screen. The screen is a 2-D representation of 3-D motion. As such, motion not parallel to the plane of the screen can produce an error in any angles measured directly from the screen.

C. Limitations

Gait analysis is not a diagnostic technique nor does it provide treatment decisions. Gait analysis techniques provide objective data that can assist in the treatment decision-making process. However, gait analysis data must be interpreted and the ability to do this requires an appreciation for the methods of calculation and signal processing used in the data collection. Also, knowledge of the expected normal data is necessary because it is used as a reference from which to base clinical decisions.

As mentioned previously, not all individuals are candidates for gait analysis. There is typically a minimum height requirement necessary to obtain valid data. The smaller the person being tested, the greater the impact of marker placement errors on the data. There are also limitations associated with the testing of obese patients. Marker motion on skin surfaces over obese areas will include a significant skin movement component that compromises the final data. Also, difficulty in palpating bony landmarks (e.g., the anterior superior iliac spine) in obese patients may require the clinician to estimate their location. A patient must also be able to ambulate independently with or without the use of walking aids. Typically, gait analysis is not suitable for patients who are capable only of body transfer or exercise ambulation. Finally, patient cooperation is necessary to carry out a long test and to tolerate the placement of joint markers and EMG equipment. Difficulties are common with small children and those who have behavioral or developmental problems.

D. Gait Analysis as a Research Tool

The techniques employed in gait analysis also function naturally as a research tool (38–41). Since the majority of data collected is assimilated and processed by computer, it lends itself to computational and statistical methods that are employed in research. Research in gait analysis usually follows one of two related directions: the documentation of a particular gait disorder or the evaluation of treatment. Documentation of a particular gait disorder through the collection and assessment of gait analysis data improves our understanding of the mechanisms behind the associated motion and ultimately the treatment decisions.

The evaluation of treatment is one of the more common forms of gait analysis research (31, 35, 39–41). This process has led to the development of new operative procedures that have ultimately changed the course of treatment. An example of this is the rectus femoris transfer now commonly used in the treatment of stiff-kneed gait in children with cerebral palsy (39, 40, 42). The study of gait patterns in patients with myelomeningocele has also led to modifications in the types of orthoses typically prescribed for these patients (35). Additionally, when treatment is evaluated in groups of patients such as those who have had selective dorsal rhizotomy (38, 43), we can better predict the outcome clinically in similar patients.

In closing, the material in this chapter was presented to afford clinicians new to the uses of gait analysis a greater understanding of the kinds of information gait analysis provides and the methods of data presentation. Although the use of computerized gait analysis is a relatively new addition to routine treatment evaluations, it has already made a profound effect on treatment protocols, especially in the area of orthopedic treatment decisions.

VI. APPENDIX: TERMINOLOGY

Planes of motion:

    Coronal plane—the vertical plane that divides the body into anterior and posterior parts.

    Sagittal plane—the vertical plane that divides the body into the right and left parts.

    Transverse plane—the horizontal plane that divides the body at right angles to the coronal and sagittal planes.

Pelvic transverse plane: The plane formed by the three pelvic markers (2 ASIS markers and 1 PSIS markers)

Pelvic sagittal plane: The plane that is perpendicular to the transverse plane and midway between the ASIS markers.

Pelvic coronal plane: The plane perpendicular to the other two planes of the pelvis.

Line of progression: A line that is parallel to the walkway along which the patient proceeds during the data collection.

Gait cycle: The period of time from one event (usually initial contact) of one foot to the following occurrence of the same event with the same foot.

Normalization of the gait cycle: Initial contact of one foot to the following initial contact of the same foot is unitized and will be represented as 100% of the gait cycle. This allows averaging of data across subjects who may not have similar gait cycle time.

Stance phase (ST): The period of time when the foot is in contact with the ground. In normal gait this represents about 60% of the gait cycle.

Swing phase (SW): The period of time when the foot is not in contact with the ground. In normal gait this represents about 40% of the gait cycle. In those cases where the foot never leaves the ground (foot drag), it can be defined as the phase when all portions of the lower extremity are in forward motion.

Double support (DS): The period of time when both feet are in contact with the ground. This occurs twice in the gait cycle, at the beginning and end of the stance phase. In normal gait, this represents about 10% of the gait cycle at the beginning and another 10% at the end of the stance phase.

Single support (SS): The period in time when only one foot is in contact with the ground. In walking, this is exactly equal to the swing period of the other limb.

Phases of the gait cycle: The stance and swing phases may be further divided into subphases as described by Perry (27). This terminology is very useful for referring to specific portions of the gait cycle (Figs. 1 and 2).

> loading response (LR) 0–10% / double support
> midstance (MST) 10–30%
> terminal stance (TST) 30–50%
> preswing (PSW) 50–60% / double support
> initial swing (ISW) 60–70%
> midswing (MSW) 70–85%
> terminal swing (TSW) 85–100%

Initial contact (IC): The point in the gait cycle when the foot initially makes contact with the ground; this marks the beginning of the stance phase.

Toe-off (TO): The point in the gait cycle when contact with the ground is terminated; this marks the beginning of swing phase. It typically occurs at 60% of the gait cycle in normal gait. For those cases where the foot never leaves the ground (foot drag), it is often assumed to be the point when all portions of the lower extremity have achieved forward motion.

Step length: The distance from one event of one foot to the following occurrence of the same event with the other foot. The right step length is the distance from the left heel to the right heel when both feet are in contact with the ground.

Stride length: The distance from initial contact of one foot to the following initial contact of the same foot. Sometimes referred to as cycle length.

Velocity: The average horizontal speed along the direction of progression measured over one or more strides (typically reported in centimeters per second).

Cadence: The number of steps per unit time (typically reported in steps per minute).

REFERENCES

1. DeLuca PA. (1991). Gait analysis in the treatment of ambulatory child with cerebral palsy. Clin Orthoped 1991; 264: 65–75.
2. Gage JR, Õunpuu S. Surgical intervention in the correction of primary and secondary gait abnormalities. Adaptability of Human Gait. In: Patla AE, ed. Amsterdam: Elsevier Science Publishers B.V. North-Holland, 1991: 359–385.
3. Gage JR, Õunpuu S. Gait analysis in clinical practice. Sem Orthoped, 1989; 4(2): 72–87.
4. Gage JR. Gait analysis for decision making in cerebral palsy. Bull Hosp Joint Dis Orthoped Inst 1983; 43: 147–163.
5. Perry J. Distal rectus femoris transfer. Dev Med Child Neurol 1987; 29:153–158.
6. Rose S, Õunpuu S, DeLuca PA. Strategies for the assessment of gait in a clinical setting. Phys Ther 1991; 71:961–980.
7. Sutherland DH, Santi M, Abel MD. Treatment of stiff-knee gait in cerebral palsy: a comparison by gait analysis of the distal rectus femoris transfer versus proximal rectus release. J. Pediatr. Orthoped 1990; 10:433–441.
8. Sutherland DH, Larsen LJ, and Mann R. Rectus femoris release in selected patients with cerebral palsy: a preliminary report. Dev Med Child Neurol 1975; 17:26–34.
9. Waters RL, Garland DE, Perry J, Habig T, Slabaugh P. Stiff-legged gait in hemiplegia: surgical correction. J Bone Joint Surg Am 1976; 61(A): 927–933.
10. Ruwe PA, Gage JR, Ozonoff MB, DeLuca PA. Clinical determination of femoral anteversion. J Bone Joint Surg. 1992; 74(A):820–830.
11. Gage JR. Gait Analysis in Cerebral Palsy. London: Mac Keith Press, 1991: 16.

12. Greenwood DT. Principles of Dynamics. Engelwood Cliffs, NJ: Prentice-Hall, 1965: 383–396.
13. Davis RB, Õunpuu S, Tyburski DJ, Gage JR. A gait analysis data collection and reduction technique. Hum. Mov. Sci. 1991; 10:575–589.
14. Winter DA. Concerning the scientific basis for the diagnosis of pathological gait and for rehabilitation protocols. Physiother Can 1985; 37(4): 245–252.
15. Yack HJ. Techniques for clinical assessment of gait. Phys Ther 1984; 64(12): 1821–1829.
16. Wells RP. The projection of the ground reaction force as a predictor of internal joint moments. Bull Pros Res 1981; 18: 15–19.
17. Winter DA. Biomechanics and Motor Control of Human Movement. 2d ed. Ontario: University of Waterloo Press, 1990: 75–114, 204–207.
18. Yank JF, Winter DA. Electromyographic amplitude normalization methods: improving their sensitivity as diagnostic tools. Arch Phys Med Rehab 1984; 65: 517–521.
19. Õunpuu, S, Winter DA. Bilateral electromyographical analysis of the lower limbs during walking in normal adults. Electroenceph Clin Neurophysiol 1989; 72: 429–438.
20. Basmajian VJ, DeLuca CJ. Muscles Alive: Their Functions Revealed by Electromyography. Baltimore: Williams and Wilkins, 1985: 30–34.
21. Kadaba MP, Wooten ME, Gainey J, Cochran GVB. Repeatability of phasic muscle activity: performance of surface and intramuscular wire electrodes in gait analysis. J Orthoped Res 1986; 3: 350–359.
22. Õupuu S, Gage JR, Davis RB. Three-dimensional lower extremity joint kinetics in normal pediatric gait. J Pediatr Orthoped 1991; 11: 341–349.
23. Winter DA, Patla AE, Frank JS, Walt SE. Biomechanical walking pattern changes in the fit and healthy elderly. Phys Ther 1990; 70: 340–347.
24. Sutherland DH, Olshen RA, Biden EN, Wyatt MP. The Development of Mature Walking. Philadelphia: Mac Keith Press, 1988.
25. Bleck EE. Orthopaedic Management in Cerebral Palsy. London: Mac Keith Press, 1987: 78.
26. Winter DA. The Biomechanics and Motor Control of Human Gait, Ontario: University of Waterloo Press, 1987: 45–55.
27. Perry J. Gait Analysis: Normal and Pathological Function. Thorofare, NJ: SLACK Inc, 1992: 9–16.
28. Winter DA. Biomechanical motor patterns in normal walking. J Motor Behav 1983; 15:302–330.
29. Inman VT, Ralston HJ, Todd F. Human Walking, Baltimore: Williams & Wilkins, 1981; 103–117.
30. Kadaba MP, Ramakrishnan HK, and Wooten ME. Measurement of lower extremity kinematics during level walking. J Orthoped Res 1990; 7: 849–860.

31. Gage JR, Perry J, Hicks RR, Koop S, and Werntz JR. Rectus femoris transfer to improve knee function of children with cerebral palsy. Dev Med Child Neurol 1987; 29:159–166.
32. Kadaba MP, Ramakrishnan HK, Wooten ME, Gainey J, Gorton G, Cochran GVB. Repeatability of kinematic, kinetic and electromyographic data in normal adult gait. J Orthoped Res 1990; 7:849–860.
33. Winter DA. Kinematic and kinetic patterns in human gait: variability and compensating effects. Hum Move 1984; 3:51–76.
34. Õunpuu S, Davis RB, Bell, KJ, Gage JR. The Repeatability of Joint Kinematic and Kinetic Data in Children with Cerebral Palsy Spastic Diplegia. Proceedings of the Canadian Society for Biomechanics, Quebec, 1990: 49–50.
35. Sutherland DH, Cooper L. The pathomechanics of progressive crouch gait in spastic diplegia. Orthoped Clin N Am 1978; 9(1):143–154.
36. Õunpuu, S, Davis RB, Banta JV, DeLuca PA. The effects of orthotics on gait in children with low level myelomeningocele. Proceedings of North American Congress on Biomechanics. Chicago, IL, 1992: 323–324.
37. Davis RB, Õupuu S, Tyburski DJ, DeLuca PA. A Comparison of Two-dimensional and Three-dimensional Techniques for the Determination of Joint Rotation Angles. Proceedings of International Symposium on 3-D Analysis of Human Movement 91. Montreal, Canada, 1991: 67–70.
38. Boscarino LF, Õunpuu S, Davis RB, Gage JR, DeLuca PA. The effects of selective dorsal rhizotomy on gait in children with cerebral palsy. J Pediatr Orthoped 1993;
39. Õunpuu S, Muik E, Davis RB, Gage JR, DeLuca PA. Part II: A comparison of the distal rectus femoris transfer and release on knee motion in children with cerebral palsy. J Pediatr Orthoped 1993;
40. Õunpuu S, Muik E, Davis RB, Gage JR, DeLuca PA. Part II: A comparison of the distal rectus femoris transfer and release on knee motion in children with cerebral palsy. J Pediatr Orthoped 1993;
41. Walsh J, Õunpuu S, DeLuca PA. The effect of iliopsoas surgery on sagittal plane motion of patients with spastic diplegia. Dev Med Child Neurol, 1991; 33: 7.
42. Gage JA. Surgical treatment of knee dysfunction in cerebral palsy. Clin Orthoped 1990; 253:45–54.
43. Cahan LD, Adams JM, Perry J, Beeler LM. Instrumented gait analysis after selective dorsal rhizotomy. Dev Med Child Neurol 1990; 32:1037–1043.

2

The Neural Control of Locomotion

AFTAB E. PATLA
University of Waterloo, Waterloo, Ontario, Canada

I. INTRODUCTION

Locomotion is essential for survival: it allows the animal to acquire food, evade a predator, or find a mate. Locomotion is made possible because of complex sensory, motor, and central nervous systems, and is characterized by cyclical angular movements of the limbs or other appendages resulting in translational motion of the whole body. Activation to the skeletal muscles produces the muscular torques that act on the complex chain of jointed bony levers, transferring forces to the support surface. How the nervous system organizes and controls the activation profile to the skeletal muscles is the focus of this chapter. We will draw on literature from animal and human studies to understand the generation and control of skilled human locomotor behavior.

II. FACTORS INFLUENCING THE EXPRESSION OF LOCOMOTOR BEHAVIOR

To provide a framework for our discussion, consider the modified diagram (Fig. 1) first proposed by Patla (40). These series of nested circles identify factors that influence the expression of locomotor behavior. The placement of factors in specific locations in the diagram and the use of nested circles are intentional: they represent layers of the locomotor program structure. The effector system occupies the center. Its neural

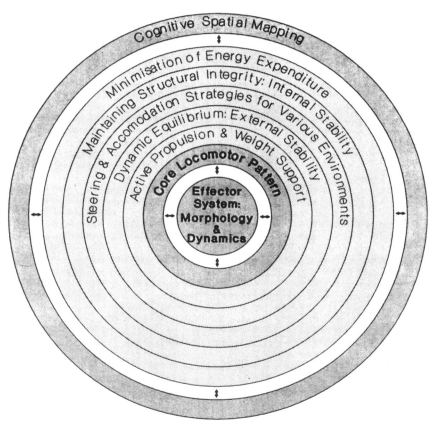

Figure 1 A schematic diagram showing the various factors that influence the expression of skilled locomotor behavior. See text for details. (Figure adapted from the original, Ref. 40.)

and mechanical interactions and the nonlinear properties of the muscle actuators are exploited by the control system in planning the activation patterns. The control system is shown as nested rings around the effector system. The innermost ring is the Core Locomotor Pattern, the skeleton around which the locomotion program structure is built. The factors listed in the three rings encircling the Core Locomotor Pattern are essential features for safe travel over various terrains, while the factors included in the next two rings are critical for the long-term integrity and viability of the locomotor apparatus. The outermost ring representing cognitive spatial mapping makes purposeful goal-directed travel beyond a local circumscribed environment possible. We begin our deliberation at the center and move outward.

III. THE EFFECTOR SYSTEM: MORPHOLOGY AND DYNAMICS

The effector system, which includes the muscles, tendons, ligaments, and skeletal structure, should occupy a prominent role in any locomotor control scheme. Knowledge of the structure that is to be controlled is essential for the design of the control system, as any engineer knows. Evolution has engineered the muscle and skeletal morphology to meet specific demands of different forms of locomotion. This is evident when we compare the changes that accompanied the transition to bipedal walking in humans. Owen Lovejoy (36) has catalogued several such modifications. Changes in muscle architecture and the corresponding new function include the following: (1) increase in size of the gluteus maximus muscle responsible for the stabilization of the upright torso in the anterior–posterior direction compared to the minor role its plays in the chimpanzee; (2) reorientation of the anterior gluteals in humans to prevent the tipping of the trunk toward the unsupported side in each step compared to its propulsive function in the chimpanzee; and (3) similar changes in the role of the hamstring muscles from propulsion to primarily controlling the limb extension in the swing phase. Concomitant with these alterations, the skeletal system has also undergone some major symbiotic changes. For example, the shorter ilium in humans serves to lower the trunk center of mass (hence lower moment of inertia about the hip joint), thereby reducing the demands on the gluteus maximus muscle for controlling the pitching motion of the trunk. Other skeletal changes include modification in the internal structure of the femoral neck and shock-absorbing arch in the foot (36). Clearly the human musculoskeletal morphology is best suited for bipedal locomotion.

Consider next the movements generated by the activation patterns during locomotion. It is well recognized that muscles provide unique power-to-weight ratio unmatched by any motor that humans have created. The force output of the muscle is not only dependent upon the activation, but also on the length of the muscle, velocity of contraction, and past history of the activation. These factors that modulate the force output are highly nonlinear and interact with each other providing a complex dynamic actuator. It is not surprising, therefore, that identifying the relationship between the activation profile (as reflected in the electromyographic signals) and force output has met with limited success, particularly for multiarticular movements such as locomotion (35). Even if we are able to predict the force output accurately from measured EMG profiles, determination of the movements generated by muscle action is not as simple as those predicted by the literature on functional anatomy. Modeling the muscle action in multiarticular movement (72) has demonstrated that muscles act to accelerate all joints, even those not spanned by the muscles. For example, depending on the body posture activation of the soleus muscle can serve to extend the knee in addition to producing the ankle extensor torque as predicted by functional anatomy (72).

The complex action created by active muscle involvement is due to inertial dynamics that introduce nonlinear coupling between limb segments due to Coriolis and centrifugal effects. During the swing phase of locomotion, for example, these gravity- and motion-dependent torques can contribute substantially to the motion of the limb, minimizing the need for active muscle involvement (58). In fact, many researchers have argued that during normal locomotion, the swing phase trajectory is primarily dictated by the pendular dynamics of the swinging limb (3, 29, 30); the initial conditions set at the end of the stance phase coupled wih the compound pendulum dynamics produce major aspects of the limb trajectory. Minimal active muscular effort is required; when muscular effort is used, such as at the end of the swing phase, it serves to control rather than to generate the limb movement. Recently, McGeer (27), modeling locomotion using synthetic wheels for legs, has shown that such a physical model can walk downhill without any motor. The gradient provides energy that is lost at each impact of the foot with the ground. When knees were introduced in a later version of McGeer's model (27), reasonably stable passive walking ability was preserved provided the model legs had feet like humans. Although passive dynamics are exploited during normal locomotion, the control system can override these effects to actively control the swing limb trajectory as observed during obstacle avoidance (45, 43).

In addition to the mechanical interactions between joints due to bifunctional muscles and inertial dynamics, the neural connections via afferent pathways between muscles may play an important role in the control of locomotion (51). These neural couplings between muscles are not responsible for generation of locomotor activation patterns via reflex chaining; rather, they may be useful in modulation of the locomotor patterns.

To summarize, the effector system morphology and dynamics are powerful shapers and contributors to the locomotor movements. Whether or not there is explicit representation of these dynamics in the nervous system, the locomotor control system is cognizant of these features, having evolved together, and capitalizes on these aspects to simplify its task.

IV. THE LOCOMOTOR CONTROL SYSTEM

To appreciate the organization and features of the locomotor control system, we need to examine the factors that define skilled locomotor behavior. These are shown as nested rings around the effector system (Fig. 1). As we discuss each factor, we will identify neural substrates, the sensory systems, and the efferent/afferent pathways (shown in Fig. 2) that are necessary for the expression of the particular factor. Figure 3 lists the locomotor capabilities of a cat transected at various levels along the neuraxis (41). Figures 2 and 3 will help in our understanding of the neural control of locomotion.

A. Core Locomotor Pattern

Numerous studies using different experimental techniques, such as isolation of the neural substrate, deafferentation, and fictive preparations (effector system immobilized) have shown in a variety of animal species that the generation of basic locomotor rhythm does not rely on input from the periphery (12). This basic locomotor rhythm, which I have termed the Core Locomotor Pattern, can be released when triggered through a simple unpatterned input (21). In mammals, several regions along the neuraxis have been identified as sites for providing input to release and sustain the Core Locomotor Patterns stored at the spinal cord level (Fig. 2) (21, 20). These Core Locomotor Patterns produced by the spinal cord provide reasonably complex activations (beyond simple

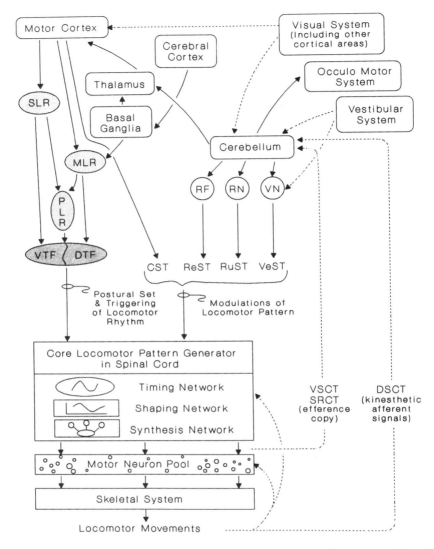

Figure 2 A simplified diagram showing various efferent (solid arrows) and afferent (dashed arrows) connections in the locomotor control system. For clarity only known and key aspects are shown. Legend description: SLR, subthalamic locomotor region; MLR, mesencephalic locomotor region; PLR, pontine locomotor region; VTF, ventral part of the caudal tegmental field; DTF, dorsal part of the caudal tegmental field; CST, cortico–spinal tract; REST, reticulospinal tract; RUST, rubrospinal tract; VEST, vestibulospinal tract; VSCT, ventral spinocerebellar tract; SRCT, spinoreticulocerebellar tract; DSCT, dorsal spinocerebellar tract; RF, reticular formation; RN, red nucleus; VN, vestibular nuclei.

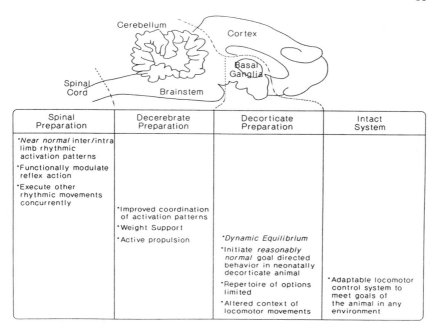

Spinal Preparation	Decerebrate Preparation	Decorticate Preparation	Intact System
•*Near normal* inter/intra limb rhythmic activation patterns •Functionally modulate reflex action •Execute other rhythmic movements concurrently	•Improved coordination of activation patterns •Weight Support •Active propulsion	•*Dynamic Equilibrium* •Initiate *reasonably normal* goal directed behavior in neonatally decorticate animal •Repertoire of options limited •Altered context of locomotor movements	•Adaptable locomotor control system to meet goals of the animal in any environment

Figure 3 The locomotor capability of various animal preparations transected at different levels along the neuraxis is shown. Text in italics is meant to indicate insufficient evidence or incomplete expression of the particular locomotor characteristics. (Adapted from Ref. 41.)

alternation) to the muscles, controlling near-normal inter and intralimb movements, but are not sufficient to support body weight, actively propel the body, or provide stability (Fig. 3) (41). The preorganized Core Locomotor Patterns in the spinal cord simplify the control of locomotion by harnessing the large degrees of freedom, and provide a skeletal structure that is molded by the supraspinal system to produce skilled locomotor behavior (4).

In humans, the evidence for these Core Locomotor Patterns has been primarily indirect, coming from developmental studies. Young infants produce steppinglike behavior that includes appropriate inter- and intralimb coordination when propulsion and balance requirements are eliminated through external support (65, 15). Recent work on paraplegic patients has provided some direct evidence for a spinal stepping generator in humans (11). Although the form of locomotor behavior is species specific (e.g., walking vs. flying), the basic framework of the control system is remarkably similar throughout the vertebrate phylum (12, 21). Therefore, there is no reason why this general principle of organizing rhythmic behavior should be different in humans.

The neuronal structures that encode these basic locomotor rhythms do not rely on pacemaker neurons for time keeping: rhythmicity is an emergent property of neuronal networks. Besides maintaining rhythmic activation to the muscles, these spinal neuronal networks have to produce specific forms of activation for each muscle. The spinal pattern generator can be modeled as a multistage network; first stage represents the time (rhythm)-keeping aspect, while the second stage includes pattern-shaping networks (Fig. 2) (48). Since pattern recognition techniques reveal that muscle activation patterns are not independent (there are underlying common features), it is possible that the outputs of the spinal pattern generator are these features rather than the individual muscle activation patterns (48). The muscle activation patterns can be synthesized from these features (synthesis network in Fig. 2) (48). A conceptual spinal pattern generator model proposed by Patla (48) is shown in Figure 2.

Deciphering these networks in the complex mammalian nervous system is beyond the reach of current experimental techniques. Nevertheless, Grillner and his colleagues have recently identified the exact neuronal network in lamprey (belonging to one of the most primitive vertebrate groups) responsible for generating locomotor behavior (19).

B. Active Propulsion and Weight Support

When the cerebellum, the brain stem, and the spinal cord are left intact, the animal not only is able to provide improved inter- and intralimb coordination, but also is able to support body weight and actively propel itself. Dynamic equilibrium is still lacking in a decerebrate preparation, particularly in the frontal plane. Improved coordination of the locomotor patterns is made possible by the cerebellum, which receives information about the output of the spinal pattern generator, called efference copy (via ventral spinocerebellar and spinoreticulocerebellar tracts); afferent inputs generated by the locomotor movements (via dosal spinocerebellar tract); and modulates the Core Locomotor Pattern by regulating the activity in various descending pathways (vestibulospinal, reticulospinal, and rubrospinal tracts) (Fig. 2).

Weight support and active propulsion is achieved through regulation of postural tonus particularly in the extensors (antigravity muscles). The work by Mori and his colleagues (31) has identified two midpontine neuronal structures that are responsible for modulating extensor muscle tone (Fig. 2). Stimulating the ventral part of the caudal tegmental field (VTF) in the pons increases the level of extensor muscle tone, while stimulation of the dorsal portion of the caudal tegmental field (DTF) reduces the extensor muscle tone. A cat supporting its weight on the limbs can be made to change its posture to sitting and even lying down when the DTF is stimulated at different intensities. In contrast, increasing the level of VTF stimulation results in the cat going from a lying posture to squatting to standing. Mori's work was shown quite clearly that appropriate postural set is a prerequisite for eliciting locomotor behavior. For example, stimulation of the DTF can override stimulation of the mesencephalic locomotor region (MLR) (cuneiform nucleus) or subthalamic locomotor region (lateral hypothalamic area) which normally would elicit locomotion. Interestingly, increasing the intensity of stimulation to the VTF beyond a certain value can result in triggering of locomotion that has spastic characteristics. This is analogous to elicitation of stepping behavior in humans when standing posture is perturbed by a large disturbance.

Initiation (or termination) of locomotion in both bipeds and quadrupeds requires an initial standing posture. Mori's work suggests that transition from postures other than standing is achieved by regulating the activity of subcortical structures (DTF and VTF) through variations in cortical drives to subthalamic or mesencephalic locomotion regions (Fig. 2). Garcia-Rill (17) has shown that the site of termination of the output of the basal ganglia, the pedunculopontine nucleus, is equivalent to the MLR. Thus basal ganglia are also involved in initiation and termination of locomotion.

An interesting feature of the animal locomotor apparatus is the fact that there are multiple sources of propulsive power generators: the animal does not have to rely on one set of muscles to provide propulsion. This is nicely illustrated in the human locomotor system when we examine walking in patients with different neuromuscular pathologies. Cataloguing the joint power patterns in a variety of pathologies, Winter et al. (69) have shown the shift in locus of propulsive power generation depending on which muscle groups are affected by a pathology. For example, an above-knee amputee must use hip muscles on the affected side to move forward. The shifts in locus of propulsive power do not need an insult to the locomotor apparatus to be realized: witness the immediate shift from pushing against the ground to pulling the leg up when we are traveling over an icy surface. When alternate power sources are used, locomotor characteristics such as stride length and velocity are generally compromised.

C. Dynamic Equilibrium: External Stability

Ensuring stability of the moving body is an absolutely essential requirement for locomotion. Bipedal locomotion offers a far greater challenge than quadrupedal locomotion. Transition from quadrupedal to bipedal stance reduced the base of support and involves precariously balancing the large mass of the upper body containing important organs high above the ground. Quadrupedal support is a minimum requirement for maintaining static stability during locomotion: bipedal locomotion necessitates control of dynamic equilibrium. During human locomotion, the body center of mass is outside the base of support 80% of the time (68), and the upper body is moving at a reasonable velocity (ranging from 1.22 m/s to 1.42 m/s during normal walking). A moving body is said to be stable if it returns to the original or another stable state of movement when perturbed.

There are two modes of controlling the dynamic equilibrium of the moving body: reactive and proactive. As its name suggests, reactive control is useful for unexpected or unpredictable perturbations, and relies on detection of these disturbances by the sensory systems. Proactive control of equilibrium during locomotion is mediated through two submodes. One submode is responsible for predicting perturbations generated by the locomotor movements themselves, and by other movements of the upper limb interacting with the environment (such as catching or carrying an object), and taking appropriate action. The second submode is visually based, experience-guided identification of a potential threat to equilibrium in the environment (such as potholes or obstacles) during locomotion, and involves selection and implementation of appropriate avoidance strategies.

Since sensory systems are critical for both reactive and proactive control, it would be useful to discuss briefly the sensory modalities playing important roles in the control of locomotion (and other movements).

1. Major Sensory Systems for Control of Locomotion: Kinesthetic, Vestibular, and Visual

Although in other animals sensory modalities such as olfactory and auditory systems play an important role in the control of locomotion, in humans, as in most mammals, the three sensory systems, kinesthetic, vestibular, and visual, are critical for mobility. When vision is compromised in humans, olfactory and auditory systems can play a role in control of goal-directed locomotion (64). Rather than discussing the detailed anatomy of these sensory systems, which can be found in many excellent texts, we shall focus our attention on the types of information each provides for the control of locomotion.

The type of information available for the control of locomotion from the three sensory modalities are listed in Table 1. It is evident that there is considerable overlap of information about the orientation and movement of the body from these sensory systems. This redundancy serves to protect the locomotor control system from failure when one of the sensory systems deteriorates.

Table 1 Information Provided by the Kinesthetic, Vestibular, and Visual Systems Useful for the Control of Locomotion.

Sensory system	Information for control of locomotion
Kinesthetic (Afferent receptors in muscles, tendons, joints and skin)	Relative orientation of body parts (posture and body schema) Movement of body parts Muscle tension Orientation of support surface and body with reference to the support surface
Vestibular (Afferent receptors in semicircular canals and otolith organs)	Angular acceleration and deceleration and velocity (through mechanical and neural integration) of the head Linear acceleration and deceleration of the head Orientation of the head with reference to gravity
Visual (Afferent receptors in retina)	Relative orientation and movements of body parts and orientation of the body referenced to the external environment Organization and features (static and dynamic) of the external environment

One important feature of these sensory systems is the level of interdependence and integration necessary for their use in the control of locomotion. Interpretation of the vestibular system output has to be considered in conjunction with the kinesthetic output about the body posture. In a posture with head tilt, for example, the same accelerations will produce different vestibular outputs. Maintaining stability of gaze (stable image on the retina) provides the best example of interdependence and integration of sensory inputs from visual, vestibular, and kinesthetic systems by the cerebellum (Fig. 2). Vestibulo-ocular reflex and optokinetic response (to compensate for head movements), cervico-ocular reflex (driven by neck torsion) and trunk-ocular reflex (elicited by trunk twisting) all serve to stabilize gaze and require sensory information from all three modalities to function. Recent work by Pozzo et al. (52) has shown clearly that the head is stabilized (and, by inference, gaze) while subjects are walking. Pitch rotation and vertical displacement of the head covary to provide stability of the head in the sagittal plane during locomotion. Similar control of head position has been demonstrated in the frontal plane (53). This reflexive head stabilization can be suppressed during smooth pursuit eye movements tracking a moving target.

Kinesthetic and visual systems unlike the vestibular system may be subjected to sensory errors. When the support surface moves (for example, while standing on a compliant surface) the kinesthetic output can be in error because its output is referenced to the support surface. Similarly, since the visual system detects relative motion between the body and the environment, environment motion can be perceived as self motion. Vestibular system measures motion with respect to inertial and gravitational fields and hence is a very robust system. The three sensory modalities with their different frames of reference (18) help to resolve conflict when one of the sensory system outputs is in error.

It should be noted, though, that the visual system can dominate the movement response as demonstrated by the elegant studies of Lee and his colleagues (26). For example, rotation of the room in which a person in running leads to compensatory rotation of the trunk to stabilize the visual surround (26). Recent work by Lackner and DiZio (24) in a rotating room and by Pailhous et al. (50) using projected visual flow, also demonstrates the influence and dominance of visual input on the control of locomotion.

There are two unique characteristics of the visual system that have an impact on the control of locomotion. First, the focus of attention can be directed to different locations in the visual field. This has a direct impact on locomotion as demonstrated by Zohar (73). By drawing attention to obstacles using colors or stripes on the floor, the likelihood of bumping into obstacles with different parts of the body was reduced considerably. The second unique feature is the fact that the resources of the visual system are not required on a continuous basis for guiding locomotion: intermittent sampling of the environment is adequate (66, 5, 37). This is not surprising considering evolutionary pressures that required the predator or the prey to attend to other things while locomoting.

Now let us turn our attention to the different modes of maintaining dynamic equilibrium.

2. Reactive Control of Equilibrium During Locomotion

Mono and polysynaptic reflexes mediated primarily through the kinesthetic and vestibular system provide a good defense against unexpected perturbations. The most interesting feature is the functional modulation of these reflexes to provide appropriate phase and task specific response to perturbations in humans (62) and other animals (16). Stein and his colleagues have shown that the gain of the soleus reflex (electrical analogue of the monosynaptic stretch reflex) is modulated during the step cycle. It is low in the early stance and swing phases, and high during the mid-to-late stance. During early stance, when the body is rotating over the foot stretching the soleus muscle, a high reflex gain would impede forward progression and therefore would be undesirable. Similarly, during early swing, when the foot is being actively dorsiflexed for ground clearance, a high reflex gain could result in tipping. In contrast, during late stance high reflex gain could assist in the pushoff action in the presence of perturbation and therefore would be desirable. Polysynaptic reflexes such as the flexor reflex (16, 14, 71) are also modulated and gated to provide functionally appropriate response. These long latency responses are probably more effective for responding to larger unexpected perturbations applied during locomotion. It is interesting to note that the spinal cord in cats is sufficient for functionally modulating these reflexes (15) (Fig. 3). The modulation of mono and polysynaptic reflexes involves task, phase, and muscle-specific control of the reflex gain (even the sign), and has been argued to be a basic control strategy (54). When perturbation magnitude is too large to be compensated by these mono and polysynaptic reflexes, appropriate voluntary response is recruited to recover balance.

3. Proactive Control: Based on Prediction of Movement
   Generated Perturbation

Every movement, even the normal locomotor movements, perturb the
body by virtue of displacement of the center of mass and reactive moments. A pioneering study by Belenkii et al. (7) demonstrated that
postural muscles were recruited prior to those required for intended
movement. Ever since then, numerous studies have documented the
role of anticipatory or proactive control in responding to perturbations
applied to upright posture (28).

   Winter (68) has documented the joint moments that counteract the
perturbations produced by the normal locomotor movements. Pitching
motion of the trunk with acceleration and deceleration in each step cycle
is controlled primarily by the moments about the hip joint (as discussed in
the effector system section). Tipping of the upper body toward the unsupported side is primarily regulated by the hig abductors: the magnitude of
destabilization is controlled by the foot placement with respect to body
center of mass. Collapse in the vertical direction is prevented by controlling the moments about the knee joint, which have been shown by Winter
(68) to covary with the hip joint moments. By using the hamstrings to
decelerate the limb extension during the swing phase, gentle foot contact
(horizontal velocity ~0.4 m/s) is achieved and chances of slipping are
minimized. Elasticity in the tendons and compliant foot pads facilitates
this gentle foot contact (1). During normal level locomotion, as simula-
tions have shown, tripping is avoided primarily through active dorsiflexion (29). Subjects can minimize locomotor movement-related perturbation by shifting the locus of propulsive power from the ankles to the hip:
push-off action by the plantarflexors is more destabilizing than pull-off
action by the hip flexors. The elderly use less push-off and more pull-off
action to walk, probably to minimize the potential of falling (70).

   Studies examining postural responses to additional movement-
generated perturbations applied during locomotion are relatively few
(33, 22). These studies have shown that proactive responses to perturbations initiated by arm movements are functional ensuring stability and
forward progression.

   This mode of proactive control of balance suggests the presence of
a movement and body schema within the nervous system.

4. Proactive Control: Visually Mediated Avoidance Strategies

The ability to use isolated footholds and go over obstacles affords legged
locomotion unique versatility over vehicles with wheels (55). Vision is

critical for selection and implementation of these proactive strategies. Patla (42) reviewed the major issues in the visual guidance of human locomotion and classified the locomotor adaptive strategies into two categories, avoidance and accommodation. Avoidance strategies are recruited when stepping on a surface is undesirable, while accommodation strategies are employed when walking over different terrains that must be stepped on.

As outlined by Patla (42) avoidance strategies include the following: (1) selection of alternate foot placement by modulating step length and width; (2) increased ground or head clearance to avoid hitting an obstacle; (3) changing the direction of locomotion (steering) when the obstacles cannot be cleared; and (4) stopping. Clearly, avoidance strategies represent locomotor adaptations that are primarily implemented to ensure equilibrium of the moving body.

The work done in my lab has provided unique insights into the basis for selection of alternate foot placement (39), minimum time (expressed in terms of the step cycle metric) required for implementing these avoidance strategies (46, 45, 39), and the characteristics of locomotor pattern changes (38–47).

The major findings from our studies on avoidance strategies are the following:

1. Most avoidance strategies can be successfully implemented within a step cycle; only steering has to be planned one step cycle ahead.

2. Selection of alternate foot placement is guided by simple rules. Minimum foot displacement from its normal landing spot is a critical determinant of alternate foot placement position. When two or more choices meet the above criteria, modifications in the plane of progression are preferred. Given a choice between shortening or lengthening step strength, subjects chose increased step length; inside foot placement is preferred over stepping to the outside provided the foot does not cross the midline of the body. As discussed by Patla et al. (39), these rules for alternate foot placement selection ensure that avoidance strategies are implemented with minimal changes while maintaining the dynamic equilibrium and allowing the person to travel forward safely.

3. The modifications made to the locomotor pattern to implement avoidance strategies are complex and task specific. They are not simple amplitude scaling of the normal locomotor

patterns: rather both inter and intralimb muscle activation patterns show phase (of the step cycle) and muscle-specific modulations (42).

4. Both visually observable and visually inferred properties of the environment influence the avoidance strategy selection and implementation (42). We have shown, for example, that perceived fragility of the obstacle modulates limb elevation (38). When obstacle avoidance response has to be initiated quickly, subjects show a two-stage modulation of limb trajectory; initial change is in response to obstacle followed by adjustments related to the height of the obstacle (44).

Earlier work on neonatally decorticate cats suggested that loss of cortex has minimal impact on the locomotor process (21, 17), although the context in which the locomotor movements are performed is affected. For example, decorticate cats are hyperreactive and tend to escape from stimuli that would normally elicit a passing interest. Decorticate cats exhibit limited range of options in locomotor movements and have curtailed exploratory behavior. These findings have generally been from visual observation of behavior.

Recent work on animal locomotion has demonstrated direct involvement of the motor cortex when the animal is required to select appropriate footholds and avoid obstacles to maintain stability (13). During normal level path unobstructed locomotion, the cortical involvement is minimal. The outputs from the pyramidal tract neurons have been shown to encode precisely not only limb elevation to clear the obstacle, but also foot placement (13). Depending on the intensity of the cortical volley, the ongoing locomotor rhythm may be modified or reset (i.e., initiate transition from stance to swing phase). The exact mapping of the inputs received by the visual cortex and the output of the motor cortex is complex and not complete (67). Basal ganglia play an important role in visually guided adaptive strategies as evidenced by lesion studies (17). Ablation of the caudate nuclei in cats results in the animal following anything that moves, termed "compulsory approach syndrome"; while diencephalic (removal of thalamus and hypothalamus) cats demonstrate "obstinate progression," walking into obstacles and not following or attending to any environmental stimuli. Therefore, neuronal structures rostral to the brainstem and cerebellum are critical for the expression of stable locomotion behavior (Fig. 3).

D. Steering and Accommodation Strategies for Various Environments

Different terrains have to be accommodated as we travel from one place to another. These terrains may have different geometric characteristics, such as sloped surfaces or stairs, and/or may have different surface properties such as compliance (a soggy field), and frictional characteristics (icy surface) that can influence the body–ground interaction (42). Unlike avoidance strategies that normally would influence one or two steps, accommodation strategies would usually involve modifications sustained over several steps. The types of changes made to the normal locomotor rhythm may include those discussed under avoidance strategies. For example, while walking on an icy surface step length is often reduced. Other changes include a change in locus of propulsive power as found in stair climbing (propulsive power from the muscles around the hip and knee joint) compared to level walking (major propulsive power from muscles around the ankle joint) (68).

The initial planning of gait adjustments during a transition from a normal level surface to a different surface has to be visually mediated. Knowledge acquired through experience plays an important role in visual regulation of locomotor patterns. An icy surface poses a far greater hazard to a person from the tropical climes than to a native of northern countries. We have recently begun to examine the changes observed while stepping onto an altered surface (59). For example, the foot position (and body posture) at landing has to be matched to the surface geometry (A.E. Patla, unpublished observations). Once the foot contact has been made with the altered surface, other sensory modalities, in particular the kinesthetic system, can play an important role in modulation of gait patterns.

Although steering has been briefly discussed under avoidance strategies, it is explicitly included in this nested ring to highlight its importance for goal-directed locomotion. Steering, unlike other changes to gait, requires preplanning in the previous step. It is interesting, therefore, to note that steering plays a critical role in the escape and capture behavior between a predator and prey (3). Patla et al. (45) have discussed the changes necessary to force a change in the direction of locomotion. What is not known is the extent to which head and neck reflexes play a role in turning behavior. The early work by Brown (9) clearly shows that when the cat's head is prevented from moving, turning behavior is seriously affected. The work discussed by Garcia-Rill (17) suggests that the basal ganglia is involved in turning behavior.

It is evident from this brief discussion that much more work is needed to understand the features of steering and accommodation strategies necessary for goal-directed travel over varied terrains.

E. Maintaining Structural Integrity of the Locomotor Apparatus: Internal Stability

The locomotor apparatus, however functional, would not be useful if it had a high probability of mechanical failure under normal operating conditions. Structures made by humans are designed with high safety factors: the ratio of failure stress (force per unit area) to those stresses normally experienced by the structure range from four to ten. Evolutionary pressures have engineered biological structures of the locomotor apparatus (bones, muscles, tendons, and ligaments) to minimize their failure during the animal's lifetime. Biewener (8) has reviewed how the changes in form, material properties, and mass of the biological structure in animals of varying sizes have evolved to minimize failure during locomotor activities. This review shows that the organization and composition of skeletal bones, muscles, and tendons are generally similar across species. To maintain stress within the biological range during locomotion, selection has preferred instead to modify muscle mechanical advantage and limb posture as the size of the animal increases. The upright posture in bipedal locomotion affords a greater effective mechanical advantage defined as the ratio of propulsive muscle moment arm to the moment arm of the ground reaction forces (8), thus reducing the muscle force and hence skeletal stress.

Researchers interested in restoring gait in patients with spinal cord damage have observed that the recruitment of muscles during walking and running increases the compressive stress on the skeleton while reducing bending stress (32). Because the bones are designed to withstand far larger compressive stress then bending stress, this anomaly is understandable. Recently, we have shown that during sustained rhythmic activity (cycling) to exhaustion, the locus of propulsive power shifts from the muscles around the knee joint to those around the hip joint (57). This may be argued as a protective response to prevent irreversible damage to the extensor muscles around the knee joint which are recruited at high intensity during cycling.

These studies clearly illustrate that the control system selects locomotor activation patterns to ensure structural integrity of the system. Because of the large safety factor during normal locomotor activity, on a short-term basis, we can afford to use activation patterns that would increase the bending stress. But for the long-term viability of the loco-motor apparatus, the control system has to consider this factor in plan-ning the activation patterns.

It is not surprising that the sensory systems, in particular the kines-thetic system, play a critical role in minimizing damage to the tissues. Inhibitory reflexes ensure that muscle force, for example, does not in-crease beyond a limit. Flexor reflex allows the animal to withdraw the limb from a noxious stimuli that may harm some tissues. When the kinesthetic system is compromised, as in patients with diabetes, foot ulcers result from repeated loading of injured tissue (63). The variability we observe in the locomotor activation patterns may therefore be a useful strategy serving to minimize potential tissue injuries.

F. Minimizing Energy Cost of Locomotion

Moving the body through an environment requires energy. Minimizing these locomotor-related energy costs can increase the animal's endur-ance, allowing it to travel farther and longer, provide more energy for reproduction, and reduce time spent on hazardous foraging to replenish the energy sources (2). These benefits would clearly increase the chances of survival and therefore selection pressures would favor loco-motor patterns that required less energy.

Locomotor characteristics in terrestrial animals have been shown to be influenced by energy costs. Hoyt and Taylor (23) demonstrated that oxygen consumption in horses walking at different speeds has a U-shaped characteristic. The self-selected walking speeds by the horse fell around the minimum value in oxygen consumption curve, illustrating that animals choose the most economical speed of walking.

Until recently, different modes of locomotion (different gaits) were thought to be unique characteristics of terrestrial locomotion. Quadru-peds walk, trot, and gallop, while humans walk and run at different speeds. These different gaits are characterized by different sequences of foot position employed by the animal. Newer techniques that made flow visualization possible have shown that the concepts of gait can be applied to other forms of locomotion such as flying (2). The selection of a particu-lar mode of locomotion has been shown to be guided by energy costs: animals switch to a different gait to reduce their energy expenditure (2).

The body morphology is matched to the environment that the animal travels through to achieve the lower energy costs. Movements of the fish through water is energy efficient because of the shape; at cruising speed the flow is laminar resulting in lower energy costs. In long-legged animals like humans, the relative mass distribution assists in reducing energy costs. Large mass muscle is concentrated around the proximal joints reducing the inertia resulting in lower energy requirements. Elasticity in various tissues has been argued to provide energy reduction (2).

Energy minimization, like maintaining structural integrity, is important for long-term viability of the locomotor apparatus. On a short-term basis, when safety is threatened, for example, energy consideration may not influence the locomotor patterns.

G. Cognitive Spatial Mapping

Since locomotion is essential for survival, it is not surprising that animals rarely move around aimlessly: locomotion is goal directed. When the route or path is visible from a single viewpoint, no spatial knowledge of the terrain is necessary. For example, when going from one part of the room to another that is visible from the point of origin, visual input alone can guide the selection of path (even around obstacles if present). When moving in a large-scale spatial area such as a city block or town, route planning generally depends on some mental representation of the area (10, 34, 56). Cognitive spatial maps are the mental representation of large-scale areas. This ability to store and retrieve information about their living environment affords animals tremendous advantage.

This topographical knowledge is not a monolithic entity. Rather, as studies examining acquisition of spatial knowledge for travels and clinical studies of topographical amnesia show, spatial maps take various forms and are stored in different locations (56). Routes defined as a series of landmark–action pairs and general spatial representation are stored to provide flexibility in navigation. Studies, for example, on bird navigation and orangutans show that animals do not just travel on a familiar travel path; they are able to reach the goals via different, unfamiliar paths (34). We can travel from our homes or any other location to the workplace via many routes, depending, for example, on traffic patterns.

Based on animal data O'Keefe and Nadel (34) have argued that the hippocampus serves as a neural substrate for storage of these cognitive spatial maps for travel. The information contained in the spatial maps is procedural (implicit and accessible through performance) rather than declarative (explicit and accessible to conscious awareness) (60). In humans, hippocampal damage does lead to memory deficits, but the information affected is declarative and not procedural (60). Generally damage to the regions in the right hemisphere including the hippocampus have been found to affect retrieval of prestored topographical memory. Whereas there are standard accepted neuropsychological tests for assessing visuospatial abilities within the extrapersonal space, there is a noticeable lack of appropriate laboratory and field tasks that could tap into the navigational deficits in patients.

Navigation requires two other abilities besides cognitive maps. First, the navigator must be able to estimate the distance and direction traveled to update their current bearing on the map. Second, they must be able to detect orientation with respect to an external frame of reference (10, 34). Estimating the distance and direction traveled may be derived from the kinesthetic and vestibular system (through integration). Birds can use information from the stars, the sun, and the earth's magnetic fields to orient themselves. How we keep track of our position and bearing during travel from one place to another is not clear. Studies on open sea navigation by Pulawat Islanders (10) show a highly abstract method of place keeping. The work by Lindberg and Garling (25) demonstrate that conscious attention is important for keeping track of one's position in an artificial maze. It is clear that "place keeping" in humans is facilitated by visual recognition of landmarks, although visually impaired individuals rely on olfactory and/or auditory cues to recognize landmarks (64). The presence of a compass in humans similar to those found in birds has not been proven although there has been much speculation and some data (10).

In summary, cognitive spatial maps, wherever they are stored in the nervous system, play a critical role in purposeful travel.

V. SUMMARY

A framework for understanding neural control of skilled human locomotor behavior has been provided in this review. It can serve to guide future studies on human locomotion by highlighting what is known and what is not known. In addition, it can be useful for interpreting deficits in locomotor behavior observed in patients and evaluating rehabilitative strategies. The orchestration of various neural substrates toward generating and regulating locomotion, a seemingly simple activity, is fascinating and can help in our understanding of control of voluntary movements.

ACKNOWLEDGMENT

The support of Natural Science and Engineering Research Council of Canada is gratefully acknowledged.

REFERENCES

1. Alexander R McN. Three uses for springs in legged locomotion. Int J Robotics Res 1990; 9(2):53–61.
2. Alexander R McN. Optimization and gaits in the locomotion of vertebrates. Phys Rev 1989; 69(4): 1199–1227.
3. Alexander R McN. Locomotion in animals. London: Blackie & Sons, Ltd, 1982.
4. Armstrong DM. The supraspinal control of mammalian locomotion. J Physiol 1988; 405: 1–37.
5. Assaiante C, Marchand AR, Amblard B. Decrete visual samples may control locomotor equilibrium and foot positioning in man. J Motor Behav 1989; 21: 72–91.
6. Belanger M, Patla AE. Corrective responses to perturbations applied during walking in humans. Neurosci Lett 1984; 49: 291–295.
7. Belenkii YY, Gurfinkel VS, Paltsev YI. Element of control of voluntary movements. Biofizika 1967; 12: 135–141.
8. Biewener AA. Biomechanics of mammalian terrestrial locomotion. Science 1990; 250: 1097–1103.
9. Brown TG. Intrinsic factors in the act of progression in the mammal. Proc R Soc London 1911; 884: 308–319.
10. Bryne RW. Geographical knowledge and orientation. In: Ellis AW, ed. Normality and Pathology in Cognitive Functions. London: Academic Press 1982: 239–264.
11. Bussel B, Roby-Brami A, Yakovleff A, Bennis N. Late flexion reflex in paraplegic patients. Evidence for a spinal stepping generator. Brain Res Bull 1989; 22: 53–56.
12. Delcomyn F. Neural basis of rhythmic behaviour in animals. Science 1980; 210(31): 492–498.
13. Drew T. Visumotor coordination in locomotion. Curr Opinion Neurobiol 1991; 91(4): 652–657.
14. Duysens J, Trippel M, Horstmann GA, Dietz V. Gating and reversal of reflexes in ankle muscles during human walking. Exp Brain Res 1990; 82: 351–358.
15. Forssberg H. Ontogeny of human locomotor control I. Infant stepping, supported locomotion and transition to independent locomotion. Exp Brain Res 1985; 57: 480–493.

16. Forssberg H. Spinal locomotor functions and descending control. In: Sjolund B, Bjorklund A, eds. Brain Stem Control of Spinal Mechanisms. New York: Elsevier Biomedical Press, 1982: 253–271.
17. Garcia-Rill E. The basal ganglia and the locomotor regions. Brain Res Rev 1986; 11: 47–63.
18. Gibson JJ. The Senses Considered as Perceptual Systems. Boston: Houghton-Mifflin, 1966.
19. Grillner S, Wallen P, Brodin L, Lansner A. Neuronal network generating locomotor behavior in lamprey: circuitry, transmitters membrane properties, and simulation. Annu Rev Neurosci 1991; 14: 169–199.
20. Grillner S, Dubuc R. Control of locomotion in vertebrates: Spinal and supraspinal mechanisms. In: Waxman, SG, ed. Advances in Neurology, Vol. 47, Functional Recovery in Neurological Disease. New York: Raven Press, 1988.
21. Grillner S. Neurobiological bases of rhythmic motor acts in vertebrates. Science 1985; 228: 143–149.
22. Hirschfeld H, Forssberg H. Phase-dependent modulations of anticipatory postural activity during human locomotion. J Neurophysiol 1991; 66(1): 12–19.
23. Hoyt DF, Taylor CR. Gait and the energetics of locomotion in horses. Nature 1981; 292: 239–240.
24. Lackner JR, DiZio P. Visual stimulation affects the perception of voluntary leg movements during walking. Perception 1988; 17: 71–80.
25. Lindberg E, Garling T. Acquisition of locational information about reference points during locomotion: The role of central information processing. Scand J Psychol 1982; 23: 207–218.
26. Leo DN, Young DS. Gearing action to the environment. Exp Brain Res Ser 1986; 15: 217–230.
27. McGeer T. Passive dynamic walking. Int J Robotics Res 1990; 9: 62–82.
28. Massion J. Movement, posture and equilibrium: interaction and coordination. Prog Neurobiol 1992; 38: 35–56.
29. Mena D, Mansour JM, Simon SR. Analysis and synthesis of human swing leg motion during gait and its clinical applications. J Biomech 1981; 14(12): 823–832.
30. Mochon S, McMahon TA. Ballistic walking. J Biomech 1980; 13: 49–57.
31. Mori S. Integration of posture and locomotion in acute decerebrate cats and in awake, freely moving cats. Prog Neurobiol 1987; 28: 161–195.
32. Munih M, Kralj A, Bajd T. Calculation of bending moments unloading femur and tibia bones. In: Advances in external control of human extremities X. Popovic DB, ed., Belgrade: Nauka, 1990: 67–79.
33. Nashner LM, Forssberg H. Phase-dependent organization of postural adjustments associated with arm movements while walking. J Neurophysiol 1986; 55: 1382–1394.

34. O'Keefe J, Nadel L. The hippocampus as a cognitive map. Oxford: Clarendon Press, 1978.

35. Olney SJ, Winter DA. Predictions of knee and ankle moments of force in walking from EMG and kinematic data. J Biomech 1985; 18: 9–20.

36. Owen Lovejoy, C. Evolution of human walking. Sci Am 1988; 259(5): 118–125.

37. Patla AE, Martin C, Holden R, Prentice S. The effects of terrain difficulty on characteristics of voluntary visual sampling of the environment during locomotion. Soc Neurosci Abstr 1992; 18(2).

38. Patla AE, Martin C, Rietdyk S. The effect of visually inferred property of an obstacle on obstacle avoidance response during locomotion in humans. In: Woollacott M, Horak F, eds. Postures and Gait: Control Mechanisms. Portland: University of Oregon Press, 1992: 222–226.

39. Patla AE, Prentice SD, Martin C, Rietdyk S. The bases of selection of alternate foot placement during locomotion in humans. In: Woollacott M, Horak F, eds. Posture and Gait: Control Mechanisms, Portland: University of Oregon Press, 1992: 226–229.

40. Patla AE. Understanding the control of human locomotion: A 'Janus' perspective. In: Patla AE, ed. Adaptability of Human Gait: Implications for the Control of Locomotion. New York: Elsevier, 1991a: 441–452.

41. Patla AE. Visual control of human locomotion. In: Patla AE, ed. Adaptability of Human Gait: Implications for the Control of Locomotion. New York: Elsevier Publishers, 1991b: 55–97.

42. Patla AE. Understanding the control of human locomotion: A prologue. In: Patla AE, ed. Adaptability of Human Gait: Implications for the Control of Locomotion. New York: Elsevier Publishers, 1991c: 3–17.

43. Patla AE, Riedtyk S. Effect of obstacle height and width on gait patterns. XIII Int Soc Biomech Conf Proc, Perth, Australia, 1991: 455–456.

44. Patla AE, Beuter A, Prentice S. A two stage correction of limb trajectory to avoid obstacles during stepping. Neurosci Res Commun 1991; 8(13): 153–159.

45. Patla AE, Prentice S, Robinson C, Neufeld J. Visual control of locomotion: Strategies for changing direction and for going over obstacles. J Exp Psychol: Hum Percep Perform 1991; 17(3): 603–634.

46. Patla AE, Robinson C, Samways M, Armstrong CJ. Visual control of step length during overground locomotion: Task-specific modulation of the locomotion synergy. J Exp Psychol: Hum Percep Perform 1989; 25(3): 603–617.

47. Patla AE, Armstrong CJ, Silveira JM. Adaptation of the muscle activation patterns to transitory increase in stride length during treadmill locomotion in humans. Hum Movement Sci 1989; 8: 45–66.

48. Patla AE. Analytic approaches to the study of outputs from central pattern generators. In: Cohen A, Rossignol S, Grillner S, eds. Neural Control of Rhythmic Movements in Vertebrates. New York: Wiley, 1988: 455–486.

49. Patla AE. Adaptation of postural responses to voluntary arm raises during locomotion in humans. Neurosci Lett 1986; 68: 334–338.
50. Pailhous J, Ferrendez AM, Fluckiger M, Baumberger B. Unintentional modulations of human gait by optical flow. Behav Brain Res 1990; 38: 275–281.
51. Pierrot-Desilligny E, Bergego C, Mazieres L. Reflex control of bipedal gait in man. In: Desmedt JE, ed. Motor Control Mechanisms in Health and Disease. New York: Raven Press, 1983: 699–716.
52. Pozzo T, Berthoz A, Lefort K. Head stabilization during various locomotor tasks in humans. J. Normal Subjects. Exp Brain Res 1990; 82: 97–106.
53. Pozzo T, Levik Y, Berthoz A. Head stabilization in the frontal plane during complex equilibrium tasks in humans. In: Woollacott M, Horak F, eds. Posture and gait: Control mechanisms. Portland: University of Oregon Press, 1992: 97–100.
54. Prochazka A. Sensorimotor gain control: A basic strategy of motor systems? Prog Neurobiol 1989; 33: 281–307.
55. Raibert MH. Legged robots that balance. Cambridge: MIT Press, 1986.
56. Schacter DL, Nadel L. Varieties of spatial memory: A problem for cognitive neuroscience. In: Lister, RG, Weingartner HJ, eds. Perspectives on Cognitive Neuroscience. Oxford: Oxford University Press, 1991: 164–185.
57. Sirin AV, Patla AE, Wells RP. Bilateral joint contribution to total work during exhaustive cycling. Sixth Conference of the Canadian Society for Biomechanics, Quebec City, Canada, 1990: 165–166.
58. Smith JL, Zernicke RF. Predictions for neural control based on limb dynamics. Trends Neurosci 1987; 10: 123–128.
59. Spaulding SJ, Patla AE, Rietdyk S, Flanagan J, Elliott D. Effect of surface characteristics on gait modifications in individuals with age-related macular degeneration. Soc Neurosci Abstr, San Diego, 1992.
60. Squire LR, Zola-Morgan S. Memory: Brain systems and behaviour. Trends Neurosci 1988; 11(4): 170–175.
61. Squire LR. Mechanisms of memory. Science 1986; 232: 1612–1619.
62. Stein RB. Reflex modulation during locomotion. In: Patla AE, ed. Adaptability of human gait: Implications for the Control of Locomotion. New York: Elsevier Publishers, 1991: 21–36.
63. Stokes IA, Faris IB, Hutton WC. The neuropathic ulcer and loads on the foot in diabetic patients. Acta Orthopaed Scand 1975; 46: 839–847.
64. Strelow ER. What is needed for a theory of mobility: Direct perception and cognitive maps-lesons from the blind. Psychol Rev 1985; 92(2): 226–248.
65. Thelen E, Ulrich BD, Niles D. Bilateral coordination in human infants: Stepping on a split-belt treadmill. J Exp Psychol: Hum Percep Perform 1987; 13: 405–410.
66. Thomson JA. (1983) Is continuous visual control necessary in visually guided locomotion? J Exp Psychol: Hum Percep Perform 1983; 9: 427–443.

67. Van Essen DC, Anderson CH, Felleman DJ. Information processing in the primate visual system: An integrated systems perspective. Science 1992; 255: 419–423.

68. Winter DA. The biomechanics and motor control of human gait: Normal, elderly, and pathological. Waterloo, Ontario: University of Waterloo Press, 1991.

69. Winter DA, Olney SJ, Conrad J, White SC, Ounpuu S, Gage JR. Adaptability of motor patterns in pathological gait. In Winters JM, Woo SL-Y, eds. Multiple Muscle Systems: Biomechanics and Movement Organization. New York: Springer-Verlag, 1990: 680–693.

79. Winter DA, Patla AE, Frank JS, Walt SE. Biomechanical walking pattern changes in the fit and healthy elderly. Phys Ther 1990; 70(6): 340–347.

71. Yang JF, Stein RB. Phase dependent reflex reversal in human leg muscles during walking. J Neurophysiol 1990; 63: 1109–1117.

72. Zajac FE, Gordon ME. Determining muscle force and action in multiarticular movement. Exercise Sport Sci Rev 1989; 17: 187–230.

73. Zohar D. Why do we bump into things while walking. Hum Factors 1978; 20: 671–679.

3

An Overview of Neurological Diseases Causing Gait Disorder

LEWIS SUDARSKY

Veterans Affairs Medical Center, West Roxbury, and
Harvard Medical School, Boston, Massachusetts

I. INTRODUCTION

Gait disorder is a common presenting feature of neurological illness at any age. Delay in learning to walk may be the manifestation of a developmental disorder. After the skill has been mastered, gait becomes a characteristic feature of the older child and young adult. Just as a limp marks a wounded animal, an abnormality of gait at this age indicates an injury to musculoskeletal or neurological systems. Gait is a fundamental motor skill, and its decomposition is a sensitive indicator of neurological disease. The clinical examination of the nervous system is not complete until the gait has been observed.

Gait disorders are particularly common among the elderly, the fastest growing segment of the population. Community-based studies suggest a prevalence of 15% in the population over 65, higher in the population over 85 (28). One-fourth of 79-year-olds use mechanical aids for walking (21). A large number of the elderly live alone, and loss of mobility is a factor in many nursing home admissions (35). Gait instability also contributes to the risk for falls (45, 37, 30). Many elderly in the community voluntarily limit their activity because of concern about mobility and fear of falling (16). Chapter 11 more fully analyzes falls in the older adult.

II. UNDERSTANDING THE DIVERSITY OF GAIT DISORDERS

Neurological illnesses frequently have an impact on gait because the performance calls on a number of motor, sensory, and integrative systems. Among neurological patients, there is an almost overwhelming diversity of gait disorders. This heterogeneity reflects the complexity of the task and the large amount of anatomy involved; there are many possible failures.

Gait can be broken down into two principal component tasks: locomotion and balance. The nervous system must manage both simultaneously to produce a stable gait. The neural control of locomotion is the subject of Chapter 2. Locomotion requires the phasic activation of the leg muscles. Motor instructions coordinate the timing of muscle activation, the advance position of the limbs, the loading and unloading as weight is redistributed. The second task is the maintenance of dynamic equilibrium, a constraint that must be addressed to prevent instability and falls.

In animals, locomotion depends on the activity of a spinal pattern generator (14, 29). The independent capacity for spinal stepping has not been found in humans (34); bipeds are presumably more reliant on higher command centers in the brainstem and diencephalon. In the monkey, automatic walking can be expressed by electric stimulation of the midbrain tegmentum (mesencephalic locomotor region) or posterior subthalamus (11). It is unclear how basal ganglia circuits and cortical projections to these regions mediate control. Higher centers may be responsible for initiation and modulation of gait, and may be relatively inactive during steady ambulation on a flat surface (2). Instructions for gait in the primate are passed along nonpyramidal pathways in the ventral spinal cord (19).

Dynamic equilibrium is maintained when the center of gravity is over the base of support on the average over time. This relationship is maintained by postural supporting responses, known in the older literature as righting reflexes. Nashner and others (26) have studied static balance and a variety of postural adjustments that occur in response to a perturbation. Similar protective adjustments occur during walking (27). When we misstep, rescue or stumbling reactions protect us from falls. Locomotion is stable by design; it is unclear to what degree postural reflexes participate when walking at a constant velocity across a flat surface (6). Gait initiation, changes in momentum, and walking on uneven surfaces provide a greater challenge to the maintenance of equilibrium. Control of balance is highly dependent on afferent information from the visual system, the vestibular system, and proprioceptive input from the lower limbs. Recent studies suggest that muscle spindle afferents may play a role in kinesthetic sense and balance (36).

III. THE PRINCIPAL PATTERNS OF GAIT DISORDER AND THEIR CAUSE

Gait disorders of various description are observed in the community as well as in acute care hospitals, psychiatric institutions, chronic care facilities, and nursing homes. The spectrum of illness reflects the population under consideration. As many as 40% of nursing home patients are nonambulatory. Many have cognitive impairment, and it is often impossible to establish a specific diagnosis for their failure. In the community, a large number of gait problems are due to arthritis and orthopedic deformity, a minor degree of which may have a profound effect on gait. Common foot disorders affecting gait are reviewed in Chapter 11. A different spectrum of illness is encountered in a hospital or a doctor's office.

Our 1983 experience provides an introduction to this common problem in diagnosis by enumerating some of the frequently observed conditions. This study represents the perspective of neurology office practice, patients over 65 referred for undiagnosed disorder of gait. The study excluded patients with limb deformity, hemiparesis, obvious and known Parkinson's disease, and patients on neuroleptic drugs. Table 1 includes our more recent experience, cases seen in the past year.

In approximately 10–15% of older patients, no etiologic factors can be identified after careful evaluation and study. These patients are sometimes referred to as having as "essential senile gait." The terminology is deeply embedded in the literature (8, 18), although controversy exists about the nature of this problem. Do these patients represent a

Table 1   Classification of Gait Disorder in 75 Elderly Patients, Based on Principal Etiologic Diagnosis

	1980–1982	1990	Total	Percent
Myelopathy	8	6	14	18.4%
Parkinsonism	5	2	7	9.2
Hydrocephalus	2	3	5	6.6
Multiple infarcts	8	5	13	17.1
Cerebellar degeneration	4	1	5	6.6
Sensory deficits	9	6	15	19.7
Toxic/metabolic	3	0	3	3.9
Psychogenic	1	2	3	3.9
Other	3	0	3	3.9
Unknown cause	7	1	8	10.5

Source: Ref. 43.

spectrum of unsuccessful aging or is this simply a diagnostic wastebasket? It is doubtful that senile gait is a distinct morbid entity.

A. Spastic Gait

Spasticity denotes a state of increased stretch reflexes and velocity-dependent resistance to movement. This state reflects a disorder of "upper motor neurons" in the corticospinal tract. Spinal spasticity and cerebral spasticity differ slightly in their manifestations; painful muscle spasms are more common with spinal disorders. In ambulatory patients, the gait is stiff-legged with bounce, and a tendency to circumduct and scuff the feet. In extreme instances, the legs cross (scissoring). Shoes often reflect an uneven pattern of wear across the outside.

Myelopathy from cervical spondylosis is a common cause of gait disorder in the elderly—18% in our combined series (40). Spondylitic bars and ligamentous hypertrophy narrow the canal, causing mechanical compression and vascular compromise (48). Some degree of standing imbalance and bladder dysfunction (urgency, incontinence) accompany a mild spastic paresis of the legs. MR imaging has improved the ease of diagnosis, although it sometimes demonstrates advanced pathology in the cervical spine in minimally symptomatic patients. There are a variety of approaches to surgery in the cervical spine, although no consensus has emerged regarding the role of surgery in the elderly patient. The natural history is quite variable; some patients stabilize, while others progress.

Acute exacerbation sometimes follows a fall. Other causes of myelopathy in the elderly include B_{12} deficiency and degenerative disease (primary lateral sclerosis, hereditary spastic paraplegia).

Among younger patients, demyelinating disease and trauma are the leading causes of myelopathy. The prevalence of multiple sclerosis is 69 per 100,000 population in North America (23). In patients with chronic progressive myelopathy of unknown cause, thorough workup with laboratory and imaging tests often establishes a diagnosis of multiple sclerosis (31). Spinal cord injury may be incomplete, leaving the patient ambulatory. Motor vehicle and diving accidents, commonly alcohol-related, are the usual causes at our institution. Retrovirus infections are increasingly recognized as a cause of myelopathy. Tropical spastic paraplegia related to HTLV-1 is endemic in parts of the Caribbean and South America. Vacuolar myelopathy from AIDS is a growing problem worldwide. Myelopathy is sometimes due to a structural lesion, such as tumor or arteriovenous malformation.

With cerebral spasticity, involvement of the upper extremities with flexed posture is often observed, annd dysarthria is usually present. Common causes include vascular disease (stroke) and multiple sclerosis. In the cerebral palsy population, a mild spastic diplegia is the most frequently observed syndrome.

B. Extrapyramidal Disorder

Parkinson's disease (PD) is common, affecting 1.5% of the population over 65. The flexed attitude in posture and festinating gait are highly characteristic and distinctive. Of patients presenting with a bradykinetic/rigid syndrome, 10–15% will turn out to have something other than idiopathic PD (32, 22). The causes of atypical parkinsonism include progressive supranuclear palsy, olivopontocerebellar atrophy (OPCA), striatonigral degeneration, and coricobasal ganglionic degeneration. These diagnoses should be considered, particularly in patients *presenting with postural instability* or those unresponsive to levodopa. Gait disorders associated with extrapyramidal disease are reviewed in Chapter 6.

Drug-induced parkinsonism is increasingly recognized in ambulatory practice as a cause of impaired gait and balance. It is particularly common in a chronic care setting. Neuroleptic drugs are known to impair postural support responses and contribute to the risk for falls (9, 4). The disorder often takes 2–3 months to resolve, after the offending medication has been discontinued (39) (see Chap. 10 for a more complete discussion).

Hyperkinetic movement disorders may also produce a characteristic and recognizable disturbance in gait. Tardive dyskinesia is the cause of many odd and stereotypical gait disturbances seen in chronic psychiatric hospitals. The gait in Huntington's disease is defined by the unpredictable occurrence of choreic movements which give a dancing quality. In primary generalized dystonia (dystonia musculorum deformans), muscular spasm produces a dysfunctional posture of the legs: typically adduction and inversion, sometimes with torsion of the trunk.

C. Frontal Gait Disorder (Gait Apraxia)

Frontal gait disorder, sometimes characterized as "gait apraxia," is also more common in the elderly and has a variety of causes. Typical clinical features include a wide base of support, short stride, shuffling on the floor, and difficulty with starts and turns. Many exhibit a peculiar difficulty with gait initiation, descriptively characterized as the "slipping clutch." In studies seeking clinicopathological correlation, lesions are usually found in the deep frontal white matter (25).

Communicating hydrocephalus in the adult often presents with a gait disorder. Other features of the diagnostic triad (mental change, incontinence) may be absent in the initial stages (1, 12). Such patients now account for 6.6% of our experience with gait disorders in the elderly. For some, the gait is strikingly parkinsonian; others have a more typical frontal gait disorder. Radiological studies (CT, MRI) demonstrate ventricular enlargement, and sometimes show a halo of edema fluid in the periventricular white matter. A dynamic test is necessary to confirm the presence of hydrocephalus. The response to lumbar puncture, with removal of 30–50 cc of cerebrospinal fluid (CSF), has been used as a screening procedure (47).

Another common cause of the frontal gait disorder is vascular disease, particularly small vessel disease related to hypertension. In our series, 17% of the patients had multiple infarcts by CT or MR. Parkinsonian features are sometimes observed with basal ganglia lacunes, a condition known as "atherosclerotic parkinsonism." There is controversy regarding the entity, as patients with basal ganglia lacunes are often asymptomatic. Gait disorder is frequently seen in hypertensive patients with ischemic lesions of the deep hemisphere white matter (Binswanger's disease). The clinical syndrome consists of mental change (variable in degree), dysarthria, pseudobulbar affect, hyperreflexia in the limbs, and a gait disorder (3). The gait has been characterized by Thompson and Marsden (44) as "a parkinsonian-ataxia with relative sparing of the upper half of the body."

D. Cerebellar Gait

Dysfunction of the midline cerebellum has a dramatic impact on gait and postural control. The gait is characterized by a wide base, lateral instability of the trunk, erratic foot placement, and decompensation of balance when attempting to walk tandem. Cerebellar patients have well-characterized abnormalities in balance on platform tests (5, 15). They show considerable variation in their tendency to fall in the real world. Cerebellar dysfunction and its effect on posture and gait is reviewed in Chapter 5.

Posterior fossa tumors of childhood can present with an ataxic gait. Patients with multiple sclerosis are often considerably unsteady. Inherited and sporadic forms of cerebellar degeneration are described. Olivopontocerebellar atrophy is the most commonly recognized syndrome, but many other types are encountered (13). In OPCA, atrophy of the cerebellum and brainstem can be appreciated by CT or MRI. Other causes of cerebellar atrophy include toxins (alcohol, possibly phenytoin) and paraneoplastic cerebellar degeneration. Chronic alcoholics with anterior vermis atrophy experience primarily truncal ataxia (46).

E. Sensory Ataxia and Disequilibrium

Gait disorder in many patients is primarily a reflection of impaired balance. These patients exhibit a tendency to fall, and may present with a fall-related injury. Such patients should be investigated for a disorder of peripheral sensory systems or central postural control mechanisms. There is no consistent relationship in our experience between the degree of imbalance patients exhibit and the fear they express. Some unstable patients are quite timid, while others lurch about and are physically active.

Patients with chronic imbalance due to a disorder of sensory afferent systems are now the largest single group, approaching 20% in our series. Balance depends on high-quality information from the visual system, the vestibular system, and proprioceptive afferents. When this information is degraded, standing balance is impaired and gait instability results. The sensory ataxia of tabetic neurosyphilis is a classic example. The contemporary equivalent is the patient with neuropathy affecting large fiber afferents. The stance is such patients is destabilized by eye closure (Romberg's test). Patients have been described with imbalance from bilateral vestibular loss caused by disease or by exposure to oto-toxic drugs.

Drachman and Hart (10), in their approach to the dizzy patient, describe a syndrome of imbalance from multiple sensory deficits. Such patients, often elderly and diabetic, have disturbances in propriocep-tion, vision, and vestibular sense that impair postural support mecha-nisms. Cataract surgery with external lenses has been a factor in the decompensation of some such patients.

F. Neuromuscular Disease

Patients with neuromuscular disease often have an abnormal gait, al-though it is not usually the presenting feature. With distal weakness (peripheral neuropathy), the step height is often increased to compen-sate for foot drop, and the sole of the foot may slap on the floor during weight acceptance. Neuropathy may be associated with a degree of sen-sory imbalance, as described above. Patients with myopathy or muscular dystrophy have primarily proximal weakness. Weakness of the hip girdle may produce a degree of excess pelvic rotation (waddle).

G. Toxic and Metabolic Disorders

Intoxication with alcohol is certainly the most common cause of acute gait disturbance in western societies. Chronic toxicity from medications and metabolic disturbances can also impair motor function and gait. Static equilibrium is disturbed, and such patients are easily displaced back. This is particularly dramatic in patients with chronic renal disease and those with hepatic failure, in whom asterixis may impair postural support. Sedative drugs, especially neuroleptics and long-acting benzo-diazepines, affect postural reflexes and increase the risk for falls (33). It is important to recognize these disorders because they are treatable. The effects of medications on gait and mobility are discussed in Chapter 10.

H. Psychogenic Gait Disorder

Psychogenic disturbances of gait are among the most spectacular disor-ders encountered in neurology. Odd gyrations of posture (astasia–abasia) and dramatic fluctuations over time may be observed in the hysterical pa-tient (20, 17). Some patients with extreme anxiety walk with exaggerated caution, as if walking on a slippery surface. Depressed patients primarily exhibit slowness, a manifestation of psychomotor retardation (38).

I. Other Identifiable Causes

Head and spinal injuries can produce a neurological deficit with impaired ambulation. A few patients presenting with gait disorder have a mass lesion: primary CNS tumor or metastatic cancer. Subdural hematoma should be ruled out in the patient with subacute evolution and a history of falls.

IV. EVALUATION OF GAIT DISORDERS

The approach to the patient with gait disorder depends on the pace of the illness. Most of the disorders reviewed above evolve slowly over a period of several years, without a recognizable event. A stepwise or sudden progression suggests vascular disease. Headache or back pain may indicate a structural lesion, particularly if the decompensation is more subacute. (Patients with an acute inability to walk present a problem of substantially different character and should be evaluated emergently.)

In the history from the patient with a chronically progressive disorder of gait, there are several common themes. Gait and bladder control may show a parallel decompensation, particularly with subcortical or spinal lesions. First awareness of a balance problem often follows a fall. This may result in loss of confidence and fear (the "timid" gait). Pain with walking suggests the presence of arthritis or lumbar spinal stenosis. It is always important to review the use of alcohol and medications that might influence gait and balance.

As the list of possible diagnoses is lengthy, information on localization derived from the neurological exam can be helpful to narrow the search. Even in the absence of a specific localization, we can separate patients into broad categories: (1) those with motor control disorders; (2) patients with impaired balance; (3) patients with diffuse encephalopathy; (4) a few patients with neuromuscular disease; and (5) those with arthritis and orthopedic deformities.

A. Observation of the Failing Gait

Observing the gait provides an immediate sense of the patient's degree of disability. By timing the patient as he walks a fixed distance and recording the number of steps, three main parameters of gait can be derived: the cadence (number of steps per minute), velocity, and stride (distance traversed between contacts of the same foot).

Characteristic patterns of abnormality are sometimes observed. Parkinson's disease produces flexion of the trunk, a lack of accessory movement, festination, retropulsion, and a tendency to turn en bloc. Some patients have freezing and start hesitation, which are less specific. Cerebellar patients have excess lateral instability of the trunk, erratic foot placement, and decompensation when attempting to walk a narrow base. Patients with spastic paraparesis have a stiff-legged circumduction.

It is more often difficult to make a diagnosis from observation (or from gait analysis) because many failing gaits are fundamentally similiar. Characteristic abnormalities are typically overwhelmed by nonspecific adaptive responses that accompany gait impairment (6). Widened stance, short steps, and increased double limb support are commonly defensive reactions, irrespective or diagnosis. Anxiety and fear of falling may color the performance. More is gained from the neurological exam in such patients than from watching them walk.

B. Experience with MRI

Magnetic resonance imaging has been a great help in diagnosis. Cranial MRI is an exquisitely sensitive test for patients with vascular disease and multiple sclerosis. In patients with ventricular enlargement from hydrocephalus, periventricular halos are often observed. CSF flow study can help distinguish true dynamic from ex vacuo hydrocephalus.

Many elderly patients with frontal gait disorders have lesions in the periventricular region and cetrum semiovale. Masdeu et al. (24) noted the frequency of white matter lesions in CT and MRI scans of elderly with recurrent fails. A few white matter lesions are sometimes seen in asymptomatic elderly, and further clinicopathological correlation is required.

REFERENCES

1. Adams RD, Fischer CM, Hakim S, et al. Symptomatic occult hydrocephalus with "normal" cerebrospinal fluid pressure: a treatable syndrome. N Engl J Med 1965; 273:117–26.
2. Armstrong DM. The supraspinal control of mammalian locomotion. J Physiol 1988; 405:1–37.

3. Babikian V, Ropper AH. Binswanger's disease: a review. Stroke 1987; 18:2–12.

4. Beckley DJ, Bloem BR, Singh J, Remler MP. Scaling of long latency responses in patients on chronic neuroleptic medication. Neurology 1991; 41 (Suppl):192.

5. Bronstein AM, Hood JD, Gresty MA, Panagi C. Visual control of balance in cerebellar and Parkinsonian Syndromes. Brain 1990; 113:767–770.

6. Conrad B. Pathophysiology of Gait Disorders, presented at Xth International Symposium of the Society for Postural and Gait Research, Munich, 1990.

7. Conrad B, Benecke R, Carnehl J, Hohne J, et al. Pathophysiological aspects of human locomotion. In Desmedt JE, ed. Motor Control Mechanisms in Health and Disease. New York: Raven Press, 1983:717–26.

8. Critchley M. On senile disorders of gait, including the so-called "senile paraplegia." Geriatrics 1948; 3:364–70.

9. Dietz V, Pharmacological effects on posture and gait: significance of dopamine receptor antagonists in postural control. In Brandt T, ed, Disorders of Posture and Gait. Stuttgart: Thieme Verlag, 1990:340–345.

10. Drachman DA, Hart CW. An approach to the dizzy patient. Neurology 1972; 22:323–34.

11. Eidelberg E, Walden JG, Nguyen LH. Locomotor control in Macaque monkeys. Brain 1981; 104:647–663.

12. Fischer CM. Hydocephalus as a cause of disturbances of gait in the elderly. Neurology 1982; 32:1358–63.

13. Greenfield JG, The Spinocerebellar Degenerations. Oxford: Blackwell, 1954.

14. Grillner S. Locomotion in vertebrates: central mechanisms and reflex interactions. Physiol Rev 1975; 55:247–304.

15. Horak F. Comparison of cerebellar and vestibular loss on scaling of postural responses. In Brandt T, ed, Disorders of Posture and Gait. Stuttgart: Thieme Verlag, 1990:370–3.

16. Imms FJ, Edholm OG. Studies of gait and mobility in the elderly. Age Ageing 1981; 10:147–156.

17. Keane JR. Hysterical gait disorders: 60 cases. Neurology 1989;39:586–9.

18. Koller WC, Glatt SL, Fox JH. Senile gait: a distinct neurologic entity. Clin Geriatr Med 1985; 1:661–9.

19. Lawrence D, Kuypers H. The functional organization of the motor system in the monkey II. Brain 1968; 91:15–33.

20. Lempert T, Brandt T, Dietrich M, Huppert D. Psychogenic disorders of stance and gait in neurology. In Brandt T, ed, Disorders of Posture and Gait. Stuttgart: Thieme Verlag, 1990:431–4.

21. Lundgren-Lindquist B, Aniansson A, Rundgren A. Functional studies in 79 year olds. Scand J Rehab Med 1983; 15:125–131.

22. Marsden CD, Parkinson's disease. Lancet 1990; 335:948–52.
23. Martyn C, The epidemiology of multiple sclerosis. In Matthews WB, ed, McAlpine's Multiple Sclerosis. 2d ed. London: Churchill Livingston, 1991:3–40.
24. Masdeu JC, Wolfson L, Lantos G, et al. Brain white matter changes in the elderly prone to falling. Arch Neurol 1989; 46:1292–6.
25. Meyer JS, Barron DW. Apraxia of gait: a clinicophysiological study. Brain 1960; 83:261–84.
26. Nashner LM. Adapting reflexes controlling the human posture. Exp Brain Res 1976; 26:59–72.
27. Nashner LM. Balance adjustments of humans perturbed while walking. Neurophysiol 1980; 44:650–664.
28. Newman G, Dovenmuehle RH, Busse EW. Alterations in neurologic status with age. J Am Geriatr Soc 1960; 8:915–17.
29. Orlovsky GN, Shik ML. Control of locomotion: a neurophysiological analysis of the cat locomotor system. Int Rev Physiol 1976; 10:281–317.
30. Overstall PW, Exton-Smith AN, Imms FJ, Johnson AL. Falls in the elderly related to postural imbalance. Br Med J 1977; 1:261–4.
31. Paty DW, Blume WT, Brown WF, et al. Chronic progressive myelopathy. Ann Neurol 1979; 6:419–24.
32. Rajput AH, Offord KP, Beard CM, Kurland LT, Epidemiology of parkinsonism: incidence, classification and mortality. Ann Neurol 1984; 16: 278–82.
33. Ray WA, Griffin MR, Schaffner W et al. Psychotropic drug use and the risk of hip fracture. N Engl J Med 1987; 316:363–9.
34. Riddoch G. The reflex functions of the completely divided spinal cord in man, compared to those associated with less severe lesions. Brain 1917; 40:264–402.
35. Rippeto R. Social disabilities created by gait disturbances in the aged. Geriatrics 1967; 22(4):175–81.
36. Roll JP, Roll R, Quoniam C, Hay L. Muscle proprioception: a powerful sensory input for postural adaptation in man, II. European Congress on Gerontology, Madrid, September 11–14, 1991.
37. Rubenstein LZ, Robbins AS, Josephson KR et al. The value of assessing falls in an elderly population, Ann Intern Med 1990; 113:308–316.
38. Sloman L, Berridge M, Homatidis M et al. Gait patterns of depressed patients and normal subjects. Am J Psych 1982; 139:94–7.
39. Stepan PJ, Williamson J. Drug-induced Parkinsonism in the elderly. Lancet 1984; 2:1082–3.
40. Sudarsky L, Ronthal M. Gait disorders among the elderly patients: a survey study of 50 patients. Arch Neurol 1983; 40:740–3.
41. Sudarsky L, Simon S. Gait disorder in late-life hydrocephalus. Arch Neurol 1987; 44:263–7.

42. Sudarsky L. Geriatrics: gait disorders in the elderly. N Engl J Med 1990; 322:1441–6.
43. Sudarsky L, Ronthal M. Gait disorders in the elderly: assessing the risk for falls, II. European Congress on Gerontology, Madrid, September 11–14, 1991.
44. Thompson PD, Marsden CD. Gait disorder of subcortical arteriosclerotic encephalopathy: Binswanger's disease. Movement Disord 1987; 2:1–8.
45. Tinetti ME, Speechley M, Ginter S. Risk factors for falls among the elderly persons living in the community. N Engl J Med 1988; 319:1701–7.
46. Victor M, Adams FD, Mancall EL. A restricted form of cerebellar cortical degeneration occurring in alcoholic patients. Arch Neurol 1959; 1:579–688.
47. Wikkelso C, Anderson H, Blomstrand C, Lindgvist G. The clinical effect of lumbar puncture in normal pressure hydrocephalus. J Neurol Neurosurg Psych 1982; 45:64–9.
48. Yu YL, duBoulay GH, Stevens JM, Kendall BE. Computer-assisted myelography in cervical spondylotic myelopathy and radiculopathy: clinical correlations and pathogenetic mechanisms. Brain 1986; 109:259–78.

4

Vestibulopathy and Gait

DAVID E. KREBS

MGH Institute of Health Professions, Massachusetts General Hospital;
Harvard Medical School; and Massachusetts Institute of Technology,
Boston, Massachusetts

JOYCE LOCKERT

MGH Institute of Health Professions, Massachusetts General Hospital,
Boston, Massachusetts

I. INTRODUCTION

Vestibulopathy impairs one of the three primary sensory modalities responsible for balance information. Even when the visual and proprioceptive sensory systems are intact, many vestibulopathic subjects are
unsteady as they walk, climb stairs, and transfer from a bed or chair.
Common complaints of patients with vestibulopathy include sensations
of abnormal movements, dizziness, or vertigo, and visual disturbances
such as nystagmus or oscillopsia. Major functional impairments experienced by vestibulopathy pateints are gait instability and unsteadiness

during transitional movements such as arising from a chair or getting out of bed. Instability worsens as other sensory inputs are removed such as while walking at night or standing with eyes closed.

Many patients with vestibulopathy exhibit severe dynamic instabilities. To date, however, most investigations of balance or instability amongst vestibulopathic patients have studied standing activities alone. The relationship between results of static standing balance tests and dynamic stability during activities of daily living including gait are unknown for any balance disabled humans, including those with vestibulopathy. Gait studies most often focus only on lower extremity kinematics or time-distance variables. Lower extremity and temporodistance measurements can reveal only fragments of human locomotion, while whole-body (center of gravity) control, head motions, and other indicators of global impairment may be overlooked.

We review here the vestibular physiology and diagnostic testing and their effects on gait and mobility of patients with vestibulopathy, and report the results of investigations currently underway at the Biomotion Laboratory at Massachusetts General Hospital, Boston, Massachusetts. To our knowledge, no prior vestibulopathic gait research has been reported using full-body three-dimensional kinematic and kinetic analysis. Common findings for temporal variables, center of gravity control, base of support characteristics, and control of head, arms, and trunk are presented. Finally, our preliminary results are summarized on the effects of vestibular rehabilitation on gait and locomotor activities of daily living (ADL) stability.

II. VESTIBULAR SYSTEM: ANATOMY AND NORMAL FUNCTION

A. Anatomy

Within each temporal bone of the skull is located a bony labyrinth that contains the membranous labyrinth. Within the membranous labyrinth the sensory organs of the vestibular apparatus are located. The membranous labyrinth contains the cochlear duct, the utricle and saccule, and three semicircular canals. The cochlea is the primary sensory organ for hearing and will not be discussed here.

1. Utricle and Saccule (Otoliths)

Located on the wall of both the utricle and saccule (known collectively as the *otoliths*) is a small sensory region called the macula. Each maculae is covered by a gelatinous layer in which small calcium crystals, called otoconia, are embedded. Hair cells are located within the macula. The hair cells project cilia up into the gelatinous layer.

The saccular and utricular maculas sense linear acceleration of the head and are known collectively as static labyrinth organs. The saccule detects vertical linear accelerations of the head in the saggital plane. The utricle responds to horizontal linear accelerations of the head. As gravity is a form of linear acceleration, the otoliths are also sensitive to tilts of the head with respect to gravity.

2. Semicircular Canals

The primary function of the semicircular canals is to sense head angular accelerations (velocity changes). The semicircular canals are maximally sensitive to higher frequency motion as occurs in locomotion, and less sensitive to low-frequency motion as occurs during static standing. The three semicircular canals (superior, posterior, and lateral) are positioned at right angles, with one lying in each of three planes. Head acceleration sensitivity of each canal is maximal in response to head accelerations in the plane of that canal.

The canals are filled with endolymph fluid. Each canal has an enlargement called the ampulla which contains small crests, cristae, covered by a gelatinous cupula. Hair cells, similar to those found in the macula, are located in the ampulla, with cilia extending up into the cupula.

3. Hair Cells

The hair cell is the basic sensory element of the labyrinth receptor organ. Present in the maculas, cristae of the semicircular canals, and cochlea, its primary function is to transduce mechanical force into electrical nerve action potentials. Two types of hair cells exist in humans (type I and type II), differing in their neural connections. Type I hair cells communicate with a single large nerve terminal, while Type II hair cells communicate with multiple nerve terminals.

Each hair cell has a large number of small cilia and one very large cilia, called the kinocilium. Stimulation of all the sensory organs of the inner ear requires displacement of the cilia by a mechanical force, created initially by an acceleration or sound. Displacement of the cilia is transduced into an electrical response carried to the brain via the eighth cranial nerve.

4. Vestibular Nuclei

Afferent signals from the labyrinths ascend the eighth cranial nerve to the vestibular nuclear complex and to the flocculonodular lobes of the cerebellum. The vestibular nuclear complex receives input from the vestibular nerve (1), the contralateral vestibular nuclear complex, cerebellum, reticular formaton, spinal cord, and other sensory systems, including somatic, visual, and auditory modalities (2,3). Therefore, efferent signals from the vestibular nuclear complex reflect input from all these sensory systems. Due to convergence of various sensory inputs at the vestibular nuclear complex, damage to another sensory system could produce signs of vestibular dysfunction, even though the individual possesses intact labyrinthine sensory input (4).

B. Vestibular Sensory and Motor Functions

The vestibular system functions as both a sensory and a motor system. As these roles function interdependently, separating these two roles is difficult. During functional tasks, sensory information relayed to the central nervous system (CNS) from vestibular sensory organs is constantly being influenced and altered by vestibular originated motor signals. In addition to influencing its own perceived information, the vestibular system works in conjunction with the visual and somatosensory systems, as well as cognitive input, to provide the central nervous system with accurate information regarding positions and movement of the head in space. The vestibular reflexes, vestibulospinal, vestibulo-ocular, and vestibulocolic reflexes work in conjunction with other descending motor systems to control whole-body equilibrium and gaze stability during head movements, posture, and locomotion.

The vestibulospinal reflexes (including the vestibulocolic reflex) affect whole-body equilibrium by mediating facilitation and inhibition of skeletal extensor muscles. Maintaining a steady visual image on the retina during rotations of the head is achieved by the vestibulo-ocular reflexes (VOR).

1. Vestibular Efferents

Vestibular efferent cells originate from cells located between the abducens and superior vestibular nuclei in the brainstem, and synapse on cilia in the vestibular end organs. Though research on the role of vestibular efferents is quite limited, Goldberg and Fernandez (5) hypothesize that a feedforward or descending command exists to alter the response magnitude of the labyrinthine nerve cells. This feedforward command would have functional importance in preventing oversaturation of signals from the semicircular canals during high-speed head rotations and preventing understimulation inhibited by omnidirectional head motion (6). The feedforward may be triggered by set rates of vestibular stimulation. Presumably, once the CNS receives a cognitive command to walk or move about, vestibular efferents would act to modulate the expected vestibular input as compared to input actually experienced during walking.

2. Vestibulo-Ocular Reflexes

Through mediation by the vestibulo-ocular reflexes, head rotation in one direction causes an oppositely directed compensatory rotation of the eyes in the orbit. Therefore, eye orientation in space (angle of gaze) remains relatively constant.

Stimulation of a semicircular canal results in eye movement in the plane of that canal. This is achieved by the semicircular canal-ocular reflex. If the stimulation to the semicircular canals is of such a large magnitude that it cannot be compensated for by the motion of the eye in the orbit, a slow, vestibular induced eye deviation in the direction opposite to the head rotation is interrupted by a quick movement in the direction of head rotation. The combination of slow backward eye motion followed by quick forward motion is called nystagmus. Overall gaze stabilization during saccadic eye motion is still possible because eye velocity during the slow component of nystagmus is approximately equal and opposite to that of head velocity (7).

The pathways from the maculas to the extraocular muscles, otolith-ocular reflex, are less clearly defined than those from the semicircular canals. Selective stimulation of different parts of the utricle and saccule result in mostly vertical and vertical-rotatory eye movements (8). Each of the vertical eye muscles appears to be related to specific areas of the maculas so that groups of hair cells whose kinocilia are oriented in opposite directions excite agonist and antagonist muscles. Therefore, rotation of the head to one side results in eye movement toward the opposite side to maintain stable gaze. Otolith-ocular reflexes are slower than semicircular canal-ocular reflexes. However, if head rotation exceeds that which can be compensated for by motion of the eye in its orbit, otolith-ocular reflexes are still capable of producing nystagmus.

3. Vestibulospinal Reflexes

Vestibulospinal reflexes influence spinal anterior cell activity through three major pathways: the lateral vestibulospinal tract (LVST), the medial vestibulospinal tract (MVST), and the reticulospinal tract (RST). The cerebellum is highly active with each of these pathways.

The LVST originates from the lateral vestibular nucleus and extends throughout the length of the spinal cord. It synapses directly with alpha and gamma motoneurons in the medial portions of the anterior horn cell. Alpha motoneurons are responsible for generation of rapid, forceful muscle contraction, while gamma motoneurons function to ensure smooth continuous control of muscle contraction. Many of the LVST neurons have axonal branches that project to both the cervical and lumbosacral areas of the spinal cord (9).

The MVST originates from neurons in the medial and inferior vestibular nuclei. Fibers of the MVST terminate primarily on the upper cervical and thoracic motoneurons, having a primarily inhibitory effect on most neurons. MVST function interacts with that of the neck vestibulo-ocular reflexes. Connections to inhibitory cervical motoneurons and thoracic motoneurons have been identified (1, 10).

Fibers of the reticulospinal tract traverse the length of the spinal cord and terminate in the seventh and eighth laminae of the gray matter. Both excitatory and inhibitory impulses are relayed by the reticulospinal tract to alpha and gamma motoneurons (11, 12).

C. Diagnostic Testing

Patients with vestibulopathy are categorized as having unilateral or bilateral vestibular dysfunction, hypofunction, or zero (absent) vestibular function by clinical evaluation and diagnostic testing. These tests may include electronystagmography, sinusoidal vertical axis rotation, visual-vestibular rotation, and posturography data.

1. Electronystagmography (ENG)

Eye movements are recorded by taping electrodes on the skin around the eyes and recording the corneoretinal potential. Test conditions include evaluation for spontaneous and gaze nystagmus, rapid eye movements (saccades), slow eye movements (pursuit), optokinetic nystagmus, positional nystagmus, and caloric (hot and cold water or air) stimulation (13).

2. Sinusoidal Vertical Axis Rotation (SVAR)

Rotational testing is performed with individuals seated on a chair attached to a motorized platform that rotates side to side (left and right). During rotation, induced eye movements are recorded. Parameters analyzed are gain (ratio of slow-phase eye-movement response to stimulus magnitude); phase (relationship between eye-movement onset and rotational velocity); and eye-movement response symmetry to clockwise and counterclockwise rotation. No gain response at all rotational frequencies (.01 to 1.0 Hz) tested signifies "no detectable vestibular function;" such results are rare (<5% at our institution).

3. Visual-Vestibular Interaction Rotation (VVI)

The VVI is also performed on the rotary chair to investigate interactions between the VOR and vision. This test is designed to evaluate brainstem and cerebrocortical pathology which may lead to balance deficits.

4. Posturography

Posturography is intended to assess vestibulospinal integrity by measuring the motor and sensory abilities of subjects to stand during various visual and proprioceptive perturbations. The individual, wearing a parachute-type harness to prevent falling to the floor, stands on a platform (Equitest™) configured with a strain gauge force plate under each foot. The platform is controlled by a computer to measure "sway" [actually the anteroposterior travel of the Center of Pressure (CP) of the ground reaction force] in the anteroposterior direction, horizontal (shear) forces, response strength (vertical force), right/left symmetry of response, and latency of response (ms from external perturbation initiation to the subject's active response). The platform and visual surround can be configured to sway in toes up and down directions in response to the individual's sway in those directions (sway-referencing). Posturography conveys little diagnostic information, but can be used to document the patient's responses to visual and proprioceptive inputs on standing balance, and to assess changes in standing balance due to treatment effects.

III. VESTIBULOPATHY EFFECTS ON LOCOMOTOR MOBILITY

A. Clinical Categories of Vestibulopathy

Vestibulopathic symptoms can be caused by the vestibular system reacting too little, asymmetrically, or inappropriately to stimuli (13). Patients with bilateral vestibulopathy complain of gait instability, unsteadiness on movement, such as arising from bed or a chair, oscillopsia, increased instability in the dark, and sensations of abnormal movement such as dizziness or vertigo. Disease processes causing bilateral vestibulopathy include ototoxicity, inner ear degenerative disease, bilateral inner ear infections, hypothyroidism, Pagets disease, autoimmune inner ear disease, and idiopathic inner ear damage. Bilateral vestibulopathy subjects have abnormal electronystagmography (ENG) responses on both sides, and sinusoidal vertical axis rotation (SVAR) abnormalities. Patients with bilateral vestibular hypofunction (BVH) have bilaterally decreased caloric responses and decreased gains at all frequencies of SVAR testing. Patients with bilateral vestibular dysfunction (i.e., bilateral vestibulopathy other than bilateral hypofunction) have positional nystagmus that occurs while the head is rotated or laterally flexed in the left and right ear down positions, during Hallpike maneuvers, or a unilateral reduced caloric response plus positional nystagmus with the contralateral ear down. Patients with unilateral vestibulopathy (UVH) may complain of instability, unsteady "veering to one side" gait, dizziness, and vertigo which may be predominantly with the head turned toward the damaged side. On vestibular testing, they show damage only to one side, including a unilaterally reduced caloric response, positional nystagmus with one ear down and/or abnormalities on rotational testing (mildly decreased low-frequency gains, increased phase leads, and asymmetrical rotation-induced nystagmus) (13). Disease processes causing unilateral vestibulopathy include poorly compensated labyrinthitis, vestibular neuritis, benign paroxysmal positional vertigo, post-traumatic vestibulopathy, as well as idiopathic vestibulopathy.

B. "Gait Laboratory" Analysis

The MGH Biomotion Laboratory employs an 11-segment whole-body model to assess posture and balance (14). We analyze the full-body kinematics (linear and angular motion) and kinetics (forces that cause these motions) during standing and locomotor activities of daily living (15,16). We have recently applied these tests to vestibulopathic patients before and after rehabilitation. We present here results from the pre-rehabilitation tests (except where explicitly noted), to provide insight to vestibulopathic gait in the absence of rehabilitation.

Patients with vestibular dysfunction were recruited from the Jenks Vestibular Diagnostic Laboratory of the Massachusetts Eye and Ear Infirmary and form neurologists at the MGH. Excluded from our studies are subjects with evidence of other disease processes that might affect balance, such as a prior stroke, Meniere's disease, perilymph fistula, other central nervous system pathology, peripheral neuropathy, severe arthropathy, orthopedic deformities, or severe visual impairment (17). A comparison group of well subjects was recruited from the lab staff and neighborhoods and communities in the Boston area. All subjects agreed to be studied by written consent and no monetary compensation was offered.

Sample groups consisted of 20 subjects with vestibulopathy (mean age: 57, range 25–82), including 16 subjects with bilateral vestibular hypofunction, and 4 subjects with unilateral vestibular dysfunction. Most of the results reported here, however, stem from those subjects whose data have been fully processed at this time. The control group consisted of 26 well subjects (mean age: 52, range 26–88), without neuromusculoskeletal dysfunction, and (among those > age 65.) who were independently exercising at least 3 times per week. Thus, the control group is an especially "fit" group, whose members can be expected to be healthier than groups that include "usual aging" unselected, and possibly subclinically impaired, elder subjects.

Our system is described in detail elsewhere (14–28), and briefly recounted here. Simultaneous bilateral whole-body kinematic data are collected with a motion analysis system using Selspot II hardware (Selective Electronics, Partille, Sweden) and analyzed with TRACK™ (Telemetered Rapid Acquisition of Kinematics) kinematic data analysis software package (M.I.T., Cambridge, MA) and software developed in our lab. Light-emitting diode arrays are mounted on eleven body segments: right and left feet, shanks, thighs and arms; as well as the pelvis, trunk, and head. The TRACK algorithm enables photostereogrammetric reconstruction of three-dimensional positions of serially illuminated infrared LEDs. The system calculates the six degree of freedom position of each body segment within an 8 m³ viewing volume. System precision is within 1 mm of linear displacement and within 1 degree of angular displacement. Knowing the precise position of body segments and given estimates of body segment masses allows precise estimation of center of gravity (CG) position, velocity, and acceleration. Floor reaction forces are acquired from two Kistler™ force platforms and processed on the same computer. Another program determines individual foot and combined center of pressure with accuracy of less than 3 mm. Kinematic and kinetic data are sampled at 153 Hz and digitally filtered.

C. Standing Stability Tests Results

"Static" standing stability is often assumed to require the ability to maintain upright posture by maintaining the ground reaction forces' center of pressure (CP) position within the base of support (27). Postural tests, such as Equitest™ posturography, are based on this static CP/CG position assumption. A subject's balance is thereby scored according to ability to maintain the body mass' normally small amplitude, low-frequency displacements (28). The relationship between the results of standing posturography balance tests and dynamic stability during activities of daily living including gait are unknown for any balance-disabled humans despite the growing use of standing posturography to assess patients with balance disorders (18).

Standing "still," of course, is not truly static. The body's center of gravity is in constant motion. Posturography assumes that the body behaves as an inverted pendulum (i.e., one rigid link rotating around a frictionless pin joint at the floor, with all of the body weight located at the whole-body center of gravity). Static imbalance is marked by center of pressure's approach to or beyond the boundaries of base of support. Lesser center of gravity excursion presumably reflects better static balance control (19). These assumptions are clearly untenable for locomotor ADL analysis.

In our laboratory, standing activities are conducted with arms folded across the chest, with the subject in the center of the lab's viewing volume, on the force plates. Subjects are instructed to stand as still as possible. During the standing activities, the center of pressure from the force plates and center of gravity from full-body kinematics are determined for quantitative comparison of fore/aft and mediolateral CP and CG excursion. Figure 1 shows CG vs. CP excursions for a bilateral vestibular hypofunction subject and an age- and height-matched normal control subject during semitandem, eyes open, "static" stance. In general, vestibular subjects sway slightly more than normal subjects with eyes open in uncompromised quiet standing, but with eyes closed or during tandem standing, vestibulopathic subjects sway much more than normals. In addition, Azen et al. (20) found that, compared with normal controls, bilateral vestibular hypofunction subjects evince greater head displacements during quiet standing with eyes closed.

D. Gait Stability

Stability during gait and locomotion can be quantified in a variety of ways. We believe that temporal variables, center of gravity, base of support, and upper body kinematics best quantify the unsteadiness experienced by vestibulopathic subjects.

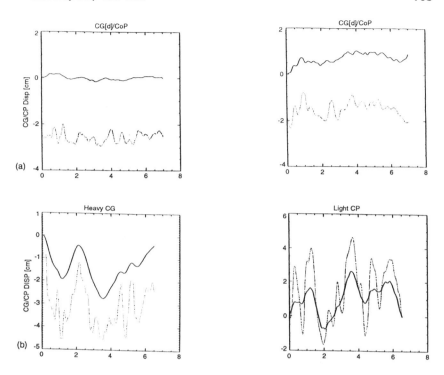

Figure 1   Center of gravity (CG, dark line) and center of pressure (CP, dashed line) vs. time representing A/P displacement (first column) and medial/lateral displacement (2nd column) for (a) one normal subject and (b) one age- and height-matched BVH subject during semitandem standing. Note scale differences between (a) and (b). Offsets between CP and CG are for illustrative purposes: in reality all appear like the right lower figure.

1. Temporal Variables

To quantify their dynamic ADL dysfunction, two trials each of preferred pace gait and paced gait (120 steps/min) over a 10-M walkway were conducted. We also collect similar data from stair ascent and rising from a chair. Preferred pace gait should reflect movement strategies under self-selected "optimal neuromotor control." Paced gait at 120 steps/min permits valid cadence-controlled within- and between-subject comparisons. Cycle time, double support, and stance duration have previously been reported to vary inversely with balance control (21, 22), Pozzo described increases in stance phase and stride lengths during free speed gait of vestibulopathic patients, but reported no numerical data (23). Table 1 provides descriptive temporodistance values for our subjects during preferred paced (free speed) gait.

Cycle time   Average cycle times during preferred pace gait ranged between means of 1–1.2 s for control of all vestibular dysfunction groups (Table 1). Bilateral vestibular hypofunction subjects have slightly longer cycle times than controls. When subjects were directed to walk to a pace of 120 steps/min, cycle times for vestibulopathy subjects decreased to approximate the control group's values, while cycle times for control subjects remained relatively unchanged. Thus, we conclude that control subjects choose approximately 120 steps per min as their preferred pace, while subjects with vestibulopathy prefer to walk at a slower cadence.

Double support and stance phase durations   Spending relatively more time in stance and double support increases vestibular (and other balance-impaired) subjects' mechanical stability. During both preferred and paced gait trials, slightly greater double support times are noted in the bilateral vestibular hypofunction group, compared to the control group (Table 1). Double support times of unilateral hypofunction subjects tend to be similar to those of control subjects. During the faster, 120 steps/min paced gait, no change is noted with duration of either double support or stance phases of the control group. However, vestibulopathic subjects tend to increase their walking velocity by reducing their overall cycle time and decreasing stance phase duration, while the double support period remains unchanged relative to their slower, preferred pace.

Table 1   Temporal Values for Cycle Time, Double Support, and Stance Duration ($\overline{X}$ ± s.d., in seconds) During Free Speed Gait for Normal Controls and Vestibulopathic (VSP) Subjects. In addition, bilateral vestibular hypofunction (BVH) and unilateral vestibular hypofunction (UVH) subgroups' values are provided separately.

Group	n	Cycle time	Double support	Stance
Normals	26	1.11±.08	.36±.04	.70±.06
VSP	16	1.16±.13	.42±.09	.77±.18
BVH	13	1.17±.14	.44±.12	.79±.20
UVH	3	1.14±.11	.36±.05	.70±.09

2. Center of Gravity Control

We define stability as the ability to control whole-body momentum (mass × velocity) during standing and locomotion. Dynamic stability can be characterized in vestibulopathy patients and other individuals with stability impairments in terms of center of gravity velocity and displacement. The key difference between static balance and dynamic stability is the former assumes stability requires the CG to remain within the base of support, while dynamic stability encompasses CG displacements outside the base of support such as occurs during gait. During human locomotion, the body's mass must be displaced outside its base of support. In gait, the CG could only be within the base of support during the brief double support phase. Winter's (24) and our data (25,26) suggest that even in normal gait and activities of daily living, the CG is never located directly above the ground reaction forces' CP (as measured by the force plates). During the gait cycle, we have examined values and timing of the maxima of CG forward velocity [anterior/posterior (A/P)], CG mediolateral (M/L) velocity, and CG M/L displacement.

Center of gravity A/P velocity   Many gait laboratories report walking velocity, as calculated from stride length × stride duration. We believe that CG kinematics provide more meaningful velocity data: we calculate walking speed from whole-body CG displacement (cm) over time (s). Thus, we can examine average, maximum, and minimum forward and mediolateral velocities. Because velocity is directly related to momentum (mass × velocity, and body mass remains constant in a given test session), the maximum and minimum velocities represent locomotor CG control parameters directly related to momentum. Table 2 provides mean and standard deviation values for maximum walking velocities (A/P and M/L) and M/L CG displacements during a typical stride. All groups attained maximum A/P momentum (velocity) during the double support phase of gait and minimum A/P momentum during mid single support phase (29). During preferred pace gait, maximum A/P velocities of the bilateral vestibular hypofunction group are considerably less than those of control subjects. Control subjects showed minimal variation between preferred pace and 120 step/min paced trials. Vestibulopathic subjects' paced (faster) gait more closely resembled control subjects than their preferred speed trials. These data indicate that stability-impaired vestibulopathy subjects prefer a slower gait velocity than controls, but when velocity is voluntarily increased in paced gait, maximum A/P velocity approaches control values (29). Our findings of equal cycle times between controls and all vestibulopathy groups (Table 1), but decreased A/P velocity in the vestibulopathic groups (Table 2) suggest vestibulopathic subjects use shorter stride lengths, supporting Pozzo's observations (25). Shorter stride lengths prevent the CG from straying far from the base of support, thus increasing stability at the expense of mobility.

Center of gravity lateral velocity During preferred pace gait, all vestibulopathy subject groups (bilateral and unilaterals) show CG maximum lateral velocities larger than the control subjects with unilateral vestibular dysfunction subjects demonstrating the greatest CG maximum lateral velocity compared to controls. Control subjects show no major change in lateral velocity between preferred pace and 120 step/min paced gait. Maximum lateral momentum (velocity) is greater in vestibulopathic subjects during paced gait compared to their slower, preferred pace gait.

Center of gravity mediolateral excursion During preferred speed gait, bilateral vestibular hypofunction subjects demonstrate slightly greater CG mediolateral excursions than control subjects, while unilateral vestibulopathy subjects demonstrate decreased CG mediolateral excursions (Table 2). Both differences are small as compared with control subjects' values. These differences become more pronounced during paced gait suggesting a decreased ability of the bilateral vestibular hypofunction subjects to allow CG excursion. Apparently, BVH patients prevent normal M/L excursions to inhibit the potentially destabilizing effects of having the CG travel close to the limits of the base of support during gait.

Table 2 Center of Gravity (CG) Kinematics ($\overline{X} \pm$ s.d.). Velocity maximums for anteroposterior (A/P) and mediolateral (M/L) CG travel (cm/s), and mediolateral CG displacements (cm), during free speed gait for normal controls and vestibulopathic (VSP) subjects. In addition, bilateral vestibular hypofunction (BVH) and unilateral vestibular hypofunction (UVH) subgroups' values are provided separately.

Group	*n*	Max Ap velocity	Max M/L velocity	M/L excursion
Normals	26	135.3±15.4	15.4±6.2	5.1±3.1
VSP	16	112.2±21.5	16.7±7.5	5.2±2.5
BVH	13	108.0±20.3	16.6±7.8	5.5±2.3
UVH	3	129.6±18.9	18.2±6.7	4.0±3.2

3. Base of Support (BOS) Kinematics

A wide base of support (BOS) has long been believed to be a hallmark of unsteady gait. Certainly, static standing stability decreases when BOS is narrowed, such as in tandem stance. No study to date has reported BOS values as determined by three-dimensional kinematics during gait analysis. Most studies have defined base of support or stride width as the mediolateral distance between either the center of the heels or the medial malleoli (21,30,31,32). We define base of support as the mediolateral distance between the longitudinal midline of the feet.

The literature includes several contradictory studies on BOS in the elderly. In a comparison of free and fast speed-walking patterns in men, Murray found that stride width increased with faster walking speeds in normal subjects (33). In a study of effects of age on variability and gait, Gabell and Nayak (21) report stride width decreased with increasing age, but variability of stride width values increased. They suggest increases in mean step width are a method of compensating for instability, and that an increase in step width variability indicated a lack of appropriate compensation. In 1989, Heitman and Gossman (31) studied the relationship between step width and balance performance in elderly, female "fallers" and nonfallers. No significant differences in step width mean or variability was found between fallers and nonfallers. However, a significant negative correlation was reported between clinical balance tests and step width variability. In a 1990 study of treadmill gait, Gehlsen and Whaley (32) reported gait profiles on two groups of elders, with and without a history of falls. A significant increase in mean heel width was noted in the group with a history of falls during higher speed gait.

All previous studies have defined base of support (stride width) by taking measurements only during the double support phase of gait when both feet are in contact with the ground. However, the majority of the gait cycle is spent in single limb stance, during which BOS reaches a minimum. Our data indicating a relative increase in the time vestibulopathic subjects spend in double support bolsters the argument that unsteady subject attempt to avoid single limb support that affords a minimum of stability from the BOS. We measure interfoot distance (BOS) throughout the gait cycle, and therefore report here both swing phase (single limb support phase) BOS and the more traditionally reported double support (at heelstrike) BOS values.

Examples of typical BOS graphs are shown in Figure 2. The ususal pattern seen with nonpathological "normals" resembles a sinusoidal wave

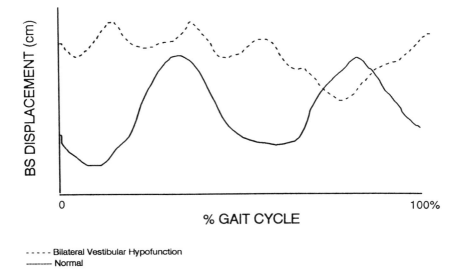

% GAIT CYCLE

- - - - - Bilateral Vestibular Hypofunction
———— Normal

Figure 2   Recreation of base of support values plotted over one full gait cycle for normal and BVH subjects.

form. Maximum BOS typically occurs during single limb stance. BOS values steadily increase at and immediately following toe-off, apparently to allow the swing limb to clear the stance limb. Subjects with bilateral vestibular hypofunction exhibit BOS graphs quite different from normal (control) subjects. An erratic, variable curve shape is seen often with more frequent curve reversals. Vestibulopathic subjects' timing of a maximum BOS is more variable than those of normals, occurring sometimes during single limb stance and sometimes during the double support phase of gait.

Base of support range   Base of support range (maximum minus minimum BOS values occurring in succession within a stride) is one method of identifying base of support variability. During preferred pace gait, BVH subjects show slightly smaller BOS ranges than control subjects (Table 3). BOS range increases during paced gait compared to unpaced gait for all vestibulopathy subjects while BOS ranges for control subjects remain relatively unchanged.

Base of support (BOS) at heel strike   The initiation of double support phase of gait (heelstrike) is a crucial event. By this time, com-

Table 3 Base of Support Kinematics ($\overline{X} \pm$ s.d., in cm) During Free Speed Gait for Normal Controls and Vestibulopathic (VSP) Subjects. In addition, bilateral vestibular hypofunction (BVH) and unilateral vestibular hypofunction (UVH) subgroups' values are provided separately.

Group	n	Range	Heelstrike	Single limb stance
Normals	26	6.67±4.71	13.32±6.98	13.45±6.69
VSP	16	5.63±3.08	13.51±5.65	14.95±4.94
BVH	13	5.31±3.15	13.29±6.35	14.41±5.17
UVH	3	6.76±2.75	14.31±1.86	16.84±3.78

pensations for instability must have been expressed to determine the double support BOS value. While no major difference in the BOS values of vestibulopathic and control subjects is noted during preferred pace gait, increases in BOS are noted in all bilateral and unilateral subjects during 120 step/min paced gait (Table 3). The greatest increase is noted in subjects with zero vestibular function.

Base of support during single limb support As the condition of double foot contact no longer exists during single limb support, the term "stride width" may be a more appropriate descriptor of the mediolateral distance between the longitudinal midline of the foot segments. The time when the body's vertical CG is at its maximum (mid single limb support) is when compensation for instability may be expressed as changes in stride width value. As noted at heel strike, stride width is greater in BVH and UVH subjects than in controls. During more rapid walking (paced gait), stride width of BVH and UVH subjects increases as compared with preferred pace gait, although the control group's paced/preferred BOS values do not differ (Table 3).

Our overall findings suggest that when required to walk faster than they prefer, vestibulopathy subjects demonstrate increased variability of base of support as shown by increased base of support range. Greater BOS values are also noted at heelstrike and mid single limb support, suggesting kinematic compensation for instability occurs at these times.

4. Head, Arms, and Trunk (HAT) Kinematics

During both preferred and paced gait, vestibulopathy subjects demonstrated altered kinematics of the head, arms, and trunk. Our findings generally agreed with those of Pozzo et al. (23) in a recent study of head kinematics during locomotor tasks in patients with bilateral vestibular deficits. Figures 3 and 4 depict a typical gait cycle for one bilateral vestibular hypofunction subject and a matched normal (control) subject.

Head During gait, vestibulopathic subjects tend to hold their heads more stiffly than normals, usually in a position of slight forward flexion or lateral tilt. This is possibly in an effort to reduce extraneous stimuli that might exaggerate illusions of movement of the surrounding environment.

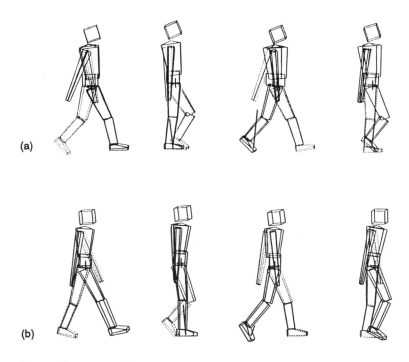

Figure 3 Lateral view of computer-generated model of (a) one normal control group subject and (b) one matched BVH subject during a single gait cycle. These "snapshots" are taken at heelstrike, midstance, toe-off, and midswing, and represent the actual body segment in space kinematics. At heelstrike, the BVH subject shows greater trunk flexion, which positions the center of gravity in a more stable region of the base of support. Note decreased armswing, head and trunk transverse plane rotation in the BVH subject. Bold + represents the whole-body center of gravity.

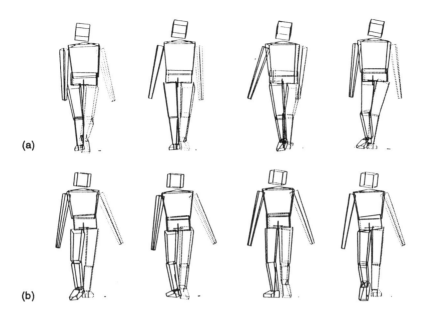

Figure 4   Anterior view of the subjects shown in Figure 3.

Vestibulopathic subjects appear to be "setting" their gaze to a fixed point in the room or on the floor, presumably to maximize the visual signal-to-noise ratio. Frequently our patients comment that they "must see the ground to know where it is," despite their intact proprioception.

Arms   Vestibulopathic subjects tend to hold their upper limbs fairly rigidly, allowing little arm swing during gait. Frequently, these subjects abduct their arms away from their sides, analogous to a tight-rope walker attempting to stabilize the trunk by positioning the arms outstretched. Arm swing during gait was often asymmetrical.

Trunk   The trunk possesses the largest mass of any body segment and its control is crucial for dynamic stability. Krebs et al. (15) recently reported normal upper body kinematics relative to the pelvis and to global/gravity coordinates. Those data suggested that trunk/pelvis coordination may be used to reduce potentially destabilizing antigravity trunk motions during daily activities. As with their head and arms, vestibulopathy subjects tend to hold the trunk stiffly and demonstrate reduced trunk rotations during gait.

IV. VESTIBULAR REHABILITATION

Currently, we are investigating the efficacy of vestibular rehabilitation on locomotor ADL stability of vestibulopathy patients. Tests performed to monitor patient changes during and after different phases of the rehabilitation program include: sinusoidal vertical axis rotation; posturography; kinemtic and kinetic analysis of standing, gait, stair ascent, and chair rise; and timed clinical balance tests.

Preliminary results among subjects completing the study indicate that, following vestibular rehabilitation, subjects decrease their relative double support and stance durations, and increase their average walking velocity during preferred pace gait. Lateral momentum (mediolateral velocity × mass) increases substantially following vestibular rehabilitation. Paced gait results are similar to free gait, but the changes were slightly less. These gait parameter improvements cannot be explained by velocity changes alone: coupled with the greater lateral velocity, we suggest that the patients do not simply improve their walking speed; they allowed more CG dynamics, and became more stable.

It is important to note that these preliminary data represent only total gains from the rehabilitation programs, that the sample is small and the variability large, so no unqualified conclusions are to be drawn from these preliminary results. However, we are encouraged by the findings to date, and will continue our studies for at least the next several years.

Many patients with vestibulopathy recover adequate function in the first 2 months following the vestibular insult to enable them to perform normal, if nonstressful, ADL (34). Our data suggest that vestibular rehabilitation may benefit the group of patients who do not recover adequately. Vestibular rehabilitation is essentially an exercise program aimed at remediating the dizziness, gaze instability, and balance disturbances in patients with vestibular dysfunction. Vestibular rehabilitation has two important specific features: vestibular adaptation and vestibular substitution strategies.

For patients with residual vestibular function, the vestibular system's ability to adapt to changes in demand or changes in sensory information received is key to this treatment approach (35,36). By providing stimuli that induce adaptation of the vestibular system, such as combining movement of an image across the retina with head movement, sensory and motor vestibular information processing within the CNS may be promoted (17).

For patients with no remaining vestibular function, substitution strategies are taught. In this approach, the patient is encouraged to rely upon visual and proprioceptive information to stabilize gaze and maintain postural stability. Such strategies can include enhancing the use of the cervical ocular reflex, performing corrective eye saccades, or decreasing the velocity of head movements. Activities such as practicing combined eye–head movements and body on head rotation are taught to encourage the patient to rely on these substitution strategies for posture and balance stability.

Our preliminary data and previous studies (37,38) suggest that vestibular rehabilitation does not "cure" the vestibulopathy, but rather enhances their compensation during locomotor ADL, permitting greater access to dynamically changing regions of stability as in gait. The challenge of understanding vestibulopathic gait must be met by more investigations of both the gait disorder and the effects of vestibular rehabilitation.

V. SUMMARY

To date, no reports of whole-body gait analysis in subjects with vestibulopathy are to found in the literature. Vestibulopathic patients studied in our laboratory typically walk rather tentatively and slowly, with decreased upper body movement. These findings are preliminary, and are probably not representative of all vestibulopathic subjects: too few subjects have been studied to date to draw unqualified conclusions. In general, gait analysis is not diagnostic for these subjects, but is a useful monitor of the effects of vestibular rehabilitation.

ACKNOWLEDGMENT

This work was supported in part by Grant No. H133G00025 from the National Institute of Disability and Rehabilitation Research, US DOE.

REFERENCES

1. Carleton SC, Carpenter MB. Afferent and efferent connections of the medial, inferior and lateral vestibular nuclei in the cat and monkey. Brain Res 1983; 278: 29–51.
2. Petrosini L, Troiani D, Zannoni B. Trigeminal stimulation modulates vestibular unitary activity. Experentia 1982; 38: 363–365.

3. Tickle DR, Schneider GE. Projection of the auditory nerve to the medial vestibular nucleus. Neurosci Lett 1982; 28: 1–7.

4. Cope S, Ryan GMS. Cervical and otolith vertigo. J Laryngol 1959; 73: 113–120.

5. Goldberg JM, Fernandez C. Efferent vestibular system in the squirrel monkey: Anatomical location and influence on afferent activity. J Neurophysiol 1980; 43: 986–1025.

6. Highstein SM, Baker R. Action of the efferent vestibular system on primary afferents in the Goldfish, Opaanus tau. J Neurophysiol 1985; 54: 370–384.

7. Melvill Jones G, Watt DGD. Observations on the control of stepping and hopping movements in man. J Physiol 1971; 219: 709–727.

8. Ito M. Neural design of the cerebellar motor control system. Brain Res 1971; 40: 81–85.

9. Peterson BW, Fukushima K, Hirai N, Schor RH, and Wilvox VJ. Responses of vestibulospinal and reticulospinal neurons to sinusoidal vestibular stimulation. J Neurophysiol 1980; 43: 1236–1250.

10. Wilson VJ, Yoshida M, Schor RH. Supraspinal monosynaptic excitation and inhibition in thoracic back motoneurons. Exp Brain Res 1970; 11: 282–295.

11. Peterson BW, Pitts NG, Fukushima K, Mackel R. Reticulospinal excitation and inhibition of neck motoneurons. Exp Brain Res 1978; 32: 471–489.

12. Peterson BW, Fukushima K. The reticulospinal system and its role in generating vestibular and visuomotor reflexes. In: Brain Stem Control of Spinal Mechanisms, Sjolund B, Borkland A, eds. Amsterdam: Elsevier, 1982: 225–251.

13. Baloh RH, Honrubia V. Clinical Neurophysiology of the Vestibular System. Philadelphia: FA Davis, 1990: 130–152.

14. Riley PO, Hodge WA, Mann RW. Modelling the biomechanics of posture and balance. J Biomech 1990: 23: 502–505.

15. Krebs DE, Wong DK, Riley PO, Hodge WA. Trunk kinematics during locomotor ADL," Phys Ther 1992; 72: 505–514.

16. Zachazewski JE, Riley PO, Krebs DE, Schenkman ML. "Biomechanical analysis of body mass transfer during stair ascent of normal subjects," Proceedings Book I, World Confederation For Physical Therapy 11th International Congress, London, England, 1991: 441–443.

17. Herdman SJ. Exercise strategies in vestibular disorders. Ear Nose Throat J 1989; 68: 961–964.

18. Nashner LM, McCollum G. The organization of human postural movements: A formal basis and experimental synthesis. Behav Brain Sci 1985; 8: 135–172.

19. Andres RO. Tests of balance performance in the elderly: A review. Dan. Med. Bull. 1987; 34 (suppl 4): 18–21.

20. Azen R, Krebs DE, Gill-Body KM. Head angular displacements and accelerations during standing, chair rise and gait. MGH Institute of Health Professions (MS Thesis): Boston, MA, in press.
21. Gabell A, Nayak BA. The effect of age on variability in gait. J Gerontol 1984; 39: 662–666.
22. Holden MK, Gill KM, Magliozzi MR. Gait assessment for neurologically impaired patients: Standards for outcome assessment. Phys Ther 1986; 66: 1530–1539.
23. Pozzo T, Berthoz A, Lefort L, Vitte E. Head stabilization during various locomotor tasks in humans: II. Patients with bilateral peripheral vestibular deficits. Exp Brain Res 1991; 85: 208–217.
24. Winter DA. The biomechanics and motor control of human gait: Normal, elderly and pathological. 2d ed. Waterloo, Canada: University of Waterloo Press, 1991.
25. Krebs DE, Ramirez J, Kirkpatrick R, Tucker C, Riley PO. Dynamic stability during normal gait. Proceedings of 7th East Coast Clinical Gait Laboratory Conference, Richmond, VA, 1991.
26. Lockert JD, Krebs DE, Riley PO. Base of support characteristics during gait. Proceedings of 7th East Coast Clinical Gait Laboratory Conference, Richmond, VA, 1991.
27. Horak FB. Clinical measurement of postural control in adults. Phys Ther 1987; 67: 1881–1885.
28. Krebs DE. Biofeedback in therapeutic exercise. In: Therapeutic Exercise, Basmajian JV, Wolf SL, eds. 5th ed. Baltimore: Williams & Wilkins, 1990: 109–124.
29. Kirkpatrick RJr, Tucker C, Ramirez J, Parker SW, Gill KM, Riley PO, Krebs DE. "Center of Gravity Control in Normal and Vestibulopathic Gait. In Proceedings, XIth International Symposium on Posture and Gait: Control Mechanisms, Portland OR, May 25, 1992.
30. Murray MP, Mollinger LA, Gardner GM, Sepic SB. Kinematic and EMG patterns during slow, free, and fast walking. J Orthop Res 1984; 2: 272–280.
31. Heitman DK, Grossman MR, Shaddeau SA, Jackson JR. Balance performance and step width in noninstitutionalized, elderly, female fallers and non fallers. Phys Ther 1989; 69: 923–931.
32. Gehlsen GM, Whaley MH. Falls in the elderly: Part I, Gait. Arch Phys Med Rehab 1990; 71: 735–738.
33. Murray MP, Kory RC, Clarkson BH, Sepic SB. Comparison of free and fast speed walking patterns of normal men. Am J Phys Med 1966; 45: 8–24.
34. Shepard NT, Telian SA, Smith-Wheelock M. Habituation and balance retraining therapy: A retrospective review. Neurol Clin 1990; 8(2): 459–475.
35. Cawthorne T. Vestibular injuries. Proc R Soc Med 1946; 39: 270–273.
36. Gauthier GM, Robinson DA. Adaptation of the human vestibular ocular reflex to magnifying lenses. Brain Res 1975; 92: 331–335.

37. Horak FB, Jones-Rycewicz C, Black FO, Shumway-Cook A. Effects of vestibular rehabilitation on dizziness and imbalance. Otolaryngol Head Neck Surg 1992; 106: 175–180.
38. Gill KM, Krebs DE, Riley PO. Rehabilitation of patients with bilateral vestibular hypofunction. Phys Ther 1991; 71(Suppl): S12.

5

Cerebellar Dysfunction and Disorders of Posture and Gait

LISA OESTREICH

University of Rochester, Rochester, New York

B. TODD TROOST

Bowman Gray School of Medicine, Wake Forest University, Winston-Salem, North Carolina

I. INTRODUCTION

Postural instability and disorders of gait are classic symptoms of cerebellar disease. The initial studies of cerebellar function arose from investigations by Flourens and Luciani in the eighteenth and nineteenth centuries indicating that the cerebellum was involved with regulating muscle tone and coordinating movement (1). Significant understanding of the function of the cerebellum was provided by the work of Sir Gordon Holmes, a neurologist who consulted with the British Army in France during World War I. He described the cardinal clinical features of cerebellar dysfunction following local gunshot wounds. His studies allowed him to see the relationship between the function and structure of the cerebellum. He defined the deficits associated with cerebellar damage broadly as errors of rate, force, tone, amplitude, direction, coordination, and regularity of movement. The appearance of a tremor during activity was also noted (2). These abnormalities were felt to arise from improper function of sense organs from deeper structures following Sherrington's concept of the cerebellum as "the head ganglion of the proprioceptive system" (3).

Abnormalities of gait, posture, and coordination of movement are the hallmark of cerebellar dysfunction. Clinically, without associated signs or symptoms, it is impossible to distinguish pure cerebellar lesions from those involving connections in the brainstem. Thus, it is best to think of the cerebellum proper and its connections within the brainstem as the cerebellar system. This chapter briefly describes the anatomy and physiology of the cerebellar system itself followed by clinical descriptions of those disorders which primarily affect gait.

II. ANATOMY

A. Overview

During the development of the cerebellum, it is initially divided postero-laterally separating the flocculonodular lobe from the corpus cerebelli. The larger corpus cerebelli is divided further into anterior and posterior lobes by the primary fissure. The flocculonodular lobe remains in its caudal position separated by a deep fissure. This lobe is called the vestibulocerebellum because its predominant input comes from the vestibular nuclei which receives peripheral labyrinthine afferent information (4).

The cerebellum can be divided into longitudinal zones perpendicular to the fissures based upon function and patterns of neuronal connection. The vermis is the midline zone nestled between the two cerebellar hemispheres. Each hemisphere is subdivided longitudinally with the medial strip adjacent to the vermis called the pars intermedia, and the larger cerebellar hemispheres more lateral. The cerebellar hemispheres are referred to as the neocerebellum, phylogenetically the newest part of the cerebellum (Fig. 1).

The cerebellum is connected to the brainstem by three paired fiber tracts, the cerebellar peduncles. They are anatomically divided into inferior, middle, and superior cerebellar peduncles where the input is predominantly from the cerebral sensorimotor and visual cortex, vestibular

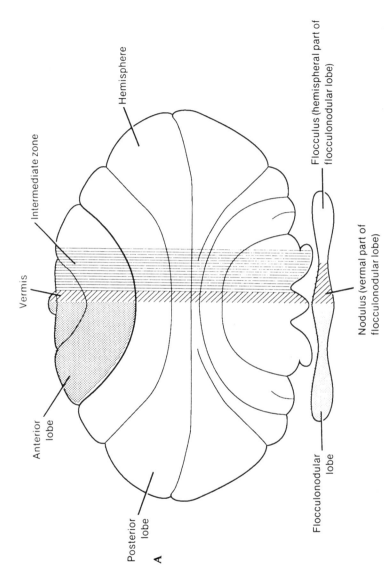

Figure 1 Diagram of the gross anatomy of the human cerebellum. Paracentral regions are outlined by hash marks; diagonal hash marks indicate the midline vermis and central region of the nodulus; vertical hash marks outline the paramedian intermediate zone of the cerebellum. (Reproduced, with permission, from Ref. 4.)

system, and spinal cord by way of the brainstem. The middle cerebellar peduncle, or brachium pontis, is the largest and is virtually exclusively afferent froom the pontine nuclei. The inferior cerebellar peduncle, or restiform body, is also primarily afferent with its cerebellar input from spinal cord and inferior olive. This supplies the cerebellum with vestibular and proprioceptive sensory input from the dorsal spinocerebellar tract and the vestibulocerebellar afferents. The superior cerebellar peduncle, or the brachium conjunctivum, contains the major efferent pathways from the cerebellum. It carries fibers from the cerebellar nuclei to the brainstem, red nucleus, and thalamus on its way to the cerebral cortex.

B. Deep Cerebellar Nuclei

The cerebellum contains deep nuclei that serve to relay information from the cerebellar cortex afferent input to the efferent system. These nuclei are paired structures. The largest and most lateral is the dentate nucleus, which is situated deep within each cerebellar hemisphere and receives its input from the cortex of each cerebellar hemisphere. Most of the fibers in the superior cerebellar peduncle originate from the dentate nucleus. Medial to the dentate nucleus is the emboliform nucleus and the globose nucleus. Collectively, they are called the interposed nucleus with its primary afferents from the pars intermedia. The most medial of the deep cerebellar nuclei is the fastigial nucleus, which receives its input from the cerebellar vermis (Fig. 2).

III. PHYSIOLOGY

A. Neuronal Circuitry of the Cerebellum in Gait Control

The cerebellar hemispheres comprise almost 90% of the human cerebellum (5). It primarily receives impulses that originate in pyramidal cells of the motor association cortex (Brodmann area 6), as well as from somesthetic areas (6). Impulses reach the contralateral cerebellar hemisphere after coursing through the pontine nuclei and the inferior olive. The cerebellum processes afferent information and returns signals to the motor cortex via connections in the ventrolateral nucleus of the thalamus. Signals are then relayed via the pyramidal tracts to the contralateral corticospinal tract to affect appendicular movement ipsilateral to the cerebellar hemisphere in the control of gait.

It has been proposed that the cerebellar hemispheres are concerned with the planning of appendicular movement rather than in its actual

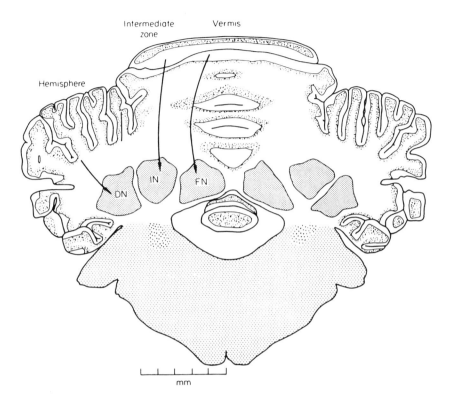

Figure 2 Section of the cerebellum and brain stem along the transverse plane. The large arrows indicate the lines of projection from the cerebellar cortex to the cerebellar nuclei. FN, fastigial nucleus; IN, interpositus nucleus; DN, dentate nucleus. (Adapted, with permission, from Ref. 5.)

execution since impulses are primarily initiated in the association cortex allowing for anticipation of a movement based upon learned experiences and sensory information from other cortical regions (7). As a movement is first executed, it is carried out slowly during the learning phase to allow intense cerebral concentration and fine-tuning by the pars intermedia. The movement then becomes preprogrammed and can be executed more rapidly in an automatic, unconscious fashion. Certain rapid movements rely on this preprogramming, such as coordination of gait while on an unsteady surface. With time, ambulation becomes more automatic (8).

The pars intermedia comprises probably no more than 5% of the human cerebellum; however, it is involved in the coordination and control of movement primarily from the motor cortex (Brodmann area 4) (5). It additionally receives impulses from pontine nuclei (particularly vestibular information), lateral reticular nucleus, and the spinal cord, which together influence postural tone. When the excitatory input enters the pars intermedia, it is relayed through the cerebellar network to the interpositus nucleus where it encounters the inhibitory influence of the Purkinje cells. There impulses can either return to the motor cortex from where they originated as they course through the ventrolateral nucleus of the thalamus, or signals can directly influence the motor neurons of the spinal cord by way of the rubrospinal tract (Fig. 3). The latter pathway allows the cerebellum (pars intermedia) a more direct influence on the motor system involved in gait (6). Since the pars intermedia has a more direct path for influencing the spinal centers via the rubrospinal tract it has been considered a controlling system by making rapid corrections of ongoing movements based on the peripheral sensory input (9). This system is regarded as a closed-loop circuit (10).

The cerebellar vermis and the fastigial nucleus are situated in the midline region of the cerebellum. This area is involved in postural reflexes affecting the main axis of the body by regulating segmental reflexes important in posture and gait (11). The vermal cortex and fastigial nucleus influence the vestibulospinal and reitculospinal efferent projections, which then regulate the tonic activity of alpha and gamma motor neurons in the spinal cord that are involved in the maintenance of gait (9).

The midline region is also responsible for phasic eye and head movements by regulating the vestibulo-ocular reflex through interactions between the flocculonodular lobe and the vestibular nuclei. This system is meant to keep the visual image on the retina during combined head and eye movement, which is important for gait stabilization (9).

Damage to the midline cerebellar region has also shown other ocular motor abnormalities including gaze-evoked nystagmus, rebound nystagmus, ocular dysmetria, and disorders of optokinetic nystagmus. Such ocular motor abnormalities, however, are also seen with diseases in other cerebellar regions (12).

B. Cellular Circuitry of the Cerebellum

The cerebellum receives two different afferent fibers, the climbing fibers, which come exclusively from the inferior olive, and the mossy fibers, which come from all other input, namely the spinal cord, reticular and pontine nuclei. Purkinje cells, however, are considered the central circuit cells since essentially all impusles are transmitted through them the only efferent cells of the cerebellum. Their impulses are inhibitory to the deep cerebellar nuclei modifying all the cerebellar activity. The climbing fibers directly innervate the dendritic tree of Purkinje cells in the cerebellar cortex, while the mossy fibers indirectly innervate the Purkinje cells by synapsing on the granule cells whose horizontal axons form parallel fibers that intersect with the Purkinje dendrites of the cerebellar cortex (5,6) (Fig. 4).

The cerebellum is kept informed of the progress of ongoing movements by inputs from the pontine nuclei, vestibular system, and somatosensory peripheral events by way of the dorsal spinocerebellar tract and the vestibulocerebellar afferents. Therefore, through the continuous excitatory and inhibitory impulses of the cerebellar circuitry, the cerebellum has an influence on the course of all movement initiated by the motor cortex. In humans this complex and multisynaptic circuit is estimated to occur in less than one-fiftieth of a second (5).

C. Cerebellar Influence on Gait

The areas of the cerebellum involved in controlling posture and gait include several of the areas of the cerebellum already discussed above but viewed in a different anatomical orientation, anterior–posterior. In particular, gait is influenced by two regions of the cerebellum, the flocculonondulus and the anterior lobe. The flocculonodular lobe receives projections predominantly from the vestibular nuclei and is therefore called the vestibulocerebellum. The anterior lobe, primarily its vermal portion and part of the pars intermedia, receives input largely from spinocerebellar pathways and is termed the spinocerebellum.

D. Gait Abnormalities due to Cerebellar Lesions

1. The Anterior Lobe Syndrome

Classically, this is seen in alcoholics where chronic alcohol intoxication and malnutrition plus an individual predisposition leads to cortical cerebellar atrophy primarily in the upper vermis and intermedia. This causes a wide-based, unsteady, staggering gait, termed ataxia. This can be associated with lower extremity ataxia as demonstrated by ataxic heel-to-knee maneuver. Ataxia, however, is essentially absent in the upper extremi-

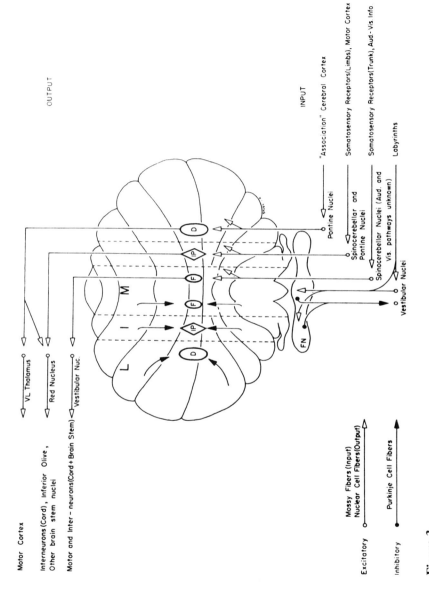

Figure 3

ties. Patients with anterior lobe atrophy, as a whole, exhibit the greatest degree of ataxia that can be measured by a sway path histogram (13). The ataxia is characteristically in an anterior–posterior direction and is the result of diminished cerebellar circuitry through the anterior lobe. Normally, the spinocerebellar tracts relay information to the cerebellum regarding the agonist–antagonist muscle activity controlled by the alpha and gamma motor neurons of the spinal cord. The ataxic gait that develops here results from an interference in the normal spinocerebellar circuitry. For similar reasons, tendon reflexes are pendular due to the lack of dampening of the reflex. The sudden tilt of the supporting platform on which a patient with anterior lobe syndrome is standing results in a large, yet slow, oscillation of the body producing a wide-based, swaying gait. Normally, the reaction is dampened and the gait remains steady. In spite of this, these patients generally do not fall (14).

The reliance on visual support is more pronounced in these patients as seen by increased sway in their gait while their eyes are closed. This specific anterior–posterior sway and visual stability differentiates this type of ataxic gait from other cerebellar ataxias.

2. Vestibulocerebellar Dysfunction

Lesions of the lower vermis involving the flocculonodular lobe, typically seen with local cerebellar hemorrhage or medulloblastomas, cause ataxia of the head and trunk while sitting, standing, and walking (11). Ataxia of the extremities is not a prominent feature. The gait disorder seen here is the result of disruption of the vestibulocerebellum and is characterized as disequilibrium. Eye movements are also abnormal, as demonstrated by nystagmus, which is initiated when the eyes attempt to correct again

---

Figure 3 Diagram of overall cerebellar organization. Transverse cortical folds comprise folia, lobules, and lobes. Shown is longitudinal pattern of projection of cortical Purkinje cells onto deep nuclei and their targets. Mossy fiber inputs often branch to reach both nuclei and cortex. Also shown is origin of mossy fibers supplying different subdivisions and modalities of information that they are likely to carry. Pontine and medullary tegmental reticular nuclei supply all of cerebellum with mossy fibers (not shown). VL, ventrolateral (nucleus of thalamus); lateral (L), intermediate (I), medial (M) cerebellar cortex; D, dentate nucleus; IP, interposed nucleus; F, fastigial nucleus. (Adapted, with permission, from Ref. 1.)

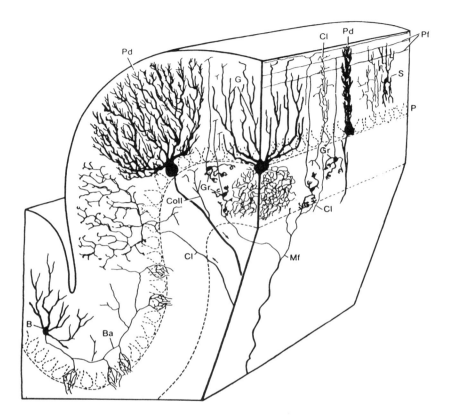

Figure 4 Semidiagrammatic representation of part of a cerebellar folium to show the main elements of the cerebellar cortex and their topographical relationships and orientation. Note especially the arrangement of the Purkinje cell dendrites (pd) and basket cell axons (Ba) in the transverse plane of the folium and the longitudinal arrangement of the parallel fibers (Pf). Other abbreviations: B, basket cell; Cl, climbing fiber; Coll, recurrent collateral of Purkinje cell; G, Golgi cell; Gr, granule cell; Mf, mossy fiber; P, Purkinje cell; Pd, Purkinje cell dendrites; Pf, parallel fibers; S, stellate cell. (Adapted, with permission, from Ref. 6.)

incorrect gaze control. The gaze-evoked nystagmus is usually horizontal with the fast phase toward the side of the lesion (12). Visual input does not improve the truncal ataxia as is seen with patients suffering from other cerebellar disorders as in the anterior lobe syndromes.

3. Cerebellar Hemispheric Lesions

A lesion in a cerebellar hemisphere, seen with tumors, vascular lesions, hemorrhage, or ischemic events, results in ipsilateral limb ataxia, hypotonia, intention tremor, nystagmus, and dysdiadochokinesis (1). The term intention tremor, often used synonymously with cerebellar tremor, is used to describe a coarse tremor that increases in amplitude as the point of termination is reached or the "intended" action is near completion. Intention tremor is brought about by decomposition of intended postural cocontractions of opposing muscles, and consists of inaccurate corrective movements toward intended positions of a limb or of the whole body. Interestingly, this tremor is considered by some to be the result of a conscious effort to correct dysmetric reactions. These lesions do not appreciably affect postural stability; however, they produce an unsteady gait. There is a tendency to lean or "stagger" toward the side of the injured cerebellar hemisphere. The ataxic gait is then more a function of the ipsilateral extremity ataxia (1). If the dentate nucleus is additionally involved, then these abnormalities are more pronounced and persistent (4).

4. Afferent Cerebellar Lesions (Friedreich's Disease)

Early in the disease, spinocerebellar afferents and the posterior columns of the spinal cord are predominantly affected. Therefore, the spinocerebellar circuitry and the proprioceptive afferents involved in the control of gait are affected. Later in the disease, the cerebellum is involved and demonstrates an ataxic gait with a significant lateral sway, particularly when the eyes are closed. The gait pattern demonstrates a larger sway than in any other group of cerebellar patients and is characteristically lateral (11). In addition, the spinal cord lesions produce increased tone, resulting in a stiff-legged, spastic-ataxic gait. Such gait disorders are frequently seen in multiple sclerosis as well as in spinocerebellar degenerations.

5. Diffuse Cerebellar Lesions

Patients with diffuse cerebellar lesions including hereditary late cerebellar atrophy, olivopontocerebellar atrophy, paraneoplastic cerebellar degeneration, and atrophy from toxic agents such as bromides and hydantoin do not exhibit a specific pattern of gait instability or characteristic cerebellar dysfunction. These patients clearly have an abnormality wide-based ataxic gait (14). In addition, they may experience bilateral limb and ocular dysmetria, dysdiadochokinesia, nystagmus, hypotonia, and a kinetic tremor (9).

IV. CONCLUSION

The cerebellum is not essential in the initiation of gait but is necessary for the coordination of the movements involved. The cerebellar control of gait is complex with three proposed roles (15). First, the cerebellum contributes to the timing of limb movements that are essential in the coordination of gait. This is achieved by the continuous modulation of the agonist–antagonist activity of limb muscles, which is controlled by the alpha and gamma motor neurons of the spinal cord that are modified by cerebellar activity. Second, the cerebellum influences interlimb coordination under the influence of the reticulospinal neurons. Third, the cerebellum is thought to influence reflex activities involved in stance and gait. It is theorized that the cerebellum modifies the degree and timing of these spinal reflexes to assist with the coordination of gait. The cerebellum, therefore, can be said to have adaptive functions to accommodate for the ever-changing motion associated with gait.

When there is a disorder of the cerebellum, gait is usually affected and is termed ataxic. The classic staggering, wide-based gait demonstrating disequilibrium is a result of damage to various regions of the cerebellum distinguishable by its clinical features. A large anterior–posterior swaying ataxia is typically seen with a lesion of the anterior lobe. Lesions of the vestibulocerebellum produce truncal ataxia. The ataxia seen with a lesion of the cerebellar hemispheres is more a function of the limb ataxia seen with these lesions. Combined cerebellar system and spinal cord lesions produce a spastic-ataxic gait. When comparing the primarily midline lesions with a lesion of the cerebellar hemispheres, the ataxia is predominantly axial, demonstrating disequilibrium, whereas the latter is appendicular, demonstrating a staggering gate.

REFERENCES

1. Brooks VB, Thach WT. Cerebellar control of posture and movement. In: Brookhart JM, Mountcastle VB, eds., Handbook of Physiology. Maryland: American Physiological Society, 1981: 877–946.

2. Holmes J. The symptoms of acute cerebellar injuries due to gunshot injuries. Brain 1917; 40:461.
3. Sherrington CS. Function of the cerebellum. Encyclopaedia Brittanica 1938; 4:3.
4. Nolte J. The cerebellum. In: Bircher S, ed. The Human Brain. St Louis: Mosby, 1988: 313–334.
5. Eccles J. Cerebellar function in the control of movement. In: Rose FC, ed., Physiological Aspects of Clinical Neurology. London: Blackwell Scientific, 1977: 157–178.
6. Brodal A. The Cerebellum. In: Brodal A, ed., Neurological Anatomy in Relation to Clinical Medicine. New York: Oxford University Press, 1981: 294–391.
7. Brooks VB. Cerebellar function in motor control. Hum Neurobiol 1984; 2:251.
8. Allen GI, Tuskahara N. Cerebrocerebellar communication systems. Physiol Rev 1974: 54:957.
9. Gilman S, Bloedel JR, Lechtenberg R. Disorders of the Cerebellum. Philadelphia: FA Davis, 1981: 1–1000.
10. Eccles JC. The dynamic loop hypothesis of movement control. In: Leibovic KN, ed., Information Processing in the Nervous System. Heidelberg: Springer-Verlag, 1969: 245–269.
11. Dichgans J, Diener HC. Different forms of postural ataxia in patients with cerebellar disease. In Dichgans J, Diener HC, eds., Disorders of Posture and Gait. New York: Elsevier Science Publishers, 1986: 207–215.
12. Troost BT. Nystagmus: a clinical review. Rev Neurol 1989; 145:417.
13. Mauritz KH, Dichgans J, Hufschmidt A. Quantitative analysis of stance in late cortical cerebellar atrophy of the anterior lobe and other forms of cerebellar ataxia. Brain 1979; 102:461.
14. Marsden CD, Merton PA, Morton HB, Hallett M, Adam J, Rushton DN. Disorders of movement in cerebellar disease in man. In: Rose FC, ed., Physiological Aspects of Clinical Neurology. London: Blackwell Scientific, 1977: 179–200.
15. Masao I. Posture. In: Masao I, ed., The Cerebellum and Neural Control. New York: Raven Press 1984: 406–424.

6

Gait Disorders in Extrapyramidal Disease

KATHLEEN M. SHANNON
Rush-Presbyterian-St. Luke's Medical Center, Chicago, Illinois

I. PATHO-ANATOMICAL CONSIDERATIONS

A. Anatomy and Physiology of the Basal Ganglia

The terms extrapyramidal motor system and basal ganglia are used interchangeably to refer to a group of deep gray matter structures believed to be important in motor control. Figure 1 outlines the important structures and their putative interconnections.

Structures of the basal ganglia play a crucial role in the transmission of information in a relay circuit between the cerebral cortex through the thalamus and back to the cerebral cortex. The apparent purpose of this circuit is to regulate cortical motor neuron activity. In the resting condition, the excitatory pathway between the thalamus and cerebral cortex is under tonic inhibition by outflow from the globus pallidus pars interna

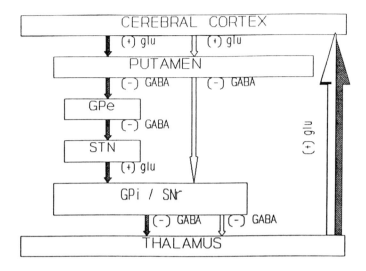

Figure 1 Schematic diagram of basal ganglia structures, interconnections, and important neurotransmitters. The open arrows indicate the "direct" pathway and the hatched arrows the "indirect" pathway (see text).

(GPi). The GPi is under the influence of two parallel pathways—"direct" and "indirect" (1). In the direct pathway, excitatory inputs from the cerebral cortex (CC) converge on the caudate and putamen (C/P). C/P outflow is inhibitory to the GPi; thus the net result is disinhibition of the excitatory thalamo-cortical pathway, and hence increased cortical activity. Activity within this pathway thus may sustain ongoing cortical motor neuron activity or initiate new motor acts (2). In the indirect pathway, excitatory inputs arrive at the C/P from the CC. Inhibitory output from the C/P terminates in the globus pallidus pars externa (GPe). Efferents from the GPe are inhibitory to the subthalamic nucleus (STN). This results in disinhibition of STN output, which is excitatory to the GPi. Since the outflow of the GPi is inhibitory to the thalamus, the net result of activity in the indirect pathway is increased inhibition of cortical activity. This might serve to slow or terminate ongoing motor activities or to inhibit the intrusion of other unwanted motor activities. The effects of activity in the direct and indirect pathway are summarized in Figure 2.

It has been hypothesized that the major role of the basal ganglia is choosing and carrying out learned motor plans by controlling the se-

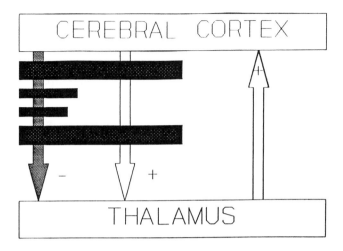

Figure 2 Simplified schematic diagram of basal ganglia indicating net effect of activity in the "direct" (open arrows) and "indirect" (hatched arrows) pathways. Activity in the "direct" pathway excites thalamus, therefore, cortex. Activity in the "indirect" pathway inhibits thalamus, therefore, cortex.

quencing of complex movements and preventing superfluous motor activity (1–4). Disorders of basal ganglia function produce inability to initiate and to carry out quickly and smoothly complex learned motor activities (akinetic-rigid disorders) or interruptions in the smooth flow of activity by involuntary movements (hyperkinetic disorders).

B. The Extrapyramidal System and Control of Locomotion

The basal ganglia do not play a role in the generation of rhythmic stepping behavior. Rather, these structures are believed to be essential in maintenance of posture and balance, initiation of gait and turning, and adaptation to changes in the walking surface and environment (5).

Understanding the role of the extrapyramidal system in normal gait is hampered by the lack of formal gait studies in most of the diseases associated with this system. Only idiopathic Parkinson's disease has been the subject of extensive gait testing. Otherwise, what is known about gait in these disorders has been gleaned from clinical observation.

C. Neuropharmacology of Extrapyramidal Disorders

Numerous neurotransmitters are known to be present in basal ganglia structures. Of these, the best understood are dopamine (DA) and acetylcholine (ACh). DA neurons arising in the substantia nigra pars compacta terminate in the C/P. The effects of DA are mediated by inhibition of cholinergic interneurons. The resulting balance between DA and ACh is such that the clinical expression of excess of one of these neurotransmitters is similar to the clinical expression of deficiency of the other.

DA enhances activity of the direct pathway and inhibits activity in the indirect pathway (6). DA deficiency (or ACh excess) leads to under-activity of the direct and overactivity of the indirect pathway (6), with difficulty in initiating and carrying out motor acts subsequent to excessive inhibition of cortical neurons. This is the presumed pathophysiological basis of parkinsonism. DA excess (or ACh deficiency) has the opposite effect and results in excessive motor activity and inability to prevent intrusion of unwanted motor activities. This is the presumed pathophysiological basis of chorea.

II. EXTRAPYRAMIDAL DISORDERS

A. Parkinsonism

Parkinsonism comprises four cardinal signs: rest tremor, bradykinesia, rigidity, and postural instability. The differential diagnosis of parkinsonism includes those conditions listed in Table 1. In a large autopsy series of parkinsonian patients, idiopathic Parkinson's disease (IPD) accounted for 60–75%, other degenerative conditions for 15%, cerebrovascular disease for 5–8%, and sequelae of encephalitis for 3% of cases (7). The presumed pathophysiological basis of parkinsonism is underactivity of the direct pathway with overactivity of the indirect pathway. The pharmacological basis of the disease is decreased dopamine activity with relative increase in acetylcholine activity.

1. Parkinson's Disease

Idiopathic Parkinson's disease is defined pathologically by loss of pigmented neurons in the substantia nigra and other nuclei and the presence of eosinophilic inclusions (Lewy bodies) in degenerating neurons (8). This degeneration results in a state of dopamine deficiency. Autopsy studies have identified a misdiagnosis rate of about 35% in IPD (9). In

Table 1   Differential Diagnosis of Parkinsonism

Neurodegenerative conditions
 idiopathic (Lewy body) Parkinson's disease
 progressive supranuclear palsy
 multiple system atrophy
 parkinsonism dementia
 corticobasal degeneration
 Huntington's disease (particularly juvenile onset)
 juvenile parkinsonism-dystonia
Acquired structural disorders
 hydrocephalus
 subdural hematoma
 brainstem tumor
Drugs and toxins
 dopamine receptor antagonists (neuroleptics, antiemetics)
 catecholamine depleters (reserpine, tetrabenazine)
 calcium channel antagonists
 alphamethyldopa
 carbon monoxide
 manganese
 MPTP

an attempt to increase the yield of clinical diagnosis of IPD, Koller has suggested including the following criteria for the diagnosis: presence for longer than 1 year of two of the cardinal signs of parkinsonism, and marked responsiveness to levodopa for a period of 1 year or more (8). Other criteria said to be highly predictive of diagnosis confirmation at autopsy are unilateral onset and rest tremor (10).

Onset of IPD is between 50 and 60 years of age in 40% of patients, and between 40 and 70 years in 80%. The most common initial complaint is rest tremor in one arm. Usually, at the time of diagnosis, bradykinesia and rigidity can be detected in the symptomatic arm and often in other extremities. In only 17% of patients are there complaints of gait disorder at onset (11). The typical mode of progression is for spread to the ipsilateral lower extremity followed by the contralateral extremities. There follows progressive deterioration in posture, balance, and gait. Untreated IPD has an extremely variable rate of progression (12). Although the rare patient survives up to 30 years, 83% of patients are dead or disabled by 15 years duration (12). Although treatment with the dopamine precursor levodopa has resulted in improved survival and longer duration of disease until onset of severe disability (12, 13), there is no evidence that this is due to an effect on the underlying disease progression.

Gait in Untreated IPD. The gait disorder of IPD is insidious. In the earliest stages of disease, gait abnormalities consist only of unilateral decrease in arm swing or shortening of stride length. As the disease advances, the posture becomes flexed, arm swing is markedly reduced, the velocity of walking slows, and the stride length shortens. With further progression, patients develop hesitation in starting to walk; initiation of gait may be with several steps in place or with several short steps. There may be an involuntary hurrying of gait (festination) which culminates in running (14). This may be accompanied by the subjective sensation of being pitched or pushed forward. It may be impossible to stop this propulsive gait without resorting to colliding with a fixed object. Turns are executed with more difficulty because postural reflexes are impaired. If the standing balance is threatened by a push, the patient may retropulse in an attempt to regain balance. Balance may be regained after a number of corrective retropulsive steps, or recovery may be impossible. In more advanced disease, there may be immediate falling without any corrective steps. Falling becomes a daily occurrence. Eventually, postural reflexes become impaired to the point that independent standing and walking are impossible and the patient becomes chair or bed bound.

Formal gait studies in IPD have demonstrated shortening of the stride length and increase in stride duration. The stance and double support duration increase and the swing phase shortens (15). Arm swing is abnormal in amplitude and timing (16). The normal pattern of heel strike disappears and there is a higher incidence of toe or mixed strike. Movements around the hip and knee are reduced in amplitude, and there is reduced vertical excursion (17) due to reduced step height. At the end of the stance phase, there is no push-off of the backward-directed leg, and the weight may shift to the forward-directed leg at the time of normal push-off (17, 18). Thus, there is little propulsive force; forward movement occurs because the trunk falls forward (17). Studies of postural reflexes have demonstrated that anticipatory and reactive postural mechanisms are impaired in IPD (19, 20).

An interesting phenomenon in parkinsonian gait is the improvement with certain sensory cues. Many different types of sensory stimuli enhance the ability to initiate gait and to lengthen stride and improve velocity. Certainly the most widely observed phenomenon is the improvement in gait initiation, velocity, and stride length induced by placement of parallel strips of paper or tape on the walking surface perpendicular to the direction of walking. A cane turned upside down with the handpiece used as a visual cue may also be useful (21). Formal studies of changes in parkinsonian gait induced by visual cues demonstrate that the stride length increases as much as 100%; the velocity increases, and there is increased mobility around the hip and knee joints. However, abnormal patterns of foot strike persist, and the propulsive force of the backward-directed leg at end stance remains poor (17). The mechanism of these improvements with visual cues is unknown. Rhythmic auditory stimuli such as music or counting aloud have a similar effect. Spouses sometimes find that stepping on the patient's foot and tapping the back of the leg or foot are effective tactile stimuli to initiate gait.

Gait in Treated IPD. A wealth of knowledge about the pharmacological basis of PD has led to its place as the most treatable extrapyramidal disorder. The central dopamine deficiency state can be improved with indirect dopamine agonists (amantadine), dopamine precursor therapy (levodopa or levodopa with aromatic acid decarboxylase inhibitor), or direct-acting dopamine agonists (bromocriptine, pergolide). Alternatively, the relative excess acetylcholine activity can be managed with anticholinergic agents (trihexyphenidyl, benztropine). Levodopa therapy dramatically improves function in PD, lessening tremor, bradykinesia, and rigidity and improving gait. The stride length and velocity increase; foot strike returns to normal, and the patient regains the ability to push off with the backward-directed leg (17). However, not all features of IPD respond with equal vigor to pharmacological treatment. Gait and postural reflexes are somewhat resistant to chronic levodopa therapy, and with progression of the underlying disease, patients become increasingly disabled by parkinsonian gait (22). In addition, treated IPD patients often have fluctuations in motor response to levodopa with reappearance of PD symptoms between medication doses ("wearing off") or at unpredictable times during the day ("on–off"). Patients also begin to have sudden spells of pronounced akinesia in the lower extremities ("freezing") that are resistant to, and may be worsened by, levodopa. Thus, gait in treated advanced PD can vary remarkably throughout the day from relatively normal to quite impaired. Levodopa also induces a wide variety of involuntary movements (chorea, dystonia, etc.), which may come and go during the day and which may be superimposed on varying degrees of parkinsonian gait.

2. Progressive Supranuclear Palsy (PSP)

Progressive supranuclear palsy usually begins in the seventh decade and is characterized by parkinsonian rigidity, axial dystonia, pseudobulbar signs, and supranuclear gaze palsy, which may be accompanied by dementia (23). In contrast to the masked face of Parkinson's disease, the patient has a startled or worried appearance with a furrowed brow and deep facial lines (4). Apraxia of eyelid opening, light sensitivity, and blepharospasm are common (24), and cause significant visual impairment. Although supranuclear gaze palsy is its hallmark, it may appear late in the disease course (25). Vertical gaze is affected initially, with restricted down gaze, but, eventually, the eyes become fixed to volitional attempts to move them. Reflex eye movements (oculocephalic or oculovestibular maneuvers) are intact (4), confirming the supranuclear origin of the gaze palsy. Gait disturbance is an early sign of the disorder, being the initial symptom in 62% of cases (23). The gait in PSP can be somewhat variable. In a series of 46 patients with PSP reported by Maher and Lees, 25 had a broad-based, unsteady gait and 21 had a parkinsonian gait (26). Parkinsonism in PSP shares some features with that of IPD. Patients may have small steps, shuffling gait, and postural reflex impairment with freezing and falling. Unlike IPD, the posture is usually more erect; there may be marked axial rigidity with an extensor posture of the neck. The broad-based, ataxic gait of the remainder of PSP patients has the flavor of carelessness. Patients may veer from side to side, cross their legs in front of each other, stagger, and fall. They may bound from sitting to standing without any attempt to establish balance. The stride length may be long, and is usually variable, and the walking velocity may be little different from normal. The major feature of both these types of gait dysfunction is that balance impairment is out of proportion to the other abnormalities.

Regardless of the type of gait, the disorder is rapidly progressive. The median time from onset to need for ambulatory assistance is 3.1 years; 8.2 years to the wheelchair-bound state (23). Death usually occurs within 10 years of diagnosis (23, 26).

There is no therapy for the progressive degeneration underlying PSP symptoms. However, 60% of patients may have modest or transient response to one or more therapeutic agents (27). Bradykinesia and rigidity may respond to dopaminergic drugs (27). However, patients with significant gait ataxia may notice that the resulting increase in walking speed without a parallel improvement in postural reflexes leads to an increased number of falls. Some patients have been reported to respond to other medications such as amitriptyline, imipramine, baclofen, and methysergide, but formal studies of these agents are scarce.

3. Multiple System Atrophies (MSA)

MSA describes a diverse group of degenerative central nervous system disorders that have in common widespread degeneration in the pons, cerebellum, pigmented brainstem nuclei, basal ganglia, and the striatum (4). MSA is generally classified into three types: Shy-Drager syndrome, olivopontocerebellar atrophy, and striatonigral degeneration.

Shy-Drager Syndrome (SDS). SDS is defined as primary autonomic nervous system failure with neurological dysfunction (28). Signs of autonomic failure, including incontinence, impotence, and orthostatic hypotension, occur early and remain prominent throughout the disease course. Patients may have one or several types of neurological dysfunction, including parkinsonism, spasticity, amyotrophy, and cerebellar ataxia. The gait of SDS may resemble IPD with start hesitation, small-stepped, shuffling gait, and postural reflex impairment. Gait may also be impaired by orthostatic hypotension, which may severely limit the ability to stand and walk. There may be other neurological features discernible in the gait including ataxia and peripheral neuropathy.

Olivopontocerebellar Atrophy (OPCA). OPCA is named for the brain regions most often affected by this disorder. Unfortunately, under this rubric fall different subtypes (dominantly inherited with or without retinal degeneration or slow saccades and peripheral neuropathy; and sporadic or recessively inherited with or without glutamate dehydrogenase deficiency) (4). OPCA has resisted rather heroic attempts to devise a classification system (29), as virtually each new family has unique clinical features. Patients may present primarily with cerebellar ataxia or may show a gait disorder similar to that of IPD. Choreic movements may be seen also, particularly in families showing a dominantly inherited form of the disease (30). The typical OPCA patient has a parkinsonian gait with hesitancy, slowness, short steps, and balance impairment. Unlike IPD, the base is widened and the gait is ataxic.

Striatonigral Degeneration (SND). The MSA that most closely resembles IPD is SND. Patients with SND differ in appearance from IPD mainly in the absence of tremor and poor response to levodopa. The gait in SND is essentially the same as that in IPD.

The diagnosis of MSA rests on an appearance which, while it may share some features with IPD, has atypical features including autonomic dysfunction, cerebellar ataxia, or poor response to levodopa. Although it may be possible to further classify many patients into the above subtypes using these clinical features, there is a great deal of overlap, and the therapeutic usefulness of such a classification remains vague. Treatment of MSA employs antiparkinsonian medications, but success is limited.

4. Lower Body Parkinsonism (LBP)

LBP is a syndrome of prominent parkinsonian gait with relative sparing of motor function in the upper extremities (31). Gait disability is the initial complaint in 90% of LBP patients, and is characterized by short, shuffling steps, freezing, and start hesitation; festination is not seen. As in IPD, gait is improved by visual and other sensory cues. Hypertension occurs in 70% and MRI scanning demonstrates multiple subcortical abnormalities, presumably of ischemic origin. The symptoms do not improve with dopaminergic therapy.

5. Other Forms of Parkinsonism

Other forms of parkinsonism are seen rarely. In general, these disorders consist of parkinsonian features combined with variable dysfunction of cognitive, motor, sensory, cerebellar, and autonomic systems. All are treated with antiparkinsonian agents, and all respond poorly to treatment.

B. Chorea

Chorea is defined as irregular, nonrepetitive, random, purposeless, movements (32). Early or mild chorea may appear to be merely excessive restlessness. The movements may be incorporated into normal motor acts that appear exaggerated. More severe chorea is readily identifiable; involuntary movements intrude on every willed action. Although other neurological features may help the clinician distinguish between the various causes of chorea, the movements themselves appear the same regardless of underlying etiology. The presumed pathophysiological basis of chorea is believed to be overactivity of the direct pathway or underactivity of the indirect pathway. The pharmacological basis of chorea seems to be excess dopaminergic or deficient cholinergic activity.

1. Huntington's Disease

Huntington's disease is an inherited neurodegenerative disease characterized by choreic movements, dementia, and psychiatric disorders. It follows an autosomal dominant pattern of inheritance with complete penetrance. The genetic basis of HD is an unstable trinucleotide repeat on the fourth chromosome (33). Although a family history is important for making the diagnosis of HD, it has been reported that 75% of patients with the typical syndrome of progressive chorea and dementia and a negative family history will go on to have definite HD (34). The disorder first becomes symptomatic for the majority of patients in the fourth and fifth decades of life. Personality changes or psychiatric disease often antedate motor abnormalities (35). The motor disorder is first apparent as mild chorea, sometimes mixed with dystonic posturing. A small number of patients overall, but a large percentage of those presenting before the age of 20, will present with a rigid-akinetic syndrome, other unusual features, and more rapid progression (36). Histopathological studies suggest that as HD progresses, cells in the direct pathway begin to degenerate. The clinical observation that virtually all HD patients come to have some features of parkinsonism (particularly bradykinesia and rigidity) lends credence to this finding (37, 38). The inexorable mental and physical deterioration leads to death, usually within 20 years of onset (35, 39). The causes of death in HD are commonly related to chronic immobility and include bronchopneumonia, aspiration, nutritional deficiencies, and chronic skin ulcers (40).

Gait in Untreated HD. Gait dysfunction is universally present in HD patients and represents the sum of involuntary choreic and dystonic movements, parkinsonism, and various features suggestive of widespread brain degeneration. Heathfield reported observational analyses of gait in 20 HD patients (39). He reported that the act of standing precipitated choreic movements of the upper extremities and trunk resulting in lordotic or scoliotic postures and the assumption of a wide base. Gait was wide-based with lurching from side to side and irregular step length and rhythm. Patients paused or rarely took steps backward, which further interrupted the rhythm of walking. Walking was accompanied variably by rigid fixation of the upper extremities against the trunk or wild choreic movements. Although the gait appeared quite unsteady, patients were believed to fall little as a result. However, Koller recently studied gait in 13 ambulatory men with HD (41). Of these patients, 85% had a history of falling; many had multiple falls every month. Falling was present in patients with and without choreic movements; 92% had evidence of gait abnormality on clinical examination. Frequently seen were poor balance, lateral ataxia, wide-based station, variability in walking speed, and difficulty with turning. (41). Features similar to parkinsonism included start hesitation, small steps, reduced associated movements, such as arm swing, and poor turns (41). Formal study in these patients demonstrated decreased walking velocity, stride length, and cadence with an increase in total gait cycle time (41).

Gait in Treated HD. Choreic movements in HD respond to treatment with drugs that have antidopaminergic properties. These include neuroleptics and catecholamine-depleting drugs (reserpine, tetrabenazine). Neuroleptics such as haloperidol and chlorpromazine have found widespread use in the treatment of HD. Unfortunately, gait disorder and falling are resistant to this therapy (41) and the functional status of treated HD patients remains poor despite improvement in chorea (42).

2. Tardive Dyskinesia (TD)

TD results from chronic therapy with drugs that have in common the potential to block the dopamine receptor. Estimates of the prevalence of TD in patients exposed to such drugs vary widely. Jeste reviewed 36 studies of TD prevalence between 1960 and 1980 in neuroleptic-treated chronically ill psychiatric inpatients. He found the overall mean prevalence of tardive dyskinesia in these studies to be 17.5% (43). Studies in outpatients are more difficult to interpret, but rates of TD have been reported to be as high as 30% in chronically treated outpatients (44, 45). It is believed that age and female gender confer greater risk of acquiring the disorder (46). The pathogenesis of chorea in TD is believed to be related to denervation sensitivity of postsynaptic dopamine receptors.

Although the spectrum of TD contains myriad involuntary movements, the most common manifestation is chorea, which may be localized or generalized. Choreic movements are often accompanied by dystonia and athetosis. When TD patients are under continuing treatment with the offending agent, parkinsonian signs may coexist with involuntary movements.

The choreic gait resembles that seen in HD to some extent. When the trunk is involved, there may be abnormalities in standing posture with exaggerated lordosis. Standing or walking precipitates an increase in dyskinetic extremity movements (47). When the patient walks, rocking, swaying, or rotatory pelvic movements may be obvious. Associated movements may be exaggerated, and the stride length may be increased and more variable than normal. There have been no formal gait studies in TD.

As with other choreic disorders, the involuntary movements are lessened by treatment with dopamine receptor blockers, but these are not recommended because of the risk of exacerbating the movement disorder. Agents that deplete presynaptic dopamine stores (reserpine, tetrabenazine) successfully control the movements in many patients. Once the offending dopamine receptor blocking drug is discontinued, the condition may gradually resolve. However, it has been estimated that in as many as 50% of TD patients, the movement disorder is permanent (48).

3. Hemiballismus (HB)

Ballism is defined as proximal violent involuntary movements. Various features of the movement disorder suggest that it is best considered a particularly violent form of chorea (49). Although ballistic movements may affect one or all four extremities, the most common clinical syndrome is the occurrence of hemiballismus, ballistic movements in the extremities of one side of the body consequent to a vascular insult in the contralateral subthalamic nucleus of Luys (50). HB is a rare clinical syndrome. The movements in HB are large amplitude, proximally predominant, and violent. They often result in soft tissue injury. Severely affected patients are bed bound. In less severely affected patients, ambulation is possible, although the patient walks with flinging movements of the affected leg. Although some authors suggest that the movements are lessened by walking, it is clear that for most patients, ballistic movements impair gait.

HB was originally believed to carry a universally grave prognosis (51), but more recent evidence suggests that most patients survive and many recover completely (52). Those with residual involuntary movements often have lower amplitude movements that are more classically choreic in appearance.

As in other choreic movement disorders, antidopaminergic medications can significantly lessen the occurrence of and disability from HB (49).

4. Other Choreas

The differential diagnosis of chorea is listed in Table 2. The extent to which gait is affected in these conditions is dependent on the extent to

Table 2 Differential Diagnosis of Chorea

Degenerative conditions
  hereditary
    Huntington's chorea
    benign hereditary chorea
    neuroacanthocytosis
    Wilson's disease
  sporadic
    senile chorea
Secondary
  drug-induced
    tardive
    acute/subacute
      anticonvulsants
      amphetamine
    oral contraceptives
  vascular
    hemiballismus/hemichorea
  systemic illness
    rheumatic fever
    hyperthyroidism
    lupus erythematosus
    acquired hepatocerebral degeneration
    chorea gravidarum

which the trunk and lower extremities are affected. The resulting gait abnormality resembles those seen in HD or TD, as described above.

C. Dystonia

Dystonia has been defined by the ad hoc committee of the Dystonia Medical Research Foundation as: "a syndrome of sustained muscle contractions, frequently causing twisting and repetitive movements, or abnormal postures" (53). Dystonic movements may affect any striated muscle except the extraocular muscles and sphincters. While the movements may be present at rest, they are nearly always exaggerated by action with the involved body part, and at times by action with other body parts. The actions required to initiate or worsen dystonic movements may be quite specific. For example, a patient with dystonic involvement of the foot may have dystonia when walking forward, but not when walking backward, or when dancing. Certain involuntary movements and postures are characteristic of dystonia, including forced eye closure, facial grimacing, jaw opening or closing, involuntary head turning, spine deformities, internal rotation of the arm, torsion of the pelvis, and plantar flexion and inversion of the foot (54). Although the classic description of dystonia includes postures that are sustained for 30 s or more, the movements may be more rapid and resemble chorea or tremor. A characteristic of dystonic movements is that they may transiently be lessened in severity by certain tricks. These include laying a finger next to the eye in dystonias of the eyelid, eating or speaking with a foreign object in the mouth in oromandibular dystonias, and lightly touching the face or cheek in cervical dystonias.

Dystonias may be classified according to several different schemes: age of onset, cause, or distribution (see Table 3). Dystonia may begin in childhood, adolescence, or adulthood. Onset in childhood has a poorer prognosis for motor function and gait. Dystonia may be idiopathic or secondary to a neurological insult. Idiopathic dystonia may be inherited or sporadic. Secondary dystonias generally are seen in the context of more widespread neurological dysfunction. Although dystonia may affect almost any body muscle, there are usually certain patterns of involvement. Focal dystonia is localized to a single body part. Segmental dystonia is confined to two or more contiguous body parts, and multifocal dystonia is confined to two or more noncontiguous body parts. Hemidystonia affects the extremities on one side of the body. Generalized dystonia is diagnosed when dystonic movements involve both legs and another body part, or the leg, trunk, and another body part.

1. Idiopathic Torsion Dystonia (ITD)

ITD is a monosymptomatic disorder characterized by the presence of dystonic movements. Although a positive family history may be difficult to obtain, particularly in adult onset focal or segmental dystonia patients, recent genetic studies suggest that dystonia is transmitted by an autosomal dominant gene with 25–30% penetrance (55, 56). The dystonia gene is believed to be located on the long arm of chromosome 9 (57).

The presentation and course of ITD depend on the age at onset and the body part first affected. Childhood onset of ITD most commonly begins with dystonia in the foot, which is precipitated by walking or running. There is rapid progression to generalized involvement in most of these patients. When childhood onset ITD begins in the face, neck, or upper extremities, progression is likely to stop with focal or

Table 3   Classification of Dystonia

By age at onset
  childhood onset, 0–12 years
  adolescent onset, 13–20 years
  adult onset, >20 years
By cause
  idiopathic
    sporadic
    familial
  symptomatic
    neurodegenerative conditions
      Wilson's disease
      GM1 (childhood or adult forms, GM2 gangliosidoses late manifestation)
      metachromatic leukodystrophy
      Lesch-Nyhan disease
      homocystinuria
      glutaric acidemia
      triosephosphate isomerase deficiency
      Leigh's disease
      Fahr's disease
      Hallervorden Spatz disease
      dystonic lipidoses
      ceroid lipofuscinosis
      ataxia-telangiectasia
      neuroacanthocytosis
      Hartnup disease
      neuronal intranuclear inclusion disease
      Huntington's disease
      idiopathic dystonia parkinsonism
      Pelizaeus-Merzbacher disease
      bilateral basal ganglia lucencies
    other
      perinatal damage
      infarction
      AVM
      tumor
      trauma
      encephalitis
      drugs (acute/chronic)
      toxins

Table 3 Continued

By distribution
focal
segmental
multifocal
generalized
hemidystonia

segmental involvement. Adult onset ITD usually begins with focal dystonic movements of the upper extremity, face, or neck and remains focal or shows progression to adjacent body segments (53).

The gait abnormality of ITD depends on the distribution of dystonic movements. Patients with dystonia localized to the cranial and cervical musculature may have normal gait. There may be a more cautious appearance to the gait in patients whose dystonic involvement of the eyes results in inability to scan the walking surface or in patients with severe cervical involvement with difficulty keeping the head and eyes forward. In a review of 42 patients with ITD (excluding those with torticollis), Marsden found that 36% of patients presented with an abnormality of gait. All had dystonic movements affecting the lower extremities. Although the most common complaint was involuntary plantar flexion and in-turning of the foot at it approached the ground, others had a bizarre gait that defied description (54). Most patients with generalized dystonia show extreme lordotic posture with superimposed torsional movements of the trunk, shoulders, and pelvis. The step height and length are variable. Walking velocity is reduced. Due to the exacerbation of dystonic posture by action of the involved part, the foot velocity and direction may appear to change in midflight. Balance is impaired by the ever-changing relationship of the body parts to one another, and falling may result.

The pharmacological basis of dystonia is largely unknown. There has been success in the treatment of childhood onset dystonia with very large doses of anticholinergic agents, or with levodopa, baclofen, or other agents. Unfortunately, not all patients respond to these agents, and while many patients may be made ambulatory again, gait is rarely normal. Adults with dystonia tend to tolerate anticholinergics more poorly than children do, and usually have less than satisfying treatment results (58). Local intramuscular injections of botulinum toxin A are useful in the treatment of focal and segmental dystonias, but dose considerations make this modality infeasible for generalized dystonia (59).

2. Dopa-Responsive Dystonia (DRD)

Dopa-responsive dystonia accounts for approximately 5–10% of dystonia in childhood and adolescence. DRD is a dominantly inherited condition with approximately 31% penetrance (60, 61). The salient clinical features are crural dystonia with onset in the first decade of life with progression to generalized dystonia in most cases. The later emergence of parkinsonism is common. Diurnal fluctuations in severity of dystonia with worsening later in the day or following periods of exercise is typical, but not universal (60). Gait disability is marked; 40% of patients in one series required a wheelchair for at least part of the day by 10 years of disease duration (60).

Treatment of dystonic and parkinsonian symptoms with levodopa is very successful. Benefit is generally marked and immediate with return of motor function to nearly normal. Unlike the response of IPD patients to levodopa, dyskinesia and wearing off are rare and not disabling despite long duration therapy (60).

3. Wilson's Disease (WD)

WD is a rare autosomal recessive disorder of copper metabolism that affects the liver, kidneys, and brain. The primary defect in WD is an inability to excrete copper into the bile with secondary deposition of copper into the tissues. Low levels of ceruloplasmin are a commonly found marker of the disease (62). An increased amount of intrahepatic copper in the presence of cirrhosis is diagnostic of WD.

Initially, copper is deposited in the liver. Asymptomatic hepatosplenomegaly may result. Other patients present with acute or chronic hepatitis. Fulminant hepatitis with hemolytic anemia and coagulopathy occurs rarely. Copper is deposited in the limbus of the cornea where it is visible as the Kayser-Fleischer ring.

The neurological presentation of WD is insidious, and may occur in patients known to have had liver disease or those without significant hapatic history. Investigation will show liver involvement in all patients at the time of neurological presentation. Almost without exception, Kayser-Fleischer rings are present to detailed investigation when neurological symptoms appear. Seizures, dysarthria, drooling, cognitive decline, and psychiatric disorders are often present. Extrapyramidal signs are common, and may be the presenting feature of the illness. The most common movement disorder in WD is tremor, but dystonia occurs with regularity. In the absence of specific decoppering therapy, there is inexorable decline to death.

The dystonia of WD usually affects the cranial and antigravity muscles. The face may be held in a grinning posture. There are constant drooling and dysarthria. There may be a retrocollic head posture and lordotic trunk. The typical gait consists of neck extension, lordosis, dystonic inversion, and plantar flexion of the lower extremities. With advanced WD, ambulation usually is not possible.

Treatment of WD involves D-penicillamine copper chelation. While D-penicillamine is quite effective at stopping the progression of the disorder, and is associated with improved survival and lessened hepatic morbidity, dystonic features of the illness fare more poorly with treatment. Occasionally patients will show some improvement of dystonic symptoms with medications such as levodopa (63).

4. Tardive Dystonia

Burke et al. reported 42 patients in whom dystonia was the primary tardive movement disorder following neuroleptic treatment (64). They found that the distribution of dystonic movements in these patients related to the age of onset of the disorder, with initial involvement in the legs and progression to generalized movements in younger onset cases. The average duration of neuroleptic exposure in this group was about 3 years, but the severity of movements did not correlate with the duration of exposure. The extent to which the lower extremities were involved determined whether gait was abnormal. Only one patient was bed bound because of dystonic movements. The treatment of tardive dystonia includes discontinuation of the neuroleptic agent if possible, and use of anticholinergic and antidopaminergic agents. As in tardive dyskinesia, the preferred antidopaminergic agents are reserpine and tetrabenazine.

5. Other Secondary Dystonias

Although dystonic movements may be a prominent symptom of the disorders that underlie secondary dystonia, signs of dysfunction of other neurological systems are usually present. The gait disorders that are seen in these patients represent the sum of these neurological deficits (cognitive, motor, sensory, cerebellar) with superimposed dystonic movements.

D. Tremor

Tremor is defined as involuntary, rhythmic alternating movement about a joint. Tremors are classified according to their presence or absence during certain motor activities, such as rest, postural, or kinetic tremors (65). Rest tremor is one of the cardinal features of parkinsonism. Although these patients commonly have gait disturbance, this is never a result of the tremor itself.

A postural tremor is one that is present during maintenance of an antigravity posture (61). All normal persons have a high-frequency (10–12 Hz) postural "physiological tremor." Under circumstances such as extreme anxiety, medical illness, and exposure to various drugs, physiological tremor may become symptomatic. Treatment of the exacerbating factors results in improvement.

Kinetic tremors occur with performance of goal-directed action of a limb (61). Such tremors are generally coarse and increase in amplitude as the target is approached. They are generally seen in patients with cerebellar disease.

1. Essential Tremor (ET)

Essential tremor is the most commonly occurring symptomatic tremor. Inherited as an autosomal dominant trait, estimates of prevalence range between 0.0005% and 1.7% of the general population and 0.33% and 6.62% of the population over 40 years of age (67). ET may begin at any age, although it is rare in infancy and childhood and becomes progressively more common with age. There may be remarkable variability in age of onset within a pedigree (68). The most commonly affected body parts are the upper extremities and head. Estimates of the frequency of lower extremity involvement range between less than 1% (69) and 31% (70). Lower extremity involvement is more likely to be seen in the later stages of the disorder (61). ET is not believed to cause gait disorder.

2. Orthostatic Tremor

Orthostatic tremor was first reported in 1984 by Heilman. The syndrome includes asynchronous, irregular movements of the trunk and proximal lower extremities that appear with standing (61) or with sustained pressure of the legs against a fixed object (62). The tremor is improved by leaning against a wall or walking and disappears when the patient is lifted from the ground (73). Prolonged standing may precipitate falling, but patients generally have normal gait and do not fall when walking (74). In some of these patients, a similar tremor can be precipitated in the upper extremities with handstands or push-ups (73). The usual age of onset of OT is in the sixth decade. Half of OT patients have a positive family history of ET and the majority have postural tremor in the upper extremities (74).

Electrophysiological studies demonstrate that the frequency of OT is 16–18 Hz, although in some patients an 8-Hz component has been described (73). OT patients do not benefit from treatment with medications that are effective in ET, but generally derive some benefit from treatment with clonazepam (74). While some authors prefer to classify OT as a clinical variant of ET (74, 75), the differences in tremor frequency and pharmacology have led others to classify it as a separate entity (73). OT should be considered in patients who complain of tremor and propensity to fall when standing, but in whom gait is normal.

3. Wilson's Disease

Wilson's disease was described in Section II.C.3. The two major extrapyramidal presentations of WD are with dystonia and with tremor. The tremor of WD may be present during rest, sustained posture, or may be seen with action. The tremor may be proximally predominant and take on a "wing-beating" character. The gait of tremulous WD patients is usually wide-based with variable foot placement. The arm swing is poorly timed and irregular in amplitude. There may be ataxia and falling (61).

The tremulous manifestations of WD are more likely to respond to decoppering therapy than are the dystonic symptoms.

III. SUMMARY

Although the extrapyramidal system is not involved in the generation of stepping movements per se, it is essential in normal ambulation. Extrapyramidal disorders disrupt the ability to generate fluid gait and to adapt to changes in the walking task as well as in the walking environment. An interesting and highly characteristic feature of extrapyramidal disorders is that the abnormalities in gait can be improved by certain internal and external cues such as changing the direction or type of ambulation or changing the sensory environment. Diagnosis rests on visual recognition of changes in movement fluidity and patterns and of the nature of involuntary movements. Fortunately, many patients with extrapyramidal disorders may benefit from specific pharmacotherapy.

REFERENCES

1. Alexander GE, Crutcher MD. Functional architecture of basal ganglia curcuits: neural substrates of parallel processing. Trends Neurosci 1990; 13: 266.
2. Young AB, Penney JB. Neurochemical anatomy of movement disorders. Neurol Clinics 1984; 2: 417.
3. Young AB, Penney JB. Biochemical and functional organization of the basal ganglia. In Jankovic J, Tolosa E, eds. New York: Urban & Schwarzenberg, 1988: 1.
4. Weiner WJ, Lang AE. Other akinetic-rigid and related syndromes. In: Weiner WJ, Lang AE, eds., Movement Disorders. A Comprehensive Survey. New York: Futura, 1989: 117.
5. Joseph J. Neurological control of locomotion. Dev Med Child Neurol 1985; 27: 822.
6. DeLong M. Primate models of movement disorders of basal ganglia origin. Trends Neurosci 1990; 13: 281.
7. Jellinger K. The pathology of parkinsonism. In: Marsden CD, Fahn S, eds., Movement Disorders. London: Butterworths, 1987; 124.
8. Koller WC. How accurately can Parkinson's disease be diagnosed. Neurology 1992; 42(Suppl 1): 6.
9. Rajput AH, Rozdilsky B, Rajput A. Accuracy of clinical diagnosis in parkinsonism—prospective study. Can J Neurol Sci 1991; 18: 275.
10. Rajput AH, Rozdilsky B, Ang L. Occurrence of resting tremor in Parkinson's disease. Neurology 1991; 41: 1298.
11. Jankovic J, McDermott M, Carter J, Gauthier S, Goetz C, Golbe L, Huber S, Koller W, Olanow C, Shoulson I, Stern M, Tanner C, Weiner W, and the Parkinson Study Group. Variable expression of Parkinson's disease: a base-line analysis of the DATATOP cohort. Neurology 1990; 40: 1529.
12. Hoehn MM, Yahr MD. Parkinsonism: onset, progression and mortality. Neurology 1967; 17: 427.
13. Hoehn MM. Parkinsonism treated with levodopa: progression and mortality. In: Birkmayer W, Duvoisin RC, eds., Extrapyramidal Disorders. Wien and New York: Springer-Verlag, 1983: 253.
14. Parkinson J. An essay on the shaking palsy. London: Whittingham and Rowland, 1817: 66.
15. Blin O, Ferrandes AM, Serratrice G. Quantitative analysis of gait in par-

kinson patients: increased variability of stride length. J Neurol Sci 1990; 98: 91.

16. Buchthal F, Fernandez-Ballesteros ML. Electromyographic study of the muscles of the upper arm and shoulder during walking in patients with Parkinson's Disease. Brain 1965; 88: 875.

17. Forssberg H, Johnels B, Steg G. Is parkinsonian gait caused by a regression to an immature walking pattern. Adv Neurol 1984; 40: 375.

18. Koozekanani SH, Balmaseda MT, Fatehi MT, Lowney ED. Ground reaction forces during ambulation in parkinsonism: pilot study. Arch Phys Med Rehab 1987; 68: 28.

19. Dietz V, Berger W, Horstmann GA. Posture in Parkinson's Disease: impairment of reflexes and programming. Ann Neurol 1988; 24: 661.

20. Traub MM, Rothwell JC, Marsden CD. Anticipatory postural reflexes in Parkinson's disease and other akinetic-rigid syndromes and in cerebellar ataxia. Brain 1980; 103: 393.

21. Dunne JW, Hankey GJ, Edis RH. Parkinsonism: upturned walking stick as an aid to locomotion. Arch Phys Med Rehab 1987; 68: 380.

22. Klawans HL. Individual manifestations of Parkinson's disease after ten or more years of levodopa. Mov Disord 1986; 1: 187.

23. Golbe LI, Davis PH, Schoenberg BS, Duvoisin RC. Prevalence and natural history of progressive supranuclear palsy. Neurology 1988; 38: 1031.

24. Jankovic J, Friedman DI, Pirozzolo FJ, McCrary JA. Progressive supranuclear palsy: motor, neurobehavioral and neuro-ophthalmic finding, Adv Neurol 1990; 43: 293.

25. Perkin GD, Lees AJ, Stern GM, Kocen RS. Problems in the diagnosis of progressive supranuclear palsy (Steele-Richardson-Olszewski syndrome). Can J Neurol Sci 1978; 5: 167.

26. Maher ER, Lees AJ. The clinical features and natural history of the Steele-Richardson-Olszewski syndrome (progressive supranuclear palsy). Neurology 1986; 36: 1005.

27. Golbe LI, Sage JI, Duvoisin RC. Drug treatment of 83 patients with progressive supranuclear palsy. Neurology 1990; 40(Suppl 1): 438.

28. Shy GM, Drager GA. A neurological syndrome associated with orthostatic hypotension. Arch Neurol 1960; 2: 511.

29. Konigsmark BW, Weiner LP. The olivopontocerebellar atrophies: A review. Medicine 1979; 49: 227.

30. Koeppen AH, Hans MB. Supranuclear ophthalmoplegia in olivopontocerebellar degeneration. Neurology 1976; 26: 764.

31. Fitzgerald PM, Jankovic J. Lower body parkinsonism: evidence for vascular etiology. Mov Disord 1989; 4: 249.

32. Weiner WJ, Lange AE. Huntington's Disease, In: Weiner WJ, Lang AE, eds. Movement Disorders. A comprehensive survey. New York: Futura 1989; 293.

33. Group THDCR. A novel gene containing a trinucleotide repeat that is expanded and unstable on Huntington's Disease chromosomes. Cell 1993; 72: 971.

34. Bateman D, Boughey AM, Scaravilli F, Marsden CD, Harding AE. A follow-up study of isolated cases of suspected Huntington's disease. Ann Neurol 1991; 31: 293.

35. Martin JB, Gusella JF. Huntington's disease: Pathogenesis and management. N Engl J Med 1986; 315: 1267.

36. van Dijk JG, van der Velde EA, Roos RAC, Bruyn GW. Juvenile Huntington disease. Hum. Gen. 1986; 73: 235.

37. Hefter H, Homberg V, Lange HW, Freund H-J. Impairment of rapid movement in Huntington's disease. Brain, 1987; 110: 585.

38. Thompson PD, Berardelli A, Rothwell JC, Day BL, Dick JPR, Benecke R, Marsden CD. The coexistence of bradykinesia and chorea in Huntington's disease and its implications for theories of basal ganglia control of movement. Brain 1988; 111: 223.

39. Heathfield KWG. Huntington's chorea. Brain 1967; 90:203.

40. Lanska DJ, Lanska MF, Lavine L, Schoenberg BS. Conditions associated with Huntington's disease at death: a case-control study. Arch Neurol 1988; 45: 878.

41. Koller WC, Trimble J. The gait abnormality of Huntington's disease. Neurology 1985; 35: 1450.

42. Shoulson I. Huntington's disease: Functional capacities in patients treated with neuroleptic and antidepressant drugs. Neurology 1981; 31: 1333.

43. Jeste DV, Wyatt RJ. Changing epidemiology of tardive dyskinesia: an overview. Am J Psychol 1981; 138: 297.

44. Chouinard G, Annable L. Factors related to tardive dyskinesia. Am J Psych 1979; 136: 79.

45. Smith JM, Kucharski LT, Eblen C. An assessment of tardive dyskinesia in schizophrenic outpatients. Psychopharmacology 1979; 64: 99.

46. Kane JM, Smith JM. Tardive dyskinesia: prevalence and risk factors, 1959–1979. Arch Gen. Psychol 1982; 30: 473.

47. Tarsy D, Baldessarini RJ. The Tardive Dyskinesia syndrome. In: Klawans, HL, ed. Clinical Neuropharmacology, volume 1. New York: Raven Press, 1976: 29.

48. Degkwitz R. Extrapyramidal motor disorders following long term treatment with neuroleptic drugs. In: Crane GE, Naranjo ER, eds. Psychotropic Drugs and Dysfunction of the Basal Ganglia. Public Health Service Publication No. 1938, Washington D.C., 1969; 22.

49. Klawans HL, Moses H, Nausieda PA, Bergen D, Weiner WJ. Treatment and prognosis of hemiballismus. N Engl J Med 1976; 295: 1348.

50. Whittier JR. Ballism and the subthalamic nucleus (nucleus hypothalamicus: corpus Luysi). Arch Neurol Psychol 1947; 58: 672.

51. Moersch FP, Kernohan JW. Hemiballismus—a clinicopathologic study. Arch Neurol Psychol 1939; 41: 365.
52. Dewey RB, Jankovic J. Hemiballism-hemichorea: clinical and pharmacologic findings in 21 patients. Arch Neurol 1989; 46: 862.
53. Fahn S. Concept and classification of dystonia. Adv Neurol 1988; 50: 1.
54. Marsden CD, Harrison MJG. Idiopathic torsion dystonia (dystonia musculorum deformans). A review of forty-two patients. Brain 1974; 97: 793.
55. Waddy HM, Fletcher NA, Harding AE, Marsden CD. A genetic study of idiopathic focal dystonias. Ann Neurol 1991; 29: 320.
56. Risch NJ, Bressman SB, deLeon D. Segregation analysis of idiopathic torsion dystonia in Ashkenazi Jews suggests autosomal dominant inheritance. Am J Hum Gen 1990; 46: 533.
57. Ozelius L, Kramer PL, Moskowitz CB. Human gene for torsion dystonia located on chromosome 9q32–34. Neuron 1989; 2: 1427.
58. Greene P, Shale H, Fahn S. Analysis of open-label trials in torsion dystonia using high dosages of anticholinergics and other drugs. Mov Disord 1988; 3: 1.
59. Brin MF, Fahn S, Moskowitz C, Friedman A, Shale HM, Greene PE, Blitzer A, List T, Lange D, Lovelace RE, McMahon D. Localized injections of Botulinum Toxin for the treatment of focal dystonia and hemifacial spasm. Adv Neurol 1988; 50: 599.
60. Nygaard TG, Marsden CD, Fahn S. Dopa-responsive dystonia: long-term treatment response and prognosis. Neurology 1991; 41: 174.
61. Nygaard TG, Trugman JM, de Yebenes JB, Fahn S. Dopa-responsive dystonia: the spectrum of clinical manifestations in a large North American family. Neurology 1990; 40: 66.
62. Scheinberg IH, Sternlieb I. Wilson's Disease. Philadelphia: Saunders, 1984: 171.
63. Barbeau A, Friesen H. Treatment of Wilson's disease with l-dopa after failure with penicillamine. Lancet 1970; 1: 1180.
64. Burke RE, Fahn S, Jankovic J, Marsden CD, Lang AE, Gollomp S, Ilson J. Tardive dystonia: late-onset and persistent dystonia caused by antipsychotic drugs. Neurology 1982; 32: 1335.
65. Hallett M. Classification and treatment of tremor. JAMA 1991; 266: 1115.
66. Koller WC. Diagnosis and treatment of tremors. Neurol. Clin. 1984; 2: 499.
67. Hubble JP, Busenbark KL, Koller WC. Essential Tremor. Clin Neuropharm 1989; 12: 453.
68. Larsson T, Sjogren T. Essential tremor. A clinical and genetic population study. Acta Psychol Neurol. Scand. 1960; 36(Suppl 144): 1.
69. Massey EW, Paulson GW. Essential vocal tremor: clinical characteristics and response to therapy. South Med J 1985; 78: 316.
70. Hornabrook RW, Nagurney JT. Essential tremor in Papua New Guinea. Grain 1976; 99: 659.

71. Heilman KM. Orthostatic tremor. Arch Neurol 1984; 41: 880.
72. Wee AS, Subramony SH, Currier RD. "Orthostatic tremor" in familial-essential tremor. Neurology 1986; 36: 1241.
73. Thompson PD, Rothwell JC, Day BL, Berardelli A, Dick JPR. The physiology of orthostatic tremor. Arch Neurol 1986; 43: 584.
74. Fitzgerald PM, Jankovic J. Orthostatic tremor: an association with essential tremor. Mov Disord 1991; 6: 60.
75. Cleeves L, Cowan J, Findley LJ. Orthostatic tremor: diagnostic entity of variant of essential tremor. J Neurol Neurosurg Psychol 1989; 52: 130.

7

Gait Apraxia

SANDER L. GLATT and WILLIAM C. KOLLER
University of Kansas Medical Center, Kansas City, Kansas

I. INTRODUCTION

Aging presents a challenge to maintain an independent lifestyle in the face of progressive disease-related physical impairment. A major determinant of the quality of life in the elderly is their ability to walk. Performance of the many activities required for daily living requires safe ambulation. However, disorders of gait are second only to dementia as the most frequent concomitants of the diseases associated with the aging process (1). In this chapter we will discuss two poorly understood clinical syndromes associated with disordered ambulation—gait apraxia and senile gait. Gait apraxia is a controversial term used to describe an ill-defined clinical syndrome associated with a variety of pathological causes related to frontal lobe injury. Senile gait is an equally controversial term for a gait disorder with a heterogeneous clinical presentation but without associated neurological deficits or known anatomic locus.

Both terms developed through a series of clinical observations made by distinguished neurologists over the past century. We will discuss this history as well as recent efforts to redefine the clinical nosology of gait disorders. Further advances require a clear clinical characterization to direct needed correlative studies in cerebral physiology and pathology.

II. GAIT MECHANISMS

Mobility is achieved through a neurological servomechanism that insures mechanical stability in all postures and positions required by one's daily activity. Mechanically, in the upright posture, this is complicated by the small base of support, between one's feet, compared to one's height. There are a number of requirements for normal locomotion, including (1) antigravity support in the upright posture; (2) balance control; and (3) forward stepping movements (2).

In the upright posture the center of gravity is located just anterior and superior to the second sacral vertebra (3). The musculoskeletal system provides antigravity support by fixing the major joints, minimizing the motor activity required to maintain the upright posture. Mechanical stability is maintained as long as the line of gravity passes within the base of support between the feet. Postural stability requires that these movements must be perceived and the gravitational forces on the body part calculated in order to perform compensatory maneuvers to return the center of gravity back over one's feet (4). Walking depends on a series of reciprocal flexion extension movements of the legs, alternating between support in extension and advancement in flexion (5). Gait has been classically studied in terms of the "walking cycle," which is the time interval between successive floor contacts of each foot. It is further divided into stance and swing phases. The stance phase occurs when the foot is in contact with the floor; the swing phase occurs when the foot is advancing to take the next position. During each walking cycle there are two periods of single limb support and two brief periods of double limb support while the legs alternate between postures (5).

The impetus to forward locomotion is achieved by pushing off on the leg in the stance phase while swinging the other leg forward. This is associated with fixation and elevation of the pelvis by the hip abductors as well as tilting the body toward the supporting limb, allowing the swinging leg to fall in a line directly anterior to the stance leg. The movement of the pelvis allows for maintenance of mechanical stability by integration of the line of gravity such that it falls through the foot of the stance leg. The "swing" leg is flexed and slightly externally rotated at the hip, flexed at the knee, and dorsiflexed at the foot. After the heel of the swing leg strikes the floor, the hip and knee extend. This phase ends as external rotation and dorsiflexion of the stance leg shifts the center of gravity forward (5). Rotatory movements of the upper body arms and shoulders are used to counterbalance the movements of the pelvis and lower extremity in order to maintain lateral stability despite alterations in the legs providing support. Movement is generated by a combination of muscular and gravitational forces. The rear stance leg pushes the body forward off its base of support where forward body momentum aided by gravity propels the body. The swing leg then hurries forward to catch the body as the forward stance leg. A mundane activity such as walking is performed safely only because of exquisitely fine control exerted by a very complicated neurological servomechanism with highly sensitive input, complex central integration, and finely graded motor effort.

Locomotor programs to direct this activity originate in central pattern generators located in the spinal cord. These areas are under the control of locomotor centers located in the brain stem regions, which in turn are responsive to cerebellar, basal ganglionic, and cortical control. Postural adjustments are directed by a variety of neurological reflexes and long loop responses (6). These are combined in a complicated scenario to produce the desired output in a preprogrammed manner depending on previous experience with the environment. These programs are readily modifiable by somatosthetic, visual, and vestibular input. This process requires accurate sensory information and considerable central processing in order to regulate, through finely graded output of both axial and appendicular musculature, the automatic programs of the spinal cord and brainstem. Malfunction in any of these areas can be reflected in abnormalities in gait and posture. We suggest that subtle disease-related neurological deficits in the elderly may be reflected as a disordered gait when clinical deficits are not evident on neurological examination.

III. GAIT APRAXIA

Macdonald Critchley was the first to call attention to the "senile disorders of gait or dysbasia of old age" (7, 8). He described a gait abnormality in the elderly with anteroflexion, short shuffling steps with legs crossing, veering from side to side, and impaired balance while examination for strength, tone, or sensation was unremarkable. Critchley (7) recognized that such gait difficulties are observed in patients with anterior cerebral artery occlusions causing frontal lobe infarction as well as diffuse small vessel disease or lacunar strokes as described by Lhermitte. He noted such patients may resemble the gait disorder seen in Parkinson's disease (9) but that the character was suggestive of an apraxia. Apraxia is defined as an inability to perform a voluntary purposeful movement with normal strength, sensation, or coordination and is generally used to refer to skilled movements of the upper extremities. Critchley (8) noted that while gait apraxia is not associated with limb dyspraxia, it is frequently associated with a truncal apraxia with difficulty changing postures or arising out of bed.

Others reported patients with similar difficulties and identified this as dyspraxia. Kremer described two patients with truncal apraxia due to widespread cerebral trauma and ascribed it to a deficit in body image (10). Pertrovici (11) described five patients with a variety of frontal lobe lesions with evidence of disordered motor activation patterns that he suggested were related to gait and truncal apraxia. Denny-Brown (12) provided the philosophical support for the concept of gait apraxia. Following Liepmann (13), who described the clinical apraxic syndromes, Denny-Brown (12) suggested that in addition to ideational apraxia, which was associated with loss of "the ideational sketch" or conceptual plan for the motor activity, and ideomotor apraxia, which involves deficits in the specifics of skill performance, there was a limb kinetic apraxia which Liepmann had suggested involved the motor cortex engrams. Denny-Brown identified the motor difficulties associated with frontal lobe lesions as being due to a kinetic apraxia with perseveration of motor activity (12). This is reflected by the grasp reflex of the hand as well as the foot grasp that is elicited when the affected foot contacts the floor. The lower limb stiffens and becomes glued to the floor; steps are small, made with difficulty, and may resemble a shuffle (12). When these disorders are bilateral, coordinated movements such as walking may be severely impaired. This has been described as the "slipping clutch" with a rapid shuffling of feet before a step may be made. This inability to inhibit the grasping response of the feet is the cause of a "magnetic apraxia" (12). Frontal lobe apraxic gait is associated with poor postural reflexes, gegenhalten or paratonic rigidity, and prominent frontal release signs (14). Particularly noted is difficulty on initiation of gait. Meyer and Barron (15) subsequently described seven patients with gait apraxia all of whom had frontal lesions. They argued that a gait disorder due to a cerebral lesion without weakness or sensory loss fulfills the definition of dyspraxia.

Behavioral neurology, which developed the modern concept of apraxia, has not agreed. Apraxia is defined as an inability to perform a voluntary purposeful movement with normal strength, sensation, or co-ordination (12). Heilman and Rothi (16) suggested limiting that definition to exclude disorders of tone, cognition, movement, or uncooperativeness. They end their introduction to a chapter describing clinical apraxic syndromes with the comment "gait apraxia is not discussed" (16). Geschwind (17), arguing against the concept of gait apraxia, noted that postural movements involving gait and balance control are performed automatically without reaching conscious awareness and are therefore not voluntary or cortical but controlled by subcortical mechanisms. He also noted that even patients with severe cortical apraxic disorders rarely have praxic difficulties with gait and balance (18).

However, the motor syndrome that accompanies frontal lobe disease does occur in the context of normal strength and sensory function. Luria describes this as the "deautomatization" of complex motor tasks and the revival of elementary automatisms with an interruption of "kinetic melodies" (19). This interruption is manifested by difficulty moving from one aspect of a complex motor task to another. Geschwind (17) argued that this deficit is due to abnormal reflex activation. Miller (20) countered that gait apraxia involves errors in force, range, direction, and speed of a learned voluntary movement indicative of an ideomotor apraxia, complicated by reflex disruption.

The term gait apraxia is deeply ingrained in clinical neurology and has been used to describe the gait disorder observed in a number of other neurological diseases. Communicating "normal pressure" hydro-cephalus presents in the elderly with a distinctive triad of a gait disturbance, dementia, and incontinence (21). The gait disorder includes elements of a gait apraxia with a magnetic short-stepped gait, poor balance control, and difficulty with turning (22). Corticospinal abnormalities with extensor–plantar responses, frontal release signs, difficulty with fine motor control in the upper extremity, and turning in bed have been reported. Recent analysis of the gait of such patients revealed there is decreased velocity and stride length with increased sway and double limb support time (23). There is a marked reduction in step height, decreased associated shoulder movements, and continuous activity in limb antigravity musculature with cocontracture instead of the normal phasic activities seen in the gait cycle (23). Paradoxically, leg movements while lying down are performed with normal agility (24). Even gait movements may be imitated. It has been suggested that similar to motor perseveration of the upper extremity due to frontal lobe lesions, stimulation of the dorsum of the foot leads to a stiffening reaction of the lower extremity. Perseveration of this reflex impairs automatic gait programs (12). The remarkable similarity to patients with frontal lobe lesions has been noted and it has been suggested that because the leg fibers lie in the medial portion of the frontal hemispheres, they are most susceptible to compression by the englarging frontal horns (21).

Similar deficits with gait apraxia have been described in Binswanger disease, presumably due to subcortical disconnection (25) and multiple subfrontal lacunar infarctions (26).

IV. SENILE GAIT

This concept derives from Critchley's (8) notion that the elderly had disturbances in ambulation without associated abnormalities on neurological examination. He described the gradual appearance of a broad-based gait with small steps associated with a diminished arm swing, a stoop posture, flexion of the hips and knees, uncertainty and stiffness in turning, occasional difficulty getting started, and a tendency toward falling. However, the clinical picture of senile gait is quite variable. Gait characteristics along with other aspects of the neurological examination in the elderly remain controversial. Some patients with senile gait present with an anteroflexed small step gait suggestive of parkinsonism, other with an entirely different appearance. The general neurological examination does not reveal neurological abnormalities of major neuroanatomic systems to adequately explain the disturbance in walking.

Koller and associates (27) described 16 patients over 60 years of age with a gait abnormality not otherwise explained by neurological evaluation and compared them to 59 subjects with normal gait. Patients with neurological diagnoses other than dementia or serious medical conditions were excluded. All subjects underwent CT scanning that was scored for infratentorial and supratentorial atrophy. Gait abnormalities in the 16 patients included: inability to tandem walk (16 patients); wide-based gait (14); poor truncal stability (12); gait dysrhythmia (11); flexed attitude (10); shortened steps (10); bradykinesia (8); loss of associated movements (5); diminished ability to advance steps (4); gait apraxia (2); and a narrowed base (1). There was no difference between groups on

CT measures of infratentorial atrophy, but small differences in third and lateral ventricular size were noted. There is likely to be overlap between clinical descriptions of senile gait and gait apraxia. However, while a small number of patients may have had elements of the magnetic apraxic gait described in Section III, none had the associated neurological deficits described by Meyer and Barron (15).

Similar patients appear to be described under other terms including idiopathic gait disorder of the elderly (28), lower body parkinsonism (29), idiopathic fallers (30), and essential gait disorder (31). Attempts to use quantitative gait analysis to characterize the gait disorder have proved disappointing. Elble and coworkers (32) used infrared computed strobo-scopic photometry to characterize gait parameters of 10 patients with senile gait as compared to 19 controls. All 10 had similar gait parameters with diminished velocity stride length, increased double support time, diminished upper and lower limb movements, decreased foot–floor clear-ance, and abnormal heel–toe–floor contact sequence. However, all these changes in parameters of gait were secondary to the slowed gait and change in stride length. This is of note because there was no difference between patients who were ultimately assigned to different diagnostic categories, including multiple infarcts and hydrocephalus. Their findings suggest that gait disturbances in the elderly appear similar because gait characteristics are heavily dependent on the change in stride length associ-ated with the cautious senile gait syndrome. On reflection, one could postulate that considering the complexity of the inputs on spinal and brainstem centers that control ambulation, there is only a limited degree to which pathological lesions can be expressed and allow for continued ambulation. While such data are similar to previous reports of age-related differences of velocity and stride length in normal populations (33), we believe that the clinical expression of a gait or balance disorder is disease related and not associated with normal aging (30).

There is little agreement or definite knowledge regarding the basic underlying cause and anatomical basis of the senile gait. Critchley sug-gested that the gait of the elderly was a manifestation of extrapyramidal dysfunction (8). Barbeau (34) suggested that disordered movements seen in senescence result from a defective striatal dopaminergic mecha-nism. Disease of the mesial frontal lobes produces a gait apraxia. Alter-natively, it has been suggested that senile gait is attributed to cerebellar disease. In recent studies of CT scans in the elderly, it was found that the cerebellar vermis selectively atrophies with age (35). Adams and Victor (36) hypothesized that the peculiar gait of the aged is due to a combined frontal lobe–basal ganglionic degeneration. Fischer (22) has offered a controversial hypothesis regarding the pathophysiology of senile gait. He suggested that the unexplained unsteady gait in late life was caused by hydrocephalus and that gait instability could be reversed by cerebrospinal fluid shunting procedures. In his study 50 patients with senile gait were found to have an increase in the size of the lateral ventricle as compared to controls. He speculated that disordered gait may be the only manifestation of normal pressure hydrocephalus. It is evident that not all patients with the syndrome respond to shunting. We believe that many such patients may have ventriculomegaly secondary to diffuse neurodegenerative and cerebrovascular lesions (37).

V. NOSOLOGY

Nutt and coworkers (38) have recently described a new schema for classifying frontal gait disorders—separating them from lower level disorders related to peripheral motor or sensory loss and middle-level disorders involving the corticospinal tract, cerebellum, or basal ganglia. They include the highest-level gait disorders: (1) cautious gait with a slowed, mildly wide-based gait; (2) subcortical disequilibrium with the gait disorder secondary to the balance disorder; (3) frontal disequilibrium with marked deficits in postural and locomotive synergies; (4) isolated gait initiation failure with start hesitation, shuffling gait, and freezing; and (5) frontal gait disorder with small shuffling steps, start hesitation, and loss of balance commonly related to multiple infarcts. There is much interest in the classification scheme of Nutt and coworkers because it is based on careful analysis of the clinical presentations of the frontal disorders of gait and allows relatively clear clinical classification. However, it is not easy for the clinician to use. The success of nosologic classification is measured by the manner with which it aids the development of testable hypotheses to further understand function and direct therapy. If the new schema provides for clearer studies of correlative physiology and pathology, then this classification would have made a contribution.

In summary, it can be said that the nosology of disordered gait remains controversial. Clearly, there are significant difficulties with both the terms, gait apraxia and senile gait. They describe clinically heterogeneous syndromes that overlap in their extremes. Behavioral neurology is not able to relate axial apraxia to their schema of apraxic cortical deficits. However, gait apraxia has a long history and has been associated ith the leading European neurologists of their day. Its widespread penetration in the neurological literature suggests that this debate will continue.

REFERENCES

1. Drachman D. An approach to the neurology of aging. In: Birren J, Sloan R, eds., Handbook of Mental Health and Aging, Englewood Cliffs: Prentice-Hall, 1980: 501.
2. Martin JP. The Basal Ganglia and Posture. Philadelphia: J. B. Lippincott, 1967.
3. Horenstein S. Managing gait disorders. Geriatrics 1974; 29: 86.
4. Martin JP. A short essay on posture and motion. J Neurol Neurosurg Psychiatry 1977; 40: 25.
5. Murray MP. Gait as a total pattern of movement. Am J Phys Med 1967; 46: 290.
6. Brooks VB. The Neural Basis of Motor Control. New York: Oxford, 1986.
7. Critchley M. The neurology of old age. Lancet 1931; 1:1221–1230.
8. Critchley M. On senile disorders of gait, including the so-called "senile paraplegia" Geriatrics 1948; 3: 364–370.
9. Critchley M. Arteriosclerotic parkinsonism. Brain 1929; 52: 23–82.
10. Kremer M. Sitting, standing, and walking. Br Med J 1958; 2: 63–68.
11. Pertrovici K. Apraxia of gait and of trunk movements. J Neurol Sci 1968; 7: 229–243.
12. Denny-Brown D. The nature of apraxia. J Nerv Ment Dis 1955; 216: 9.
13. Liepmann H. Apraxie. Ergebn ges Med 1920; 1: 516–543.
14. Meyer JS. Apraxia of gait: A clinico-pathological study. Brain 1960; 83: 261.
15. Meyer JS, Barron DW. Apraxia of gait: A clinicophysiological study. Brain 1960; 83: 261–284.
16. Heilman K, Rothi L. Apraxia. In: Heilman K, Valenstein E, eds., Clinical Neuropsychology, 2d ed. Oxford: Oxford University Press, 1985.
17. Gerschwind N. Disconnexion syndromes in animals and man. Brain 1965; 88:237–294.
18. Gerschwind N. The apraxias: Neural mechanisms of disorders of learned movement. Am Sci 1975; 63: 188–195.
19. Luria AR. Frontal lobe syndromes. In: Vinken PJ, Bruyn GW, eds., Handbook of Clinical Neurology, vol. 2, Localization in Clinical Neurology. Amsterdam: North-Holland, 1969: 725.
20. Miller N. Dyspraxia and Its Management. Rockville, MD: Aspen Publishers, Inc., 1986.
21. Adams RD, et al. Symptomatic occult hydroencephalus with "normal" cerebrospinal fluid pressure (a treatable syndrome). N Engl J Med 1965; 273: 117.

22. Fisher CM. Hydrocephalus as a cause of disturbance of gait in the elderly. Neurology 1982; 32: 1358.
23. Sudarsky L, Simon S. Gait disorder in late-life hydrocephalus. Arch Neurol 1987; 44: 263.
24. Estanol BV. Gait apraxia in communicating hydrocephalus. J Neurol Neurosurg Psychiatry 1981; 44: 305–308.
25. Thompson PD, Marsden CD. Gait disorder of subcortical arteriosclerotic encephalopathy: Binswanger's disease. Mov Disord 1987; 2: 1–8.
26. Kotsoris H, Barclay LL, Kheyfets S, Hulyalkar A, Dougherty J. Urinary and gait disturbances as markers for early multi-infarct dementia. Stroke 1987; 18: 138–141.
27. Koller WC, Glatt SL, Fox JH. Senile gait: a distinct neurologic entity. Clin Geriatr Med 1985; 1: 661–669.
28. Wall JC, Hogan DB, Turnbull GI, Fox RA. The kinematics of idiopathic gait disorder. Scand J Rehab Med 1991; 23: 159–164.
29. Fitzgerald PM, Jankovic J. Lower body parkinsonism: evidence for vascular etiology. Mov Disord 1989; 4: 249–260.
30. Wolfson L, Whipple R, Derby CA, et al. A dynamic posturography study of balance in healthy elderly. Neurology 1992; 42: 2069–2075.
31. Sudarsky L, and Ronthal M. Gait disorders among elderly patients. A survey study of 50 patients. Arch Neurol 1983; 40: 740–743.
32. Elble RJ, Hughes L, Higgins C. The syndrome of senile gait. J Neurol 1992; 239: 71–75.
33. Elble RJ, Sienko SS, Higgins C, Colliver J. Stride-dependent changes in gait of older people. J Neurol 1991; 238: 1–5.
34. Barbeau A. Aging and the extrapyramidal system. J Am Geriatr Soc 1973; 21: 145–149.
35. Koller WC, Glatt S, Wilson R, et al. Cerebellar atrophy: relationship to aging and cerebral atrophy. Neurology 1981; 23: 405.
36. Adams RD, Victor M. Principles of Neurology, 4th ed. New York: McGraw-Hill, 1989.
37. Masdeu JC, Wolfson L, Lantos G, et al. Brain white-matter changes in the elderly prone to falling. Arch Neurol 1989; 46: 1292.
38. Nutt JG, Marsden CD, Thompson PD. Human walking and higher-level gait disorders, particularly in the elderly. Neurology 1993; 43: 268–279.

8

Characteristic Patterns of Gait in Older Persons

MING-HSIA HU

National Taiwan University, Taipei, Taiwan, Republic of China

MARJORIE WOOLLACOTT

University of Oregon, Eugene, Oregon

I. INTRODUCTION

The ability to maintain normal mobility and gait function with advancing age is important for the independence and health of older people. Many physiological functions, such as visual and vibratory sensations, cardiovascular capacities, and muscle strength deteriorate with age (1–4). It has been suggested that motor functions, including balance and gait, also deteriorate with age (5,6). However, recent evidence using stringent subject selection criteria for participation in aging research have failed to find significant age effects on gait function, suggesting that pathology, rather than age, contributes to the loss of mobility in older people (7).

The question of whether age or pathology affects gait in older adults is complicated by the fact that the prevalence of pathology increases with age. Older people have sustained more minor trauma throughout their lives than younger people, and the effect of the accumulated trauma might not be exhibited as clinically diagnosed pathologies. Therefore, it is important in aging research to differentiate pure age-related changes in the system studied versus changes related to pathology. Two models for decline in nervous system function illustrate the assumptions underlying most aging research (see Fig. 1). The first model assumes that neuron function deteriorates at a steady rate with age. Thus, after a certain age, a disease such as Parkinson's disease will evolve unavoidably. The second model, on the contrary, assumes that neuron function does not decline with normal aging. Different catastrophes and diseases affect people over certain ages and cause a decline in neuron function and therefore a disease state.

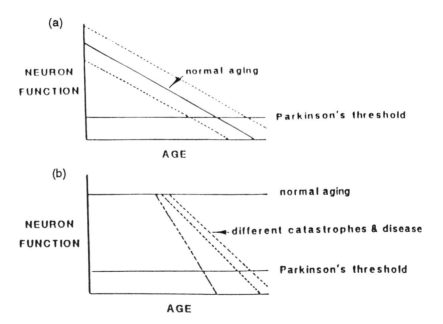

Figure 1   Two possible models to explain a decline in nervous system function with age. (a) A linear decline, with continued neuron loss across the life span. (b) Continued high-level function unless pathology causes a rapid decline in a particular brain area (Ref. 7a).

When discussing age-related changes in gait, older clinical studies have considered gait disorders, such as gait apraxia, hypokinetic-hypertonic syndrome, and marche a petit pas as changes that occur with normal aging, and disorders such as these were often called "senile gait" (8–10). However, a survey study of 50 patients with previously undiagnosed gait disorders found that a causal diagnosis could be made in approximately 84% of the patients (11). Those causes most frequently observed were myelopathy, Parkinsonism, frontal gait disorder (normal-pressure hydrocephalus, multiple strokes), cerebellar degeneration, and sensory imbalance. (Chapter 6 reviews this study in greater detail.) Thus gait disorders may not be purely an age-related phenomenon. In fact, studies with healthy older adults often failed to demonstrate significant age-related changes in gait patterns.

In addition, studies distinguishing fallers and nonfallers have demonstrated some interesting differences between these categories of older adults. Thus an increased prevalence of falling or gait disorders observed in older people may be the result of subclinical or undiagnosed pathologies rather than age alone.

The main purpose of this chapter is to review the literature on changes in the characteristics of gait in normal older adults. Age-related changes in different neural and musculoskeletal systems contributing to normal gait control, including cognitive function (fear of falling), sensory function, motor function, balance control, and muscle strength, will be reviewed. Gait control will be viewed as a mobility task requiring the integrity of the above components. The effect of age versus pathology on gait will be discussed.

II. GAIT CHARACTERISTICS IN OLDER ADULTS

The characteristics of gait patterns can be reported in many ways. Before modern techniques for gait analysis were available, researchers visually observed gait patterns or used a very simple stop watch to measure walking speed. From these observations, it has been consistently reported that there is a decrease in walking speed with age. Stride length can be calculated by counting the total number of strides over a fixed walking distance. However, stride length calculated by this method assumes bilateral symmetry and stride-to-stride consistency, which may not always be the case in subjects with gait problems. Therefore, more detailed measurements are used in the laboratory to obtain information regarding stride length, step length, step width, and joint angle excursions in young and older adults. To these kinematic measures of gait has been added the analysis of joint mechanical power generated and absorbed during walking (12), as additional parameters to examine when studying age-related decline in gait control.

The following section is divided into three parts: First, walking speed in older people will be discussed. Second, kinematic analysis of gait, including foot-fall patterns and joint rotation excursions, will be reviewed. Third, mechanical power analysis of gait patterns will be reported.

A. Studies on Walking Speed

Cross-sectional studies have repeatedly demonstrated that walking speed decreases with age. Speilberg (6), one of the first investigators to observe age-related changes in gait patterns, described the earliest stage of gait pattern change (between 60–72 years of age) as consisting of a slower walking velocity and decreased displacement amplitudes of the joints and stride. Drillis (13) observed 752 pedestrians walking on the sidewalks of New York City. Subjects were interviewed after cadence and velocity were determined using a marked distance on the sidewalk for their age, height, and weight. Drillis found that, as age increased, there was a decrease in walking velocity, step length, and step rate. These changes were similar to the first stage of change in gait in Spielberg's report.

An approach like that of Drillis allows observation of gait in a natural environment without interference by laboratory instrumentation. However, the health status of subjects, age range, and goal for walking cannot be controlled in this setting. Thus the effect of pathology cannot be isolated from the effect of age. Furthermore, whether slower walking speed was due to a decrease in stride length or a decrease in cadence was unknown. Laboratory studies are necessary to study the effect of age on walking speed, cadence, and stride length. For example, a reduction in walking speed and stride length (heel strike to the heel strike of the same foot), and an increase in stride width (between successive strides of two feet) have been reported by Murray et al. (14,15) in both older men and older women.

Gabell and Nayak (7) were interested in the relationship between age and the variability of gait. In order to isolate an age effect from a pathology effect, their older subjects were selected from 1184 older adults over 64 years of age. Older adults with any disorder likely to affect gait or balance, including all musculoskeletal, neurological, or cardiovascular disorders; severe bilateral visual impairment, or glaucoma; a history of falls or dizzy spells during the past year; and the use of a walking aid; or women habitually wearing high heels (exceeding 4 cm) were excluded from their study. Thirty-two older adults were selected to participate in the gait study after the screening process. Four gait parameters (stride time, double-support time, step length, and stride width) of older adults (66–84 years old) were compared with 32 young subjects (21–47 years of age) by using an electronically equipped walkway. It was found that step length (heel strike of one foot to heel strike of the contralateral foot) of the older adult (median = 64.34 cm, range 50.69–80.06) was shorter than that of the young adult (median = 75.55 cm, range 64.98–90.98). But the coefficient of variation (median/range) of the step length was similar between the two age groups. That is, older adults were not more variable in their step length than younger adults. However, a wider range of coefficients of variation was found in the older group than the younger group in the stride time measurement. There was no difference between age groups in the stride width or double-support time measurements. The authors suggested that step length and stride time are indications of the gait patterning function and stride width and double-support time are the indexes for balance function. Thus this study did show some age-related changes in gait patterning function (shortened step length, increased range of variability of stride time). However, the statistical analysis of coefficient of variation values did not show any differences to be significant. This paper concluded that the variability of gait patterns of *healthy* adults does not increase with age. However, the results showed that the median and range values of step length decrease with age even in healthy subjects.

B. Kinematic Analysis: Joint Angles

Footfall patterns, i.e., the walking speed, cadence, stride length, and step length, are sensitive to the effects of age. However, they do not give us insight into the possible causes of falls or trips during walking, nor can we pinpoint the body segment(s) causing the reduced stride length with age. Camera-based analysis of gait enables us to investigate the foot–floor clearance and ranges of motion during gait. Patients may have similar footfall patterns but very different joint angle change patterns during each stride. It is thus important to review studies providing joint angle information during gait to provide normative data for comparison to patients.

Murray and associates (14,15) were one of the first research groups to systematically study gait patterns of healthy older people with a camera-based analysis tool. Subjects were photographed using interrupted-light photography at 20 Hz while walking at their preferred and fast speeds. Twenty kinematic measures were made from the resulting photographs. Subjects were grouped by age (range: 20–87 for men; 20–70 for women). The results showed that walking speed, stride length, swing-to-stance duration ratio, and hip rotation amplitude decrease after 65 years of age. Cycle duration and stance duration increased after 65 years of age. Stride width increased after 74 years of age. Out-toeing and gait variability (rhythmicity of repeated strides) increased after 80 years of age. Peak heel-rise decreased after 80 years of age. They also observed small changes in toe–floor clearance patterns (increases during initial sway, decreases at end of sway), decreased knee flexion amplitude, and decreased ankle extension amplitude at push-off with age. Gait patterns showed similar changes in women, except women showed decreased stride length after age 50, and with overall smaller excursions, slower walking speed, and faster cadence. They also found a profound influence of heel height on the gait pattern in women.

At first glance, the results of Murray et al.'s studies (14, 15) appear different from the study of Gabell and Nayak (7). Murray et al. found age effects to be evident in most of the variables they investigated, including gait variability. Gabell and Nayak concluded that there was no significant age-related increase in gait variability. Since screening procedures were used in all of these studies, we can assume that pathological effects do not confound with the age effect. It is noteworthy that in Murray et al.'s studies subjects had to walk under dark conditions in order to use the interrupted-light photography (light flashes at 20 Hz). However, in Gabell and Nayak's study, subjects walked under normal lighting conditions. It has been shown that decreased sensory function, especially within the visual system, affects the balance of older subjects more than younger subjects (5, 16). Thus it is possible that the gait patterns of the older subjects in Murray et al.'s studies were affected by the lack of a normal visual environment. A second reason for the different findings between Murray et al. and Gabell and Nayak is that although the latter study concluded that there was no statistically significant age effect on variability of the gait pattern, their data showed an increased range of coefficient of variations in the older group on all four gait variables measured (Fig. 2). In addition, if one examines data from the tables presented in Gabell and Nayak's study, one sees that the basic value of step length decreased in the older group, and the range of the

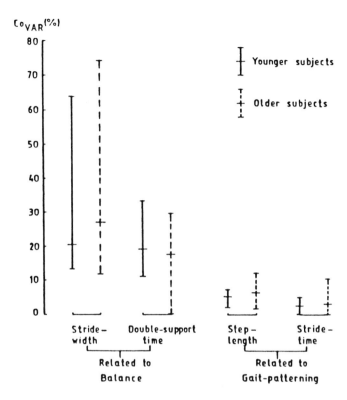

Figure 2 Ranges and medians of coefficients of variation for parameters of contributing to gait patterning and to balance in younger (n = 32) vs older (n = 32) adults (Ref. 7).

coefficient of variation of stride time increased in the older group. Thus there was a trend toward increased variability and decreased step length in Gabell and Nayak's study, although they failed to find significance statistically. Further research is needed with more subjects to understand the extent of an age effect on gait characteristics in older people. The present studies suggest that a pure age effect on gait patterns is minor in comparison with possible pathological effects.

Murray et al. (14) found that at free walking speed, minimal toe–floor clearance (in initial swing phase) increased from 1.0 cm at age 20 to 2.6 cm at age 81 (between 81 and 87). However, the toe elevation at the end of swing phase decreased from 16 cm to 12 cm between ages 20 and 87. Because decreased foot–floor clearance may cause trips during walking, it is important to know if there are changes in the patterns of stepping over obstacles with aging. In order to answer this question, Chef et al. (17) analyzed the gait of 24 young and 24 older healthy adults while they stepped over obstacles of varying heights. Obstacles of 0, 25, 51, and 152 mm in height were chosen. Zero mm (a tape on the walkway) and no obstacle conditions were used as control conditions. The 25- and 51-mm height obstacles corresponded to typical 1-in. and 2-in. height floor and door thresholds. The 152-mm obstacle height corresponded to a typical 6-in. curbstone, toy, or pet in the home. A four-camera Watsmart opto-electronic system was used to analyze the gait patterns within a 2-m range surrounding the obstacle while subjects walked at their comfortable speeds. The following seven kinematic parameters were measured: approach speed; crossing speed; stance foot toe-to-obstacle distance (before crossing the obstacle); heel strike toe-to-obstacle distance (after crossing the obstacle); step length; step width; and foot clearance from the top of the obstacle. The results showed that foot clearance increased nonlinearly with obstacle height (including the 0-mm height condition). There was no age-related change in foot clearance over an obstacle. However, 4 of 24 older subjects stepped on an obstacle (0- or 25-mm height) during the experiment, while none of the young subjects stepped on an obstacle. There were no significant age differences in any measured parameter in the obstacle-free gait condition. Older adults exhibited a significantly more conservative strategy when crossing obstacles, with slower crossing speed, shorter step length, and shorter heel strike toe-to-obstacle distance. Older adults decreased their approaching and crossing speeds to an obstacle, and kept the toe-to-obstacle distance of the stance foot (foot not crossing the obstacle) longer than the young subjects. Thus for the older adults, heel or midsole was the lowest point on the shoe as it crossed the obstacle. Compared with a toe contact, a heel or midsole contact with an obstacle during gait is more likely to cause a stumble rather than a trip, thus possibly causing less risk for a fall.

Chef et al. noted that despite the fact that white-colored obstacles were used on a black walkway to increase their visibility, the cognitive factors involved in crossing obstacles were not controlled. A few older subjects stepped on the 0- or 25-mm obstacles during the 48 walking trials experiment. Since the episodes of obstacle contact were equally distributed over the test period, inattention, rather than fatigue, was probably the cause of these incidents. Chef et al. suggested that the age-related differences in gait patterns while crossing obstacles may be partly due to the decreased total active range of joint motion in the lower extremities in the older adults. Pathological effects, on the other hand, are less likely to be a factor because older subjects with mild pathological deficits did not differ substantially in their performance from other elderly subjects without these deficits. This study showed that age differences in cognition and active range of motion might be two factors contributing to age-related changes in gait patterns while crossing obstacles.

C. Mechanical Power Analysis

Positional data obtained from a camera-based study describe patterns of locomotion, but they provide no further understanding concerning the amount of force generated by the subject. Using the method of inverse dynamics, moments of force generated at each joint and the mechanical power generated and absorbed at each joint can be calculated. The amount of power generated by muscles can also be estimated. Power generation and absorption are related to increases and decreases in rotational and translational energy. You need to increase energy to swing, and decrease energy to prepare for heel strike. It has previously been reported that older women exhibited more electromyographic activity and different activation sequences among leg muscles than younger women during walking (18). Concomitant mechanical power analysis and EMG analysis of gait are needed to understand the resultant age-related changes in gait patterns.

Winter et al. (12) compared the gait patterns of 15 healthy older adults (age range 62–78 years) to 12 young adults (age range 21–28 years). Basic kinematic data were converted into kinetic data using an inverse dynamics model. Older adults (1) were found to have significantly shorter stride length, with significantly longer double-support stance duration; (2) generated significantly less power by the plantar flexors at push-off; and (3) absorbed significantly less energy by the quadriceps femoris muscle during the late stance and early swing phase. The reduction of plantar flexor power during push-off may result in (1) a shorter step length; (2) a more flat-footed heel strike; and (3) increased double-support stance duration. The reason for a weaker push-off in the older adult may be reduced muscle strength in the ankle plantar flexors as has been reported by many researchers (3,19) or an adaptive change selected by the older adults to ensure a safer gait since high push-off power acts upward and forward and is destabilizing.

Another important finding in Winter et al.'s (12) study is that the knee–hip covariance was marginally less for the elderly than the young subjects ($p < .07$). The knee–hip covariance is calculated from the moment-of-force patterns over all the strides between the knee and the hip joints. Because the moment-of-force of the knee joint must correspond to that of the hip joint during each stride in order to maintain dynamic balance during gait, the knee–hip covariance can be used as the "index of dynamic balance" (12). Thus older adults seem to have reduced dynamic balance ability during gait. The range of the index of dynamic balance of the older subjects in Winter et al.'s study seems to fall into two modes: 10 of the older adults fell within the same range as the young subjects and 5 of them showed quite low covariances. The authors speculate that these 5 elderly subjects may have had a balance impairment not detected in their initial exams. It is thus possible that the index of dynamic balance could be used to differentiate subjects with a balance deficit from those without. A larger sample is needed to establish the norm for the index of dynamic balance.

Studies of gait patterns in healthy older adults have reported some age-related changes in gait patterns. The only consistent finding among all of the studies is a reduction in walking speed and a reduced stride (step) length with age. Many researchers have suggested that older adults adopt a safer, more conservative gait pattern. Pathology, weakness in the leg muscles, reduced sensation, and cognitive factors have been mentioned as possible causes of the various age-related changes in gait patterns. The following section will briefly review some factors that might contribute to age-related changes in gait patterns and therefore should be carefully evaluated in older people with possible gait abnormalities.

III. FACTORS INFLUENCING CHANGES IN GAIT PATTERNS IN OLDER ADULTS

A. Level of Physical Activity and Functional Capacity

A consistent finding in studies of gait in the aging is that walking speed (or stride length) decreases with age. Leiper and Craik (20) investigated the relationship of walking speed and level of physical activity in 81 healthy women (range 64.0–94.5 years). Subjects were categorized into: (1) a sedentary group (subjects who walked less than three city blocks per day, did not regularly prepare meals, and lived in a retirement community); (2) a community-active group (walked more than three city blocks per day, regularly prepared meals, and lived independently in the community); and (3) an exercise group (participated in a regular, ongoing exercise activity for more than 4 months prior to testing).

Defining the groups in this way led to a significant difference among the three physical activity groups. Women in the sedentary group were the oldest (mean = 81.3, s.d. = 5.4), followed by the community-active group (mean = 76.3, s.d. = 8.13), and those in the exercise group were the youngest (mean = 71.1, s.d. = 4.7). Thus, age was used as a covariate during the analysis of physical activity and walking speed.

Each subject was asked to walk repeatedly at different paces (very slow, slow, normal, fast, and very fast) over a portable instrumented walkway. The pressure switches of the walkway monitored foot contact of each foot during each trial. Subjects were asked to walk at their preferred pace first, then at slow and very slow paces. Following the very slow pace, subjects were asked to walk at their preferred pace again, then at fast and very fast paces.

A walking speed by activity level interaction was found. When asked to walk at their very slow pace, subjects in the exercise group were able to walk significantly slower than the sedentary and the community-active group. The exercise group was the fastest of the three groups at the very fast pace, but this relationship was not significant. The authors concluded that level of physical activity does not affect the ability to produce different walking speeds except at a very slow pace. When compared to data from young subjects in other studies, older women in this study walked slower even at the very fast pace. It is possible that subjects in the exercise group seldom practiced the type of exercise requiring quick or forceful activity, which may be important to produce a fast walking speed. The lack of a significant relationship between physical activity and walking speed may also be the result of a sampling problem. It was noted that the most inactive persons tended to be reluctant to volunteer for the sedentary group.

Why did level of physical activity affect walking speed at the very slow pace? It was observed that the very slow pace was different from the other paces in that larger portions of the walking cycle were spent in the double-support phase of the cycle and subjects commented on having a feeling of instability at this pace. Thus walking at the very slow pace may require more precise control of balance.

This study further identified age as the most important determinant of walking speed, with a small contribution from the person's weight/height ratio. In addition to age and weight/height, Bendall et al.

(21) found that walking speed is also affected by calf strength and the presence of health problems in men. Thus the presence of health problems may contribute to loss of mobility and a decline in level of gait function in older persons.

Are gait abnormalities seen in older adults due to normal aging or pathology? In a study that aimed to answer this question, Sudarsky and Ronthal (11) found that the majority of older patients with idiopathic gait disorders could actually be diagnosed by further detailed examination. Thus it appears that pathological conditions may be the underlying mechanism for changes in gait patterns observed in older people who participate in studies without a stringent screening process. For example, Spielberg (6) described the gait patterns of older adults beyond 72 years of age as showing an absence of arm–leg synergy and the presence of arrhythmical stepping patterns. These patterns more closely resemble clinically diagnosed gait disorders than changes in gait patterns accompanying normal aging in healthy older adults.

While gait characteristics of healthy older adults show few differences from younger adults, older adults with a history of falls have significantly different gait characteristics compared to older adults without a history of falls (22,23). Heitmann et al. (23) found that elderly female fallers ($n = 26$) stood for significantly shorter times with feet in tandem position with eyes open than nonfallers ($n = 84$). In addition, older female subjects with poor balance performance have increased step width during gait. Gehlsen and Whaley (22) reported that heel width (step width measured at the heel) was significantly larger in elderly persons with a history of falls when they walked at a fast speed of 6 km/h when compared to subjects without a history of falls. It is possible that subjects with a history of falls had some undiagnosed pathological conditions. Thus the health status of subjects is an important factor to consider in studies on age-related changes in gait. However, it is also possible that, after repeated falls, subjects have a fear of falling, and this fear contributes to changes in gait characteristics as well. This cognitive factor will be discussed in the next section.

B. Cognitive Function: Fear of Falling and Inattention

Many researchers have suggested the possibility that older adults walk more slowly, not because of specific constraints on walking speed per se, but because they consciously select a more conservative or safe gait (12, 14). Thus it is possible that changes in attitude toward walking, such as fear of falling or inattention, may contribute to changes in gait patterns in older adults. Chef et al. (17) suggested that inattention may be a factor contributing to changes in the way in which older adults step over obstacles while walking. Tinetti et al. (24) found that preferred walking pace, anxiety level, and depression are good predictors of the level of fear of falling in community-dwelling older persons. Subjects who reported avoiding activities due to a fear of falling tended to have a slower walking pace, higher anxiety level, and depression compared to subjects with a low level of fear of falling. Maki et al. (25) found that fear of falling affected balance performance during a spontaneous sway test and one-leg stance test. The authors commented that it was not clear whether subjects with a fear of falling had a true deterioration in postural control mechanisms, or whether the fear of falling affected the balance performance in an artifactual manner. Thus, it would be important to consider the possible effect of fear of falling on locomotion performance in older adults in future studies in this area.

C. Sensory Function

Decreased reaction time, reduced sensation, and decreased muscle strength have been reported to accompany the aging process (2,4,26–29). Lord et al. (30) reported that reduced sensation, muscle weakness in the legs, and increased reaction time are important factors associated with postural instability. Since postural instability has been shown to accompany falls during walking (31), it is important to evaluate the possible effect of sensory function changes on age-related changes in gait patterns.

Brownlee et al. (32) compared the perception of verticality and horizontality between six elderly fallers and six controls (ages ranged from 67–76 years). It was found that the visual perception of verticality and horizontality was not different between the fallers and the controls. However, 50% of the fallers indicated difficulties in the recognition of postural tilt when they stood on a tilting platform. Fallers also leaned more heavily on a supporting frame when standing on one leg when compared to control subjects. The results suggest that fallers may rely on visual cues to recognize postural deviations, thus implying impairment of their proprioceptive system. Thus intact visual function may be crucial for older persons who have a history of falls to avoid recurrent falls. However, Warren et al. (33) reported that the threshold to detect optical flow that accompanies normal body sway increases with age. If deterioration in sensory function is part of the normal aging process, we must evaluate the effect of environmental factors and training to improve stability and gait in older adults.

Simoneau et al. (34) studied the influence of environmental visual factors on gait patterns during stair descent in a group of 36 healthy women between the ages of 55 and 70. Subjects were asked to descend stairs under the following conditions: (1) stairs were painted black; (2) stairs were painted black and the subject wore a headband with a light-scattering plastic shield (the blurred condition); or (3) stairs were painted black with a white stripe at the edge of each tread. Eighteen of the subjects descended stairs with a surrounding vertically striped corridor, the remaining 18 subjects descended stairs using a visual surround with horizontal stripes. The cadence, foot clearance, and foot placement during stair descent were measured using a high-speed filming system (100 Hz). The results showed significantly slower cadence, larger foot clearance, and more posterior foot placement while subjects walked under the blurred condition as compared to the other two stair color conditions. No statistically significant differences were found between the two visual surround stripe-orientation conditions. The authors further observed that foot clearance, albeit small (ranging from 3.7–63.5 mm), was larger than that obtained during previous pilot work performed in their laboratory with young, healthy subjects. Thus older subjects walked with larger foot clearance during stair descent as compared to young adults, and gait patterns during stair descent were affected by visual conditions. We should remember that Murray et al. found age-related changes in gait characteristics including decreased toe–floor clearance while subjects walked in the dark with an interrupted-light stroboscope. It is possible that older adults are more affected by the lack of normal visual feedback during walking that young adults, and some of the age-related differences found in Murray et al.'s studies could be contributed to reduced sensory function rather than age alone.

The reduced ability of older adults to deal with altered sensory conditions during balancing has been reported in many studies (35–37). Results from these studies consistently demonstrated that older adults are able to maintain good balance when only one sensory input is altered. Older adults are significantly worse than younger adults when two sensory inputs are altered simultaneously. For example, when both vision and somatosensory inputs from the ankles and feet were simultaneously altered in the laboratory, the only appropriate sensory inputs for maintaining balance came from the vestibular system. Older adults swayed excessively or fell under conditions when both vision and somato-sensory inputs were altered or deprived. These results suggested that sensory redundancy is important for older adults to maintain balance. Furthermore, when one sensory input is inappropriate for maintaining balance, older adults are able to select and reweight sensory inputs to avoid instability, if they are given multiple training trials. Since balance is an important component of gait function, it is possible that this ability affects the characteristics of gait patterns in older adults as well (12).

D. Muscle Strength

Using an inverse dynamic technique, Winter et al. (12) reported a significant decrease in push-off power during gait in healthy older adults. It would be interesting to know whether the decreased push-off power during gait is the sole result of decreased muscle mass with age, or whether impairment of descending motor pathways constitutes an additional factor. Vandervoort and McComas (3) studied the strength of the ankle dorsiflexor and plantar flexor muscles of 111 healthy subjects aged 20–100 years. The results showed that the average values for maximum voluntary muscle strength (measured by torque generation) of the ankle muscles began to decline in the sixth decade. Older adults had smaller muscle cross-sectional areas and prolonged twitch contraction and half-relaxation times. During maximum voluntary effort, stimulation of motor nerves produced no additional torque in the majority of elderly subjects. Thus healthy older adults remained able to utilize their descending motor pathways for optimal muscle activation.

Reduction of muscle strength in other muscles has also been reported. Rice et al. (38) measured the strength of several upper and lower extremities using a simple dynamometer (a modified sphygmomanometer) in a group of 118 older adults. It was found that after the age of 75, age is the most important factor predicting strength reduction. The other factors studied were height, weight, and sum of skinfolds. The authors reported that the strength of elbow flexion, grip, knee extension, and dorsiflexion could be used as the best indicators of overall limb strength. Significant reduction in strength of both concentric and eccentric contractions of the knee extensor and flexor muscles has also been reported in a group of healthy older women (66–89 years old) as compared to younger women (20–29 years) (39). It was found that age differences are smaller for eccentric contraction than for concentric contraction.

Reduction of muscle strength in older adults has functional significance. Whipple et al. (19) found that fallers (mean age = 82.2 years) with no overt etiology had significantly smaller peak torque and power generated by the ankle and knee muscles than a group of age-matched nonfallers. Thus muscle weakness, especially in the ankle musculature, is an important factor contributing to poor balance in older adults. Fiatarone et al. (40) found that high-intensity resistance training can significantly increase the knee extensor muscle strength, muscle size, and improve functional mobility among frail older adults up to the age of 96 years. Frail older adults increased their mean tandem gait speed by 48% after an eight-week training program. Furthermore, two subjects no longer used canes to walk at the end of the study.

In summary, age-related reduction in muscle strength has been found in selected upper and lower extremity muscles. Concentric contraction is more affected in older female subjects than eccentric contraction for knee muscles. Age-related reductions in muscle strength at the ankle joint may contribute to reduced push-off power during gait and poor balance. Strength training can significantly improve functional mobility in older frail adults.

IV. SUMMARY

In this chapter, we have reviewed studies characterizing gait patterns in older adults. Generally speaking, healthy older adults have reduced walking speed, shorter stride length, and shorter step length than young adults. Many studies reported that older adults are unable to walk faster than 1.4 m/h, a speed recommended by the Swedish authority to safely pass an intersection. While walking under less than optimal sensory feedback conditions, such as when the laboratory setup required the use of interrupted-light photography, an overall reduction of joint angle amplitude and increased gait variability were also observed.

Stride width and floor clearance are two important gait parameters that distinguish between fallers and nonfallers. Changes in floor clearance with age are not consistently reported among different studies. Despite this, it was found that older adults are more likely to step on obstacles, probably due to inattention rather than a lack of ability to walk with sufficient floor clearance.

Changes in the characteristics of gait patterns in older adults are influenced by balance ability, leg muscle strength, and altered sensory feedback. Fear of falling and inattention may also be important. When evaluating gait patterns of older people, we must consider the underlying mechanisms contributing to these changes and attempt to differentiate between contributions related to pathology versus aging per se. The only consistent findings across all studies concerning age-related changes in gait pattern are reduced walking speed and stride length. Thus, when studies report additional changes in gait patterns, it would be helpful to examine further other possible influencing factors, including pathology. Only after the underlying mechanisms influencing gait pattern alterations are identified can a clinician or therapist design effective and appropriate interventions to improve gait function in older adults and thus help them achieve a safe and independent life style.

ACKNOWLEDGMENT

This work was supported by NIA grant No. 2 RO1 AG05317-04A3 to Dr. M.H. Woollacott.

REFERENCES

1. Gilcrest BA, Rowe JW. The biology of aging. In: Rowe JW, Besdine RW, eds., Health and Disease in Old Age. Boston: Little, Brown, 1982: 15.
2. Sekuler R, Hutman LP, Owsley CJ. Human aging and spatial vision. Science 1980; 209: 1255.
3. Vandervoort AA, McComas AJ. Contractile changes in opposing muscles of the human ankle joint with aging. J Appl Physiol 1986; 61: 361.
4. Whanger AD, Wang HS. Clinical correlates of the vibratory sense in elderly psychiatric patients. J Gerontol 1974; 29: 39.
5. Sheldon JH. The effect of age on the control of sway. Geront Clin 1963; 5: 129.
6. Spielberg PI. Walking patterns of old people: Cyclographic analysis. In: Bernstein NA, ed., Investigations on the Biodynamics of Walking, Running, and Jumping. Moscow: Central Scientific Institute of Physical Culture, 1940.
7. Gabell A, Nayak USL. The effect of age on variability in gait. J Gerontol 1984; 39: 662.
7a. Woollacott M. Aging, posture control and movement preparation. In: Woollacott M, Shumway-Cook S, eds., Development of Posture and Gait Across the Life Span. Columbia: University of South Carolina Press, 1989: 156.
8. Barron RC. Disorders of gait related to the aging nervous system. Geriatrics 1967; 22: 113.

9. Critchley M. On senile disorders of gait, including the so-called "senile paraplegic." Geriatrics 1948; 13: 364.

10. Steinberg FV. Gait disorders in old age. Geriatrics 1966; 21: 134.

11. Sudarsky L, Ronthal M. Gait disorders among elderly patients: a survey study of 50 patients. Arch Neurol 1983; 40: 740.

12. Winter DA, Patla AE, Frank JS, Walt SE. Biomechanical walking pattern changes in the fit and healthy elderly. Phys Ther 1990; 70: 340.

13. Drillis R. The influence of aging on the kinematics of gait. The Geriatric Amputee, Publication 919, National Academy of Science, National Research Council, 1961.

14. Murray MP, Kory RC, Clarkson BH. Walking patterns in healthy old men. J Gerontol 1969; 24: 169.

15. Murray MP, Kory RC, Sepic SB. Walking patterns of normal women. Arch Phys Med Rehabil 1970; 51: 637.

16. Pyykko I, Jantti P, Aalto H. Postural control in elderly subjects. Age Ageing 1990; 19: 215.

17. Chef H, Ashton-Miller JA, Alexander NB, Schultz AB. Stepping over obstacles: Gait patterns of healthy young and old adults. J Gerontol 1991; 46: 196.

18. Finley FR, Cody KA, Finizie RV. Locomotion patterns in elderly women. Arch Phys Med Rehabil 1969; 50: 140.

19. Whipple RH, Wolfson LI, Amerman PM. The relationship of knee and ankle weakness to falls in nursing home residents: an isokinetic study. JAGS 1987; 35: 13.

20. Leiper CI, Craik RL. Relationships between physical activity and temporal-distance characteristics of walking in elderly women. Phys Ther 1991; 71: 791.

21. Bendall MJ, Bassey EJ, Pearson MB. Factors affecting walking speed of elderly people. Age Ageing 1989; 18: 327.

22. Gehlsen GM, Whaley MH. Falls in the elderly: Part I, gait. Arch Phys Med Rehabil 1990; 71: 735.

23. Heitmann DK, Gossman MR, Shaddeau SA, Jackson JR. Balance performance and step width in noninstitutionalized, elderly, female fallers and nonfallers. Phys Ther 1989; 69: 923.

24. Tinetti ME, Richman D, Powell L. Falls efficacy as a measure of fear of falling. J Gerontol 1990; 45: P239.

25. Maki BE, Holliday PJ, Topper AK. Fear of falling and postural performance in the elderly. J Gerontol 1991; 46: M123.

26. Stelmach GE, Worringham CJ. Sensorimotor deficits related to postural stability: implications for falling in the elderly. Clin Geriatr Med 1985; 1: 679.

27. Birren JE. Vibratory sensitivity in the aged. J Gerontol 1947; 2: 267.

28. Skinner HB, Barrack RL, Cook SD. Age-related decline in proprioception. Clin Orthop Related Res 1984; 184: 208.

29. Rosenhall U, Rubin W. Degenerative changes in the human vestibular sensory epithelia. Acta Otolaryngol 1975; 79: 67.

30. Lord SR, Clark RD, Webster IW. Postural stability and associated physiological factors in a population of aged persons. J Gerontol 1991; 46: M69.

31. Lipsitz LA, Jonsson PV, Kelley MM, Koestner JS. Causes and correlates of recurrent falls in ambulatory frail elderly. J Gerontol 1991; 46: M114.

32. Brownlee MG, Banks MA,, Crosbie WJ, Meldrum F, Nimmo MA. Consideration of spatial orientation mechanisms as related to elderly fallers. Gerontology 1989; 35: 323.

33. Warren WH, Blackwell AW, Morris MW. Age differences in perceiving the direction of self-motion from optical flow. J Gerontol 1989; 44: P147.

34. Simoneau GG, Cavanagh PR, Ulbrecht JS, Leibowitz HW, Tyrrell RA. The influence of visual factors on fall-related kinematic variables during stair descent by older women. J Gerontol 1991; 46: M188.

35. Peterka RJ, Black FO. Age-related changes in human posture control: sensory organization tests. J Vestibular Res 1990; 1: 73.

36. Teasdale N, Stelmach GE, Breunig A. Postural sway characteristics of the elderly under normal and altered visual and support surface conditions. J Gerontol 1990; 46: B238.

37. Woollacott MH, Shumway-Cook A, Nashner LM. Aging and posture control: changes in sensory organization and muscular coordination. Int J Aging Human Devel 1986; 23: 97.

38. Rice CL, Cunningham DA, Paterson DH, Rechnitzer PA. Strength in an elderly population. Arch Phys Med Rehabil 1989; 70: 391.

39. Vandervoort AA, Kramer JF, Wharram ER. Eccentric knee strength of elderly females. J Gerontol 1990; 45: B125.

40. Fiatarone MA, Marks EC, Ryan ND, Meredith CN, Lipsitz LA, Evans WJ. High-intensity strength training in nonagenarians. JAMA 1990; 263: 3029.

9

Common Foot and Ankle Disorders Affecting Mobility in Older Persons

MELVIN H. JAHSS
Mount Sinai School of Medicine and Hospital for Joint Diseases, New York, New York

I. INTRODUCTION

The foot is the end organ of weightbearing. It refines the crude arcs of motion of the pelvis, hips, and knees and compensates for any abnormalities or deformities above the foot. Its proprioception is approximately four times more sensitive than at the musculotendinous junctions above the ankle level. It permits normal gait and propulsion along with the flexibility and accommodation needed on uneven surfaces and in sports activities. The foot carries up to double the body weight with running. Normally the reciprocal action between the ankle and midtarsal joints is so intricate and balanced that degenerative arthritis rarely occurs (spontaneously) unless there has been prior trauma or damage by disease process. Conversely, interruption of normal foot function by

187

injury or disease may be very incapacitating. What distinguishes humans from other primates is the development of the foot with upright planti-grade walking.

Approximately 17–20% of orthopedic consultation cases, as well as surgical, involve the foot and ankle. Considering the care tended by nonorthopedists and podiatrists, foot and ankle problems and treatment are very commonplace, especially in the elderly, where up to 80% have foot problems.

In general, the type of foot problems varies with the age popula-tion. Most common in children and infancy are congenital and neurologi-cal deformities; in young adults, injuries; and in older adults, injuries and medically induced and static disorders. In the aged, static disorders have superimposed local degenerative problems, including vascular inef-ficiency and, less serious but uncomfortable, osteoarthritic and neuro-logical symptoms. It is in the elderly that the examining physician must differentiate between the etiologies of occult foot pain. Similar pain may occur from seronegative disorders, Lyme disease, mild peripheral neu-ropathy, spinal stenosis, vascular insufficiency, or local plantar soft tis-sue atrophy. In essence, this list is almost endless, and patients often require considerable diagnostic workup (such as nuclear imaging) and specialty consultations, especially rheumatological, neurological, and vascular.

II. FOOT DISORDERS

Foot disorders in the elderly are best evaluated and diagnosed in rela-tion to the area of presenting pain and for deformity. Each area is affected by certain static, degenerative, or medical disorders or, occa-sionally, mainly by only one condition. Rapid diagnosis leads to prompt treatment that may be curative in the early stages. For example, plantar heel pain usually occurs distally and medially and is related to plantar fasciitis in the young athlete; in slightly older groups, it is caused more frequently by seronegative disorders; in the middle aged, it is more related to obesity. However, in the aged, plantar heel pain is located more posteriorly and centrally due to overlying heel fat pad atrophy (Fig. 1). At the other extreme is pain and local swelling behind and below the medial malleolus in patients past 40 years of age which, invari-ably, is due to rupture of the tibialis posterior tendon until proven other-wise. Excessive delay in treatment of this condition may result in perma-nent disability.

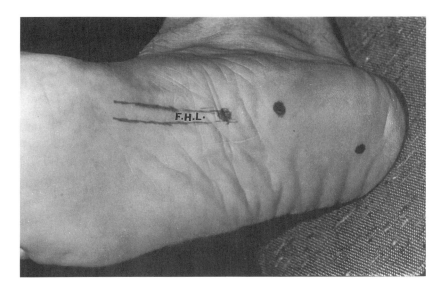

Figure 1 Tender areas (black dots) under heel: (1) posterior midheel is the site of palpable atrophy; (2) distal and medial tenderness is over the medial plantar tubercle or site of plantar fascial origin; (3) just distal to the medial tubercle is the flexor hallucis longus tendon as it enters the sole and may be irritated secondary to prolonged walking.

III. PATHOLOGICAL ANATOMY AND BIOMECHANICS OF THE SENESCENT FOOT

Normally, the foot is plantigrade and pain free with no deformities, intact neurovascular structures, and normal motion. Specific changes occur in the senescent foot which may mitigate against elective orthopedic surgery; but, on the other hand, they may require vascular surgery.

The normal foot is plantigrade (9), indicating that the plantar weightbearing load is well distributed with standing and walking and there is no area of excess weightbearing to cause pain and callus formation. Normally, with standing, equal weightbearing is shared between the heel and the metatarsal heads. In addition, weightbearing is divided equally under each of the metatarsal heads except for the first, which bears twice the amount. The foot has a moderate degree of supppleness as well as dorsiflexion–plantarflexion motion of the ankle and lateral side-to-side subtalar motion of the foot. A high arch or a high heel will throw excess weightbearing onto the metatarsal heads. If a metatarsal is shortened or tilts upward from an injury or from surgery, or if there is loss of a metatarsal head from infection or surgery, excess weightbearing will be thrust under the adjacent heads with additional pain and disability. This is termed weightbearing transfer. Minute changes in bony architecture—as little as 1–2 mm—may upset the normal pain-free homeostasis of the plantigrade foot. Aside from diabetes and rheumatoid arthritis, bony deformities of the foot in the elderly play a less common pathological role than senescent soft tissue degeneration.

The plantar skin is ten times thicker than the skin in the rest of the body and acts as a protective mechanism on weightbearing. This skin, as all senescent skin, atrophies and degenerates. Of greater significance are the metatarsal and heel plantar fat pads that normally offer a resilient cushion action of weightbearing. The heel pad buffers heel strike and weightbearing. The metatarsals are loaded to 20% above the body weight with push-off and considerably more with rapid walking and running. Gait analysis indicates that the ground impact is decreased in the elderly by a shorter stride, slower cadence, and lower swing-to-stance time ratios (2).

Histological and MRI studies of the plantar foot pads done by this author indicate atrophy of the fat cells along with degenerative changes in the fibroelastic septa that interlace about the fat and support the fat cells. With senescence, the septa split, fragment, and stain darkly (Fig. 2). Similar changes have been noted in senescent skin. Palpation reveals the metatarsal and heel pads to be thinner and excessively compressible. Plantar weightbearing pressure studies using Fuji film reveal that weightbearing is centralized to a smaller area with high-peak pressure rather than being dispersed wider at lower pressures. Coronal MRI studies on normal and atrophied heel pads, with and without simulated weightbearing, reveal that the heel pad appears as vertically aligned rectangular septa located centrally and sickle-shaped septa seen medially and laterally (Fig. 3). Upon weightbearing, the central septa compress while the lateral septa further bend and bulge out medially and laterally offering an excellent cushioning effect (Fig. 3). In general, the efficacy of the heel and metatarsal pads, with respect to shock absorption, depends not only on the integrity of the fat, septa, and septal shape but, especially, on overall thickness.

Gait analysis and the biomechanics of the foot and ankle have been studied with normal weightbearing and walking as well as running (11).

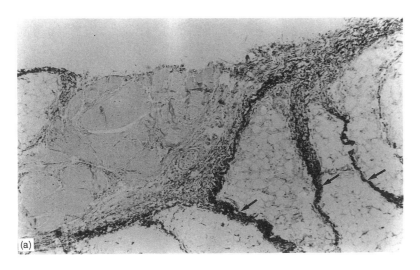

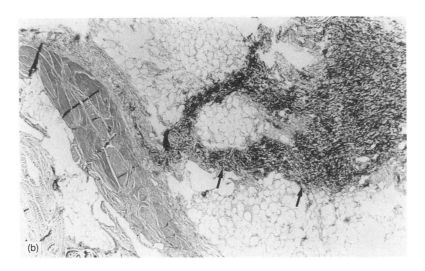

Figure 2 Histological sections of normal and abnormal (senescent) heel pads. (a) Normal pad with interlacing fibroelastic septa. Verhoeff x100. (b) Senescent pad showing atrophied fat cells with split, fragmented, and dark staining septa. Verhoeff x100. (From Ref. 3.)

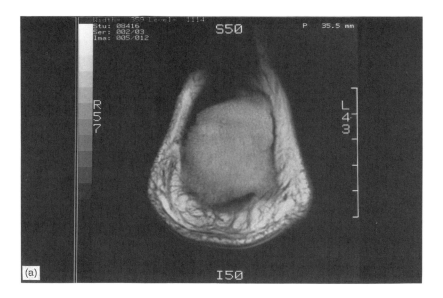

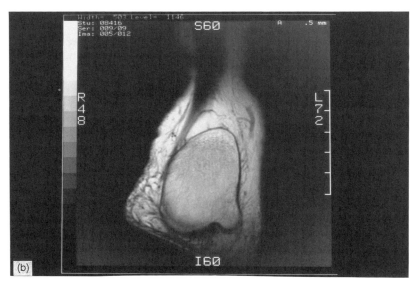

Figure 3 Nonweightbearing and simulated weightbearing coronal cut MRI studies of partially atrophic heel pad. (a) Note the normal vertically aligned rectangular fat septa centrally and the sickle-shaped septa medially and laterally. (b) Simulated weightbearing. Note the central compression of the pad plus medial and lateral bulging due to bending of the peripheral septa.

Muscle firing, EMGs, and force plate weightbearing analysis of the normal, abnormal, and postoperative foot is evolving slowly; it requires considerable research, time, expenditure, and improved accuracy and perfection of testing equipment.

IV. EXAMINATION OF THE FOOT AND ANKLE

Foot problems in the elderly relate to a multiplicity of possible etiologies. The majority of these are static and degenerative, as well as medical diseases affecting the foot such as seronegative disorders and neurovascular impairment. As noted, complaints in a specific area may be caused by many different disorders, often initially occult to the examining specialist. It is for this reason that thorough laboratory and often nuclear imaging may be necessary.

A. History

The patient's history includes the chief complaint, specific area(s) of pain, past surgical and medical treatment, any causally related medical disorders, such as psoriasis or symptoms related to seronegative disorders; what aggravates the symptoms and how they are relieved. It is best to disregard temporarily past medical information and doctors' findings that may be misleading, especially if the patient has not improved under their care. Read any laboratory reports or nuclear imaging films and decide if they are adequate or need to be redone. In my experience, 75% of MRIs are too small, too indistinct, or involve the wrong cuts or density to be evaluated adequately, especially in relation to tendon pathology about the foot and ankle.

Certain statements with respect to history often give a clue as to the possible diagnosis, thereby permitting the examining physician to hone in on appropriate further examination and workup. Numbness or pain down the lateral aspect of the foot may be due to S1 radiculopathy and may be associated with a decreased ankle jerk, or a history of back pain.

In the majority of cases, the pain or discomfort is localized fairly well, but still requires a differential diagnosis as to the underlying etiology. The most common pain is under the ball of the foot about the metatarsal heads. Is this due to excessive prominence of one of the heads or from generalized metatarsal fat pad atrophy? Is there tenderness under a prominent metatarsal head associated with an overlying callus? This would confirm too much weightbearing in this area. Is this pain about the second metatarsal head, but no callus or tenderness under the head? If the tenderness is slightly distal in the capsule of the second metatarsophalangeal (MTP) joint, the diagnosis is synovitis of this joint. If the synovitis involves a few MTP joints, seronegative disease must be ruled out. If the tenderness is localized in the second web space, the diagnosis may be a Morton's (plantar) neuroma.

B. Physical Examination

Since foot pain in the elderly may be obscure and related to systemic disorders or neurovascular insufficiency, a routine comprehensive foot and ankle examination should be done (5). Vague foot pain, occasionally severe, may be caused by an unrecognized diabetic peripheral neuropathy. Decreased or absent vibratory sense, using a 128 VPS tuning fork over the first metatarsal head, makes a presumptive diagnosis pending further workup. One should consider that such vibratory sense may be decreased as a normal finding in patients past 65 years of age and, more frequently, past 75 years. A routine sequence of examination may be as follows.

Let the patient stand barefoot, exposing both feet and ankles, to observe any local swelling or deformities, especially in relation to the patient's complaints. Is one foot flatter than the other? Any dependent vascular changes? The patient now sits on the examining table and the physician sits on a stool at a lower level directly in front of the patient. Both feet should relax normally and hand down into equinovarus. If one foot is dorsiflexed and in valgus, it may be due to subtalar pathology. This can be confirmed if there is painful limitation of subtalar motion compared to the normal foot. One should keep in mind that subtalar (side-to-side) motion is normally somewhat limited in the elderly.

Now examine and palpate the soles. Are there any calluses over prominent bones? If the complaint is plantar heel pain, is there atrophy of the heel pad on palpation? In such cases, the tenderness is usually in the midplantar heel rather than over the distal–medial calcaneal tubercle seen in younger patients from plantar fasciitis. Vague generalized heel pain may be related to seronegative disorders. Look for any skin condition such as scaling of soles from epidermophytosis, but which may be simulated by psoriasis. Check the ankle and knee jerks and test for vibratory sense. Now palpate the dorsalis pedis and posterior tibial pulses. Claudication may be simulated by spinal stenosis.

Examine for any local tendon pathology that is common in the elderly, especially the tibialis posterior. A drop foot walk may be due to spontaneous rupture of the tibialis anterior tendon, which is rare, or peroneal nerve injury, occasionally secondary to prior hip surgery or rupture from a rheumatological synovitis. Spontaneous heel cord rupture is more common and invariably treated conservatively. Of greater significance is spontaneous rupture of the tibialis posterior tendon that occurs past the age of 40 and is common as well as disabling.

The forefoot is examined now, starting with the hallux. Does the forefoot spread out with weightbearing, accentuating any metatarsus primus varsus (splay foot)? Is there a bunion? Are there arthritic changes in the first MTP joint with limitation of motion (hallux rigidus)? Is this motion painful? Are there arthritic spurs over the dorsum of the first MTP joint? With respect to the small toes, are they hammered and, if so, which joints are involved? Are there calluses overlying these toes? Any secondary infections or draining sinuses? Examine the metatarsal heads on the soles of the feet. Are some of the heads more prominent and associated with tender calluses? Is there an associated high arch? Is there any metatarsal fat pad atrophy?

C. Diagnostic Workup, Consultations, and Ancillary Needs

Once a tentative diagnosis is established on examination and history, more specific definitive diagnosis must be made to effect proper treatment and relief. A hammer toe may be secondary to static deformity, simply requiring a high toe box shoe or possibly surgery in recalcitrant cases. Multiple hammer toes with pes cavus, especially in the presence of decreased vibratory sense and small muscle (in the arch) atrophy may indicate an unsuspected Charcot–Marie-Tooth disease (Fig. 4). Neurological consultation and/or EMGs may be indicated. Synovitiss of the small toes may make one suspicious of seronegative disease or Lyme disease and requires a rheumatologic consultation. Similarly, a tenosynovitis, especially with findings of enthosopathy, also may suggest a rheumatological disorder, especially if the tibialis posterior tendon is involved. MRIs of the hindfeet, which are more discerning and accurate than the clinical examination, are then advisable.

Any drainage from under the hallux or plantar foot ulcer or hemorrhage under a callus should signal arterial insufficiency, especially diabetes (Fig. 5). Such ulcers and hemorrhages simply do not occur with neurovascular intact feet. The pedal pulses are present usually with small vessel disease and early neuropathy may be overlooked. Decreased vibratory sense in the feet is usually diagnostic, mandating

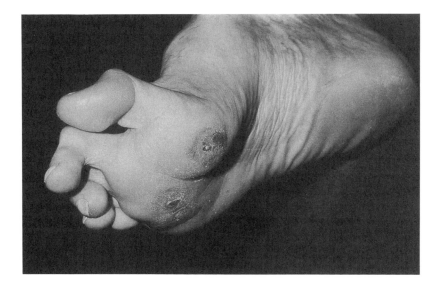

Figure 4   Charcot–Marie-Tooth disease with pes cavus and atrophy of the small muscles of the foot. Note the hammer toes and the metatarsal calluses.

EMGs. While a good orthopedic shoe store is helpful (along with appropriate orthotics), the diagnosis and specific prescription should be the responsibility of the treating physician.

V. TENDON PATHOLOGY

Aside from neurovascular deficiency, tendon pathology is the most disabling foot problem in the elderly (7). Patients with old unrecognized ruptured Achilles tendons, who do not run, have minimal disability. Spontaneous ruptures of the tibialis anterior tendon, which often occur in the sixth or seventh decades, cause mild drop foot and, usually, do not require surgical repair. A high-top shoe or low boot prevents the foot from dropping further. On the other hand, rupture of the tibialis posterior tendon, when neglected or left undiagnosed, progresses to a painful flat foot deformity (peritalar dislocation). This rupture in the younger patient is due to seronegative disease or psori-

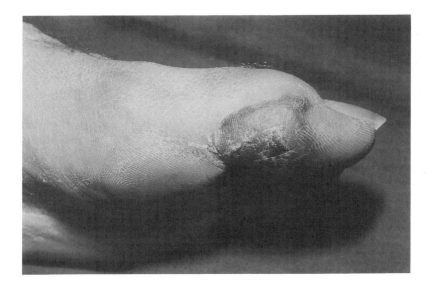

Figure 5 Spontaneous hemorrhage under a plantar callus in an area of excess weightbearing. The pedal pulses were present. The patient had an undiagnosed early diabetic peripheral neuropathy. (From Ref. 3.)

atic tendinitis. In patients over 40 years of age, the rupture is usually spontaneous and degenerative in nature.

A. Rupture of the Tibialis Posterior Tendon

In most cases there is no history of trauma. In the majority of patients, local swelling and discomfort occur spontaneously over the medial aspect of the involved ankle. Often it is neglected due to delayed diagnosis. Ordinarily, the rheumatologist or orthopedist is most familiar with this entity. There is specific tenderness over the tibialis posterior tendon behind and distal to the medial malleolus as the tendon approaches the medial navicular tubercle. At this stage, x-rays are negative (and remain so) while bone scans are "hot" over the medial malleolus. Most important is that an MRI of the hindfoot will detect early degeneration of this tendon. The MRI must be sharp, large, with T_1 coronal cuts. T_1 as well as T_2 density will reveal any peritendinitis which is more pronounced with seronegative disease (Fig. 6). Early MRI changes (1 year to 16 months) show slight heterogeneity and irregularity of the tendon. Normal tendons on MRI (T₁) are homogeneous, black, and smoothly rounded. Ultimately (2–2½ years), the tendon becomes swollen, reveals multiple areas of light grey degeneration, and, finally, is seen as an enlarged swollen area with small residual traces of tendon tissue (2½–3 years). A good MRI is extremely accurate. It details the inside and outside degenerative changes of the tendons about the ankle. Frequently, it picks up multiple tendon pathology, which may be completely unrecognizable clinically even by an astute physician. The MRI confirms the diagnosis including qualitative evaluation of the pathology, thereby permitting early and more satisfactory treatment. MRIs are cost effective as well as noninvasive.

As the tendon gradually degenerates, it elongates and eventually ruptures. Clinically, the elongation occurs in about 1½ years after onset

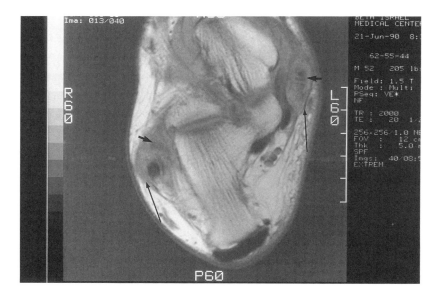

Figure 6 MRI T₁ coronal cut distal to the ankle joint. Note the severe peritendinitis about the peroneals and tibialis posterior tendons (long arrows) with almost complete degeneration of the peroneus brevis and the tibialis posterior (short arrows).

is *not* apparent on MRI but is manifested as weakness and incompetency, and inability to maintain the hindfoot in neutral. The result is gradual flattening of the arch with increasing valgus deformity of the foot and heel (Fig. 7). This is due to sequential stretching of the passive maintainers of the arch and hindfoot, namely, the spring ligament and the deltoid. The lateral aspect of the hindfoot below the lateral malleolus now becomes painful due to impingement. At first, the subtalar joint becomes stretched, ending in paritalar subluxation and, finally, the ankle becomes unstable due to undue deltoid laxity. By 2½–3 years, this severe, painful valgus deformity becomes fixed, which makes it impossible at this stage to correct fully by surgical reconstruction.

Treatment should be surgical, unless there are local or general medical contraindications. Since early diagnosis permits better surgical results, surgical delay by attempting conservative treatment is inappropriate. If surgery is contraindicated medically, a high-top sneaker or shoe or low boot with a custom-made molded leather ankle gauntlet

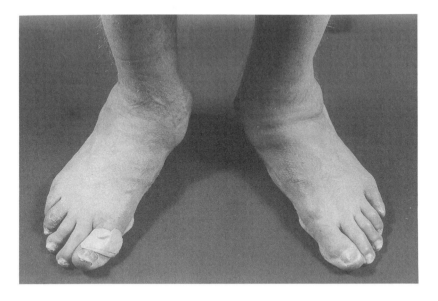

Figure 7 More advanced stage of bilateral rupture and elongation of the tibialis posterior tendons with elongations of the tendons and excessive valgus of the feet. (From Ref. 3.)

is the most effective conservative approach. Moderate relief will be obtained.

VI. SKIN AND TOENAILS

Corns and calluses occur from excess plantar or shoe pressure. Soft corns are due to similar pressure between toes. Hard painful corns develop on the top prominences of fixed hammer toes from the shoe toe box and over the lateral aspect of the fifth toe from the relatively pointed toe box in women's shoes. Orthopedic shoe stores readily provide high, wide-toe box shoes. Lamb's wool is excellent for interdigital soft corns. Calluses with painful fissures may occur about the plantar perimeter of the heels and are treated by paring down the excess callus and then using an emollient (3).

Toenail problems in the elderly may be problematical and even catastrophic in the presence of a diabetic and/or dysvascular foot. In many instances, the patient as well as the physician is unaware of an underlying diabetic condition. Under such circumstances, ingrown toenail surgery may lead to gangrene. Any sloughing, ulceration, or subungual drainage adjacent to an ingrown toenail should alert the examining physician to vascular impairment (Fig. 8). Similarly, any tender swelling and hemorrhage under a plantar callus or interdigital corn (Fig. 9) should forewarn of a pending slough under the skin. The pedal pulses should be checked and an urgent vascular consultation requested. Paring the corn or trimming back the offending toenail will uncover the underlying infection and slough/ulceration. If there is an associated peripheral neuropathy, symptoms may be minimal and misleading.

Occasionally, nail or paraungual corns are secondary to a severe hammer toe where the end of the toe presses into the ground. In the fifth toe, shoe pressure causes a painful lateral paraungual corn (Fig. 10). In addition to conservative treatment, such as callus trimming and protective devices, the orthopedist may elect to do a simple amputation of the end of the toe (terminal Syme operation).

Miscellaneous minor nail problems include chronic onychomycosis, which is best left untreated. Various nail deformities, such as onychogryposis (ram's horn deformity) (Fig. 11) require nail trimming. Older patients often are unable to cut their corns and thick nails because of limitations in bending or due to poor eyesight and limited hand strength.

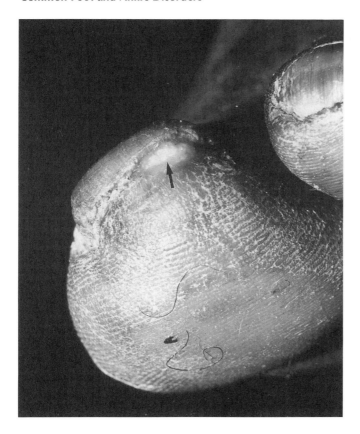

Figure 8 Subungual drainage. Patient was unaware he had diabetes. The examining physician should also look through the nail plate carefully for any abnormal changes. (From Ref. 3.)

VII. THE HALLUX AND SMALL TOES

The most common foot deformities seen in the elderly involve the hallux and small toes. Basically, these deformities have progressed slowly and become fixed over the years with one deformity leading to another. Understanding these sequential pathomechanical deformities will clarify the surgical and/or conservative elements of treatment.

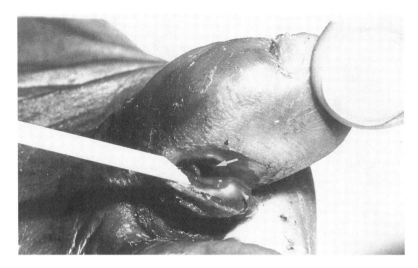

Figure 9   Soft corn under a fifth toe associated with local swelling and suspicious early infection. The corn was lifted up revealing a necrotic infected base. A dysvascular diabetic foot was diagnosed. (From Ref. 3.)

A. The Hallux

The initiating pathology, in many cases, is congenital hyperlax joints seen especially in the hand and, more subtly, in the feet. These loose joints cause flattening and widening of the forefeet on weightbearing with medial deviation of the first metatarsal from the second (metatarsus primus varus). Ligamentous laxity also causes pes planus, which thrusts the hallux into a valgus deformity (hallux valgus), which in turn accentuates the metatarsus primus varus. The problem is aggravated by high heels and pointed toe box shoes. This supports the fact that there is a ten times higher incidence of hallux valgus in women. The hallux valgus exposes the medial portion of the metatarsal head, which is the bunion. The hallux now pushes up against the second toe causing a hammer toe deformity [Fig. 12(a)]. Ultimately, the second toe dislocates dorsally over the second metatarsal head, which depresses the head, resulting in a painful plantar metatarsal callus. This callus may bother the patient more than the toe deformities especially on weightbearing. The pathological cycle is now complete. Reconstructive surgery at this point may be too extensive, especially in the elderly who have limited foot circula-

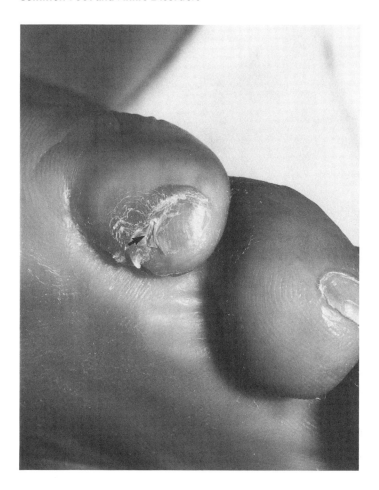

Figure 10 Hard corn over the lateral aspect of a fifth toenail from excess shoe pressure.

tion as well as limited activities. Conservative care is often quite success-ful and certainly devoid of iatrogenic complications. In fact, hallux valgus may be caused by second toe pathology or excision of the second metatarsal head. Surgical shortening and/or second toe instability allow the hallux to drift laterally [Fig. 12(b)]. The toe deformities decrease their weightbearing function, thereby thrusting added weight upon the

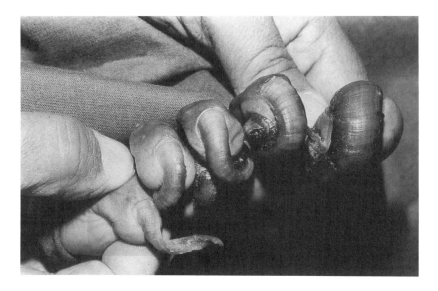

Figure 11   Onychogryposis involving all of the toenails.

metatarsal heads. This is intensified by senescent atrophy of the metatarsal fat pads. While toe surgery may improve cosmesis and facilitate
more normal shoe wear, it rarely relieves the anterior metatarsalgia and
frequently accentuates it.

B. The Small Toes

Small toe deformities, aside from inflammatory arthritis, are related to
abnormal static forces. The most common is hammering and overlapping
of the second toe and, to a lesser extent, the third and fourth toes, from a
hallux valgus deformity. As the small toes hammer, eventually, they dislo-
cate dorsally over the metatarsal heads forcing the heads plantarward,
thereby causing anterior metatarsalgia. The second most common cause
is forefoot equinus and especially high arches. The high arch (pes cavus)
causes increased pressure under the metatarsal heads. In addition, the
toes are forced dorsally and, in time, hammer further accentuating the
anterior metatarsalgia (Fig. 4). Calluses form under the metatarsal heads,
as well as dorsally over the elevated hammer toes. In the elderly, further
increase in shoe pressure over the tops of the toes cause thick corns to

develop and even breakdown of the skin with secondary infection and drainage. In addition, patients with high arches cannot tolerate low heels, which would lessen forefoot pressure in the shoe, because if they wear low heels or are barefoot, their heels simply will not reach the ground. In these patients, the forefoot is closer to the ground than the heels. Heel elevation, of course, only adds to forefoot pressure. Simple correction of the hammer toes, at any age, without correcting the high arch does not alleviate the anterior metatarsal excess weightbearing problem. If one is to compare plantar weightbearing in patients with flat feet (pes planus), the plantar stresses are dramatically opposite. There are no metatarsal calluses, since there is less pressure under the metatarsal heads. In addition, gait studies have indicated that weightbearing is also borne under the midtarsus so that body weight is distributed more evenly throughout the entire sole. Weightbearing is absent under the midtarsus and arch in pes cavus. In addition, in pes planus one does not encounter hammer toes except for those associated with the hallux valgus deformity.

VIII. TREATMENT OF TOE DEFORMITIES

Wearing a shoe that accommodates toe deformities invariably gives satisfactory relief. The main problems are usually the associated anterior metatarsalgia and, especially in women, obtaining a cosmetically appealing shoe. In some instances, the orthopedic surgeon is able to correct major deformities with less radical and yet palliative simpler procedures. For example, a hammer toe may be relieved dorsally by a high toe box shoe, but the end of the toe may dig painfully into the sole. Correcting the rigid stiff hammering may be surgically risky. On the other hand, simple excision of the nail, nail matrix, and tuft of the toe (terminal Syme amputation) is simple and routinely successful.

With respect to the bunion and hallux valgus surgery, the indication is relief of pain and not simply correction of deformity. In addition, these chronic deformities in the elderly become fixed and often arthritic. They require different surgical treatment than in the younger patient with flexible deformities. Conservative treatment depends upon the type and site of the deformities and the sites of pain. A working knowledge of the anatomy of shoes and sneakers plus their corrections and modifications is mandatory, rather than leaving the correction to a shoe store (4,6). The Prescription Footwear Association (PFA) has trained personnel in orthopedic shoe stores in most of the larger cities and also promulgates educational courses in association with orthopedic surgeons.

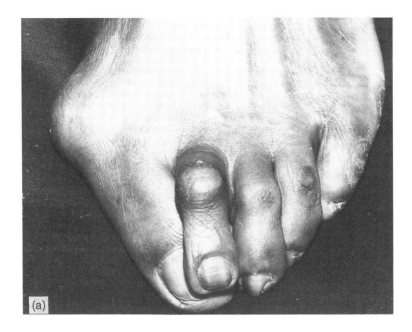

Figure 12 Hallux valgus (HV) deformities. (a) Hallux valgus, metatarsus primus varus (MPV), and hammered overlapping second toe. (From Ref. 3.)

Briefly, orthopedic shoes are well-made leather shoes with supportive lace-ups about the midfoot and are constructed to allow the addition of corrections and modifications. Thus the soles have thick leather sufficient enough to permit the addition of a metatarsal bar or a metatarsal rocker bar. The prescriber must order specifically what the patient needs. If there is a bunion, a bunion last oxford should be ordered. If there is a wide forefoot associated with the bunion (splay foot), the shoes must be wide at the ball. This will accommodate a tailor's bunion over the fifth metatarsal head. If there are hammer toes, a high toe box shoe must be ordered. With vascular impairment, a soft leather upper, or wool-lined slipper shoe, may be all that can be tolerated. If there is a draining sinus over the bunion or dorsally over a hammer toe, the patient must cut out an old shoe over the area of involvement. No local pressure is permitted and, usually, it takes 6–8 weeks to heal. In many

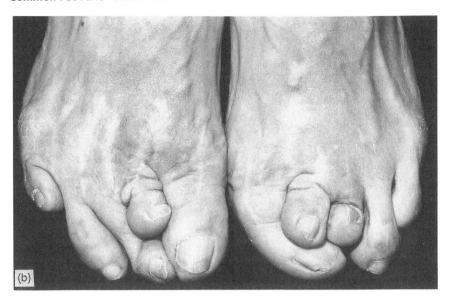

Figure 12 (Continued.) (b) Hallux valgus secondary to iatrogenic insufficient support by the second toe. (From Ref. 3.)

instances, a well-padded jogging sneaker may be more satisfactory than an orthopedic shoe. Men's sneakers are rounder and roomier in the toe box and may be excellent for both young and old women with wide forefeet and square wide toes. Numerous commercially made ortho-digital protective and shielding devices are available and may be helpful (Fig. 13).

When the deformities are severe, commercial shoes are inadequate. At this point, custom-molded shoes are required. Since the shoes are custom made, they will adapt to any severe deformity. They are best made so that adjustments are feasible. Shoe and orthotic corrections for anterior metatarsalgia are discussed in Section IX.

IX. THE METATARSALS

Anterior metatarsalgia is the most common complaint encountered in the foot in the elderly. It is static in nature due to unequal weightbearing

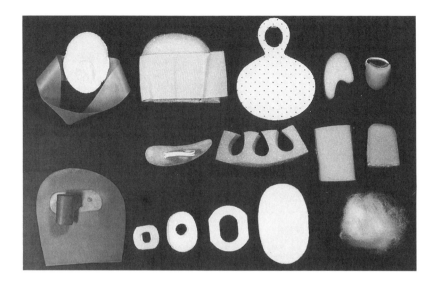

Figure 13 Orthodigital supports and shields. Top row: bunion shield, removable metatarsal pads, and toe shields. Middle row: toe crest (fits under the toes and helps end corns), toe separator, toe sleeve, and toe cap. Lower row: Budin splint (for hammer toe), toe and exostosis shields, and lamb's wool. (From Ref. 3.)

under the metatarsal heads with excess force being exerted most frequently under the more rigid metatarsals, namely, the second and third. Often it is aggravated by atrophy of the normally protective metatarsal fat pads. It must be differentiated from pain simulating anterior metatarsalgia. The pathomechanics of weightbearing under the foot and metatarsal heads has been discussed. In general, foot pain is very accurately localized, including point tenderness which facilitates differential diagnosis. In reiterating the differential diagnosis of anterior metatarsalgia, as noted in examination of the foot and ankle: excess weightbearing under a prominent metatarsal head causes local hyperkeratosis or callus formation. If there is no callus but the tenderness is $\frac{3}{16}$ in. distal to the head under the joint capsule, passive joint motion is painful and the toe is swollen and beginning to hammer, the diagnosis is a synovitis of the metatarsophalangeal joint. Approximately 30% of isolated synovitis of the second MTP, usually due to hallux valgus and/or hallux interphalangeus, is misdiagnosed as a plantar neuroma. With plantar neuromas, the tenderness is localized plantarward deep in the web space. In addition, the history is classic; pain on walking and relieved by sitting down and taking off the shoe. In my experience, plantar neuromas are not common in the elderly. In addition, they very rarely occur in blacks. Burning pain under the metatarsals is found with metatarsal fat pad atrophy and, rarely, as erythromelalgia in the elderly.

Surgical relief of localized pain under a prominent metatarsal head is not particularly reliable. Even conservative surgical corrections by metatarsal osteotomy may result in overcorrection with weightbearing transfer to an adjacent metatarsal. Nonunion of the osteotomy also may occur. In general, especially in the presence of metatarsal fat pad atrophy, conservative treatment in the form of shoe corrections and orthotics, offers the most reliable relief. If one considers simple weight-bearing distribution, the shoe/sneaker and orthotic prescription become logical. Weightbearing should be on soft surfaces. In addition, weight-bearing should be taken away from the area of excessive pressure and added to areas of minimal or no pressure, such as the medial longitudinal arch (12). The simplest correction for anterior metatarsal pain is a low-heeled rubber wedgie shoe or sneaker plus a metatarsal pad placed proximal to the middle metatarsal heads. Instead of a metatarsal pad, a Denver heel may be used which is a leather bar nailed to the outersole just proximal to the metatarsal heads. In many instances, the associated toe deformities and anterior metatarsalgia are too advanced for these mild corrections. In these cases, an extra-depth rubber wedgie shoe/ sneaker should be ordered along with a moderate density custom-molded polyethylene full-length orthotic. With diabetes and rheumatoid arthritis, a soft density should be used. Since this type of soft orthotic is compressible, it must be made thick enough to be effective; hence the need for the extra-depth shoewear. The orthotic is usually $\frac{3}{16}$ to $\frac{1}{4}$-in. thick and incorporates a metatarsal raise, a longitudinal arch, and "wells" or depressions under the offending calluses. If the callus is predominantly under the first metatarsal head, a sesamoid pad should be substituted for the metatarsal pad. With severe deformities, extra-depth shoewear will not be sufficient because they are not deep enough to accommodate severe hammer toes and very prominent bunions plus the orthotic. In such cases, a custom-molded shoe is the treatment of choice along with the thick, soft custom-molded removable orthotic (Fig. 14).

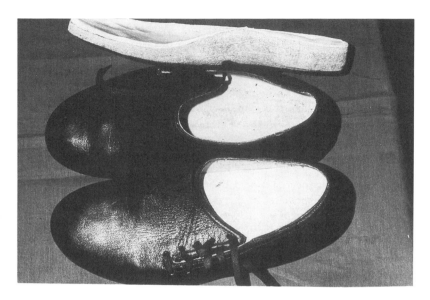

Figure 14 Custom-molded shoe. The shoes are deep enough to contain thick, soft polyethylene foam custom-molded orthotics and any hammer toes. Rubber wedgies disperse and lessen ground impact. The shoes are laced on the side to avoid any dorsal prominences. (From Ref. 3.)

X. LISFRANC'S JOINT AND THE MIDTAURUS

Minor problems involving Lisfranc's joint (tarso–metatarsal joints) are much more frequent in the elderly due to progressive osteoarthritis of this joint (8). Usually it starts and predominates in the first metatarsal medial cuneiform joint. This joint gradually becomes thicker dorsally, medially, and, ultimately, plantarward where the bony prominence becomes painful on weightbearing (Fig. 15). To a lesser extent, the arthritis tends to spread laterally across Lisfranc's joint. Similar changes may be present on the opposite foot. Subtalar motions are not involved; the foot moves normally. This osteoarthritis may occur secondary to an old unrecognized (often untreated) Lisfranc fracture-subluxation. The bony proliferation should be differentiated from a diabetic Charcot joint, which is most common in this location. Treatment may involve excision of a painful prominence or excision with arthrodesis. In most cases, relief is

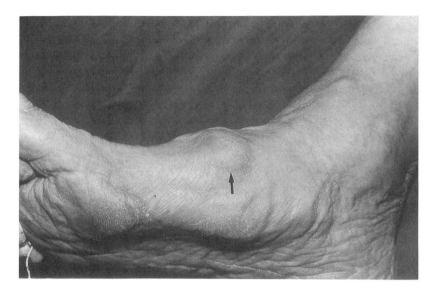

Figure 15 Osteoarthritis of the first metatarsal medial cuneiform joint. (From Ref. 3.)

obtained conservatively via appropriate shoes and orthotics since this condition is not too painful.

XI. THE HINDFOOT AND ANKLE

Disorders of the hindfoot are relatively common in the elderly and basically involve spontaneous tendon ruptures, especially the tibialis posterior and plantar or, occasionally, posterior heel pain. Degenerative subtalar arthritis secondary to pes planus is surprisingly mild. Similarly, spontaneous ankle osteoarthritis is relatively rare unless there has been prior hindfoot or ankle fracture.

With respect to plantar heel pain, it is more frequently located in the midplantar heel where palpable atrophy is present and the underlying calcaneal surface is more apparent (see Fig. 1). In younger patients, the tenderness usually is more distally and medially under the medial calcaneal tubercle, although elderly patients may also have pain in this area. X-rays are not helpful, since a plantar heel spur may be present without pain or pain may exist without the spur. The plantar heel pain is not too severe in the elderly, perhaps because of decreased activities, slower cadence, and less forceful heel strike. Many patients wear sneakers or rubber-soled wedgies or hard orthotics, all of which are not helpful and probably detrimental. Many etiologies have been postulated or appear to be related to plantar heel pain. The most familiar to rheumatologists is rheumatoid arthritis and seronegative disorders where fluffy periostitis and subcortical erosions may be present on x-ray. This is rare and more common diagnoses are plantar fasciitis, anterior calcaneal bursa, nerve entrapment of the medial calcaneal nerve or of the nerve to the abductor digiti quinti. In either case, treatment is conservative and the same regardless of the possible etiology. The heel is unloaded. Low heels, rubber wedgie shoes, and sneakers all tend to throw the weight-bearing posteriorly, thereby aggravating the condition. Soft heels accentuate heel weightbearing. While heel cups may offer some relief, they are most often insufficient. The most reliable conservative shoe modification is called the Steindler heel spur correction. It consists of ordering an orthopedic oxford with a long medial counter and scaphoid. This exerts pressure under the arch and lessens heel pressure. The heel in the shoe is gouged out and filled with sponge rubber. Finally, both heels are elevated posteriorly $\frac{3}{16}$ of an inch to throw weight more on the forefoot (Fig. 16). In most cases, relief is obtained in 6–8 weeks. The shoe should be worn at least 3 months or as long as necessary. Surgical intervention is rarely necessary. Cortisone injections are not advisable as they may cause atrophy and anti-inflammatory medication is ineffective. Pain in the the back of the calcaneus occurs in middle and old age and may be associated with posterior heel spurs, Achilles bursitis, or a "pump bump." The latter is painful enlargement of the posterior superior process of the calcaneus. However, it occurs more frequently in younger age groups. Treatment consists of the use of soft heel counters, open heels, and/or $\frac{3}{16}$-in. posterior heel elevations.

The second most common, and most disabling, hindfoot condition is tendon rupture about the ankle, especially the tibialis posterior. This has been detailed in Section V.

Stiff, painful hindfeet secondary to old, congenital deformities with superimposed surgery, such as club foot, may have secondary osteoarthritis of the subtalar joint and/or ankle. Old trauma involving the hindfoot and ankle also may lead to stiff painful hindfeet. Arthrodesis may be needed. Total ankle joint replacement has not been perfected as of this time. Conservative management is to immobilize the hindfoot

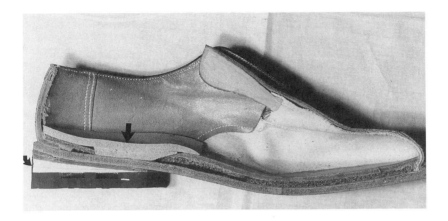

Figure 16   Sagittal section of a shoe revealing the Steindler heel spur correction. (From Ref. 6.)

and substitute a rolling forward motion for the stiff hindfoot and ankle joints. This consists of the use of high-top shoes or sneakers plus posterior pitched heels with a long sole rocker on the affected side.

XII. TRAUMA TO THE FOOT AND ANKLE

Fractures of the foot and ankle, in most instances, are treated by open reduction and internal fixation to obtain anatomic reduction in order to avoid late traumatic arthrosis. Mild fractures, such as those involving the calcaneus, without joint involvement, or occasionally the lateral malleolus or styloid process of the fifth metatarsal usually do not require surgery. On the other hand, seemingly mild fractures and injuries may be more serious than they appear clinically or on x-ray. A stress x-ray of the ankle or Lisfranc joint may indicate sufficient instability to warrant surgery. Similarly, a CAT scan done on a seemingly innocuous hindfoot fracture may reveal unsuspected joint injury requiring major reconstruction.

XIII. THE RHEUMATOID AND SERONEGATIVE FOOT

Inflammatory arthritis, in the past, was limited to rheumatoid arthritis, but during the past 10 years seronegative disorders have taken equal or more prominence, especially with respect to foot involvement (1). To this may be added Lyme disease and HIV infection, which cause similar symptoms. Seronegative disorders, Lyme disease, and HIV infections as related to the foot frequently are overlooked. Lyme disease is not as prevalent in the elderly and HIV is relatively rare.

Seronegative arthritis is approximately three times as common as rheumatoid arthritis in the experience of the orthopedic foot surgeon, but with the exception of psoriatic arthritis, are uncommon in older adults.

The seronegative diseases (especially psoriasis) commonly involve ankle tendons, most frequently the tibialis posterior. Except for psoriasis, joint involvement is minimal. In psoriasis, the forefoot is mainly involved (14,16). It may simulate rheumatoid arthritis or may exhibit more psoriatic joint changes (Fig. 17). The deformities are managed either conservatively and/or surgically. The main deformities are severe stiff hallux valgus, metatarsus primus varus, advanced rigid hammer toes, and anterior metatarsalgia.

Rheumatoid arthritis invariably involves the feet and tends to be bilaterally symmetric (Fig. 18). Tendons are involved much less frequently. Most patients with long-standing rheumatoid arthritis become quite stoic and readily tolerate their severe bunions, hallux valgus, and hammer toes by purchasing more comfortable and forgiving shoes or sneakers. However, as the deformities progress and the metatarsal fat pads atrophy, unrelenting painful anterior metatarsalgia develops with tender bony metatarsal heads being palpable just under the plantar skin (Fig. 19). In spite of adequate shoes and orthotics, they are unable to walk more than three or four blocks without pain. Now is the time to excise the metatarsal heads (Hoffmann operation) which, with appropriate shoe wear, once again makes ambulation bearable. In the earlier stages, before the painful anterior metatarsalgia develops, extra depth shoes or sneakers with soft, thick, polyethylene foam custom-molded orthotics offer considerable relief. Ultimately, with severe deformities, the shoes must be custom made along with the orthotics. Surgery on the hallux valgus is not necessary except for a simple exostectomy–bunionectomy to relieve the large sharp exostoses that will not fit comfortably into a shoe. Similarly, hammer toes rarely need correction. In addition, due to small vessel disease, which is often present, plus poor local soft tissues, small toe surgery may lead to local gangrene. When the Hoffmann procedure is done, simple manipulation of the small toes will straighten them due to the very soft underlying bones that freely "give" without any sequelae.

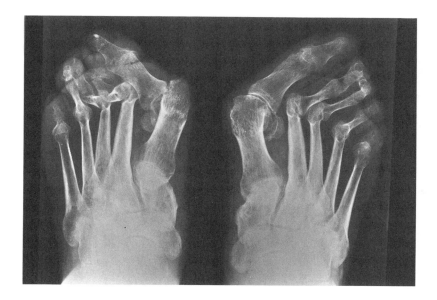

Figure 17 Psoriatic arthritis of feet with mixed psoriatic and rheumatoid changes. The osteoporosis is more typical of rheumatoid arthritis as well as involvement of the MTP joints. The spontaneous fusion of the right second PIP joint combined with tuft absorption and pencil and cup deformity of the left fifth MTP joint is found with psoriatic arthritis. The dislocation of the left hallux may be found with either type of arthritis. (From Ref. 3.)

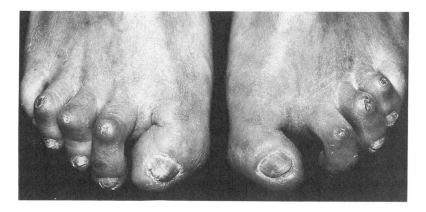

Figure 18 Rheumatoid arthritis involving all the toes with small toe hammering and hallux interphalangeus.

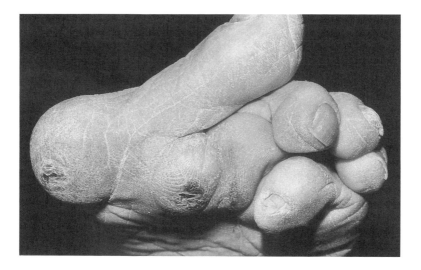

Figure 19 Advanced stage of rheumatoid forefoot involvement. The hallux is fixed in valgus and extension while the small toes have varying types and degrees of fixed hammering. Of greater significance is the severe depression of the metatarsal heads appearing just under the skin. There is severe atrophy of the metatarsal fat pads and calluses under the prominent metatarsal heads. (From Ref. 3.)

The second most common surgical need is a triple arthrodesis for severe and painful hindfoot involvement, which in most cases is associated with advanced hindfoot valgus. Total ankle joints, while working best on the rheumatoid patient, have not proven satisfactory in long-term followup.

XIV. METABOLIC DISORDERS INVOLVING THE FOOT

The most common metabolic disorder involving the foot is gout, which may be primary or secondary to chronic renal disease, or antihypertensive medicines. The classic example is acute gout involving the first MTP joint. In more severe cases, gouty tophi may destroy the joint along with draining tophaceous sinuses (Fig. 20). In acute gout, the onset is within hours, and the joint is extremely tender and very painful

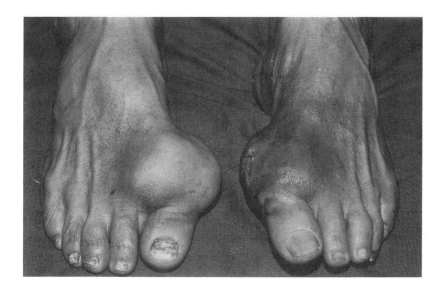

Figure 20 Advanced gouty tophaceous arthritis of the first MTP joints with draining sinuses on the right. There was severe joint destruction on x-rays. (From Ref. 3.)

on motion. Treatment is medical, and the best results are obtained with very early treatment.

Many other medical disorders affect the foot and ankle, including blood dyscrasias and even porphyria, which, ultimately, are diagnosed by extensive medical workup.

XV. THE DYSVASCULAR FOOT

The dysvascular foot may occur without any other foot problems or may occur in combination with all of the previously mentioned foot pathology. When considering any foot surgery, especially in the elderly, vascular consultation is advisable even in the presence of normal pedal pulses. The vascularity of the foot is normally limited with poor subcutaneous tissue and limited underlying vascular muscle. For example, even in young healthy patients, surgery on the heel cord has a 20% incidence of soft tissue and skin complications.

XVI. THE DIABETIC FOOT

The problems with the diabetic foot are unique and consist of small vessel disease, large vessel disease, and peripheral neuropathy with its sequelae (13). Insulin-dependent diabetes is more severe, occurs at earlier ages, and exhibits the neurovascular complications earlier along with life-threatening systemic complications.

Small vessel disease involving the foot is invariably present. The extent of vessel involvement may be appreciated on routine x-rays of the foot (Fig. 21). This small vessel disease is responsible for local foot infarcts with limited necrosis, ulcers, and infection. Prompt debride-

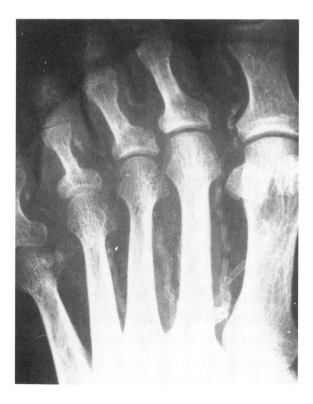

Figure 21   Diabetic sclerosis of the intermetatarsal and digital arteries as seen on routine x-rays. (From Ref. 3.)

ment, local care, antibiotics and, if necessary, limited resections, such as a toe, may be necessary. The rest of the foot may be surprisingly viable with brisk bleeding.

It must be stressed that the diabetic foot frequently has associated large vessel disease with a poor prognosis. This must be ruled out in cases of poor healing or any pending surgery, however minor. The presence of pedal pulses or even Doppler readings may be misleading. The development of a spontaneous trophic ulcer, or a pending ulcer with hemorrhage and swelling under a skin pressure area, or a subungual infection mandates the consideration of diabetes. If the pain is too minimal in association with the objective findings, peripheral neuropathy should be ruled out as well. To perform ingrown toenail surgery without vascular workup may lead to gangrene. On the other hand, surgical revascularization of the foot abets ulcer and soft tissue healing, may avoid amputation or, at least, minimize the level of amputation and increase the success rate for needed minor surgery, including debridement and skin grafting (10).

One major foot problem is peripheral neuropathy. With increase in the life span of diabetic patients, peripheral neuropathy is encountered more frequently, especially with insulin-dependent diabetics of more than 10 years history. Subjective symptoms may be minimal. In most cases, rapid presumptive diagnosis is made by noting decreased or absent vibratory sense in the feet using a 128 VPS tuning fork. Peripheral neuropathy is often manifested by mild tingling or numbness in the toes associated with soft tissue (intrinsic muscles) and fat pad atrophy of the soles of the feet. Commonly, there is present a relatively pain-free trophic ulcer due to the small vessel disease and neuropathy. Peripheral neuropathy is complicated not only by trophic ulcers, but eventually by Charcot feet.

With respect to stroke patients with spastic equinovarus and claw toes, appropriate gait training rehabilitation and bracing is necessary (15). Tendon surgery may be advisable, namely tibialis anterior transfer (SPLATT procedure) for the equinovarus, and flexor tenotomies for the claw toes. In the elderly, poliomyelitis may be encountered occasionally, but usually surgery and bracing were done in childhood, and treatment is now limited to appropriate light-weight shoe wear and soft orthotics. Peripheral nerve injury may occur secondary to total joint surgery of the hip or knee. It usually consists of foot drop from sciatic or peroneal nerve injury, often with spontaneous recovery. Peripheral neuropathy has been discussed in relation to diabetes. Atrophy of the soles of the feet, including the intrinsic muscles and fat pads, is found in association with peripheral neuropathy. Secondary plantar ulceration is common.

Pain emanating from discogenic disease or spinal stenosis is seen very frequently in middle and older age. In addition, spinal stenosis may simulate intermittent claudication and/or sciatica. Lumbar radiculopathy frequently presents itself as pain over the dorsolateral aspect of the lower leg or foot (S1 nerve distribution) with minimal or no low back symptoms. There may be vague pains, tingling, or numbness going into the toes. MRI of the low back usually confirms the diagnosis.

Finally, we come to neurosis and anxiety, which are very common in relation to foot pain and disability. Approximately 15 % of my patients exhibit anxiety, neuroses, or conversion hysteria in regard to their feet. They present themselves with a list of vague nonanatomical complaints and often repeated prior unsuccessful surgical foot operations. In addition, they bring with them bags of shoes, shoe corrections, and orthotics and ask to have them examined and discussed. Most of these patients have normal feet on examination or complain about questionable or miniscule findings in their feet. Extensive objective workup invariably is negative.

REFERENCES

1. Calin A. Spondylarthropathies. Orlando, FL: Grune & Stratton, Inc., 1984.
2. Evanski PM. The geriatric foot. In Jahss MH (ed.), Disorders of the Foot and Ankle: Medical and Surgical Management, 2nd ed. Philadelphia: WB Saunders Co, 1991: 1643–1653.
3. Gibbs R. Skin Diseases of the Feet. St. Louis: Warren H Green, 1974.
4. Gould N. Shoes and shoe modifications. In Jahss MH (ed.), Disorders of the Foot and Ankle: Medical and Surgical Management. Philadelphia: WB Saunders Co, 1991: 2879–2920.
5. Jahss MH. Examination. In Jahss MH (ed.). Disorders of the Foot and Ankle: Medical and Surgical Management. Philadelphia: WB Saunders Co., 1991: 35–51.
6. Jahss MH. Shoes and shoe modifications. In American Academy of Orthopedic Surgeons, Atlas of Orthotics. St. Louis: CV Mosby, 1975: 267–279.
7. Jahss MH. Tendon disorders of the foot and ankle. In Jahss MH (ed.). Disorders of the Foot and Ankle: Medical and Surgical Management. Philadelphia: WB Saunders Co, 1991: 1461–1513.
8. Jahss MH. Geriatric aspects of the foot and ankle. In Rossman I (ed.), Clinical Geriatrics, 2nd ed. Philadelphia: JB Lippincott Co, 1979: 638–650.

9. Jahss MH. The plantigrade foot. In Frankel VH (ed.), Instructional Course Lectures, American Academy of Orthopedic Surgeons, St. Louis: CV Mosby, 1982: 200–217.
10. Kaufman JL, Leather RP. Vascular diseases of the foot. In Jahss MH (ed.). Disorders of the Foot and Ankle: Medical and Surgical Management. Philadelphia: WB Saunders Co, 1992: 1787–1827.
11. Mann RA. Biomechanics of the foot. In American Academy of Orthopaedic Surgeons, Atlas or Orthotics, 2nd ed. St. Louis: CV Mosby Co, 1985.
12. Milgram JE. Padding and devices to relieve painful feet. In Jahss MH (ed.). Disorders of the Foot and Ankle: Medical and Surgical Management. Philadelphia: WB Saunders Co, 1992: 2834–2878.
13. Sammarco GJ. The Foot in Diabetes. Philadelphia: Lea & Febiger, 1991.
14. Sherman MS. Psoriatic arthritis. Observations on the clinical, roentgenographic and pathological changes. J Bone Joint Surg 1952; 34A:831–852.
15. Water RL, Garland DE. Disorders of the lower extremity in the stroke and head trauma patient. In Jahss MH (ed.). Disorders of the Foot and Ankle: Medical and Surgical Management. Philadelphia: WB Saunders Co, 1992: 1117–1121.
16. Wright V. Psoriatic arthritis. A comparative radiographic study of rheumatoid arthritis and arthritis associated with psoriasis. Ann Rheum Dis 1961, 20:123–132.

10

Adverse Effects of Medications on Gait and Mobility in the Elderly

DENNIS J. CHAPRON
School of Pharmacy, University of Connecticut, Storrs, and University of Connecticut Health Center, Farmington, Connecticut

Physicians and other health-care providers must be ever vigilant for potential adverse effects that certain medications can have on gait and mobility in their elderly patients. The elderly appear to be particularly vulnerable to drug-induced gait disorders. Aging per se has been shown to increase postural sway and slow its support responses as well as impair the integration of sensory information (1). From a pharmacological point of view, advanced age has been shown to impair the body's ability to metabolize or excrete numerous medications, thereby augmenting and prolonging their effects (2,3). Aging organ systems may also respond in an exaggerated manner to even normal serum concentrations of certain medications. Furthermore, the polymorbidities (arthritis, Parkinson's disease, symptomatic osteopenia) that commonly occur with advancing age can have an adverse impact on mobility. Thus the triad of sluggish or maladaptive control systems for maintaining balance, increased propensity for exaggerated drug effects, and increased prevalance of disabling pathology make the elderly uniquely susceptible to drug-induced gait disorders. It is not surprising that the use of certain drugs or polypharmacy has been shown to be an independent risk factor for falling episodes in this age group (4–6).

Drugs can be the sole cause of a new-onset gait disorder or they may exacerbate a preexisting problem. Drug-induced mobility disorders may reflect the noxious effects of a single medication or may point to a synergism between certain drug combinations. Accompanying complaints of dizziness, lightheadedness, stiffness or weakness, falling episodes, difficulty in initiating movement, and unsteadiness in a setting of polypharmacy should immediately alert the attending physician to the possibility that a drug may indeed be the culprit. These adverse drug responses are almost always reversible and provide for a great deal of gratification for the physician who discovers them and for the patient who is relieved of their effects.

Drugs potentially involved in iatrogenic gait disorders represent diverse pharmacological classes making a physiological systems approach a logical and facile way of investigating this problem. Figure 1 displays some common physiological systems which, when purturbed by medications, can result in problems of gait and mobility. A comprehensive description of selected drugs involved follows.

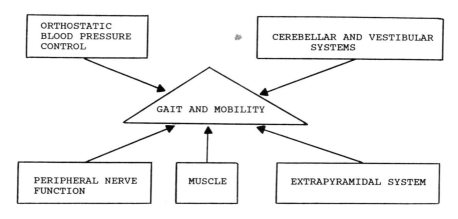

Figure 1   Selected physiological systems that may be compromised by medication and result in problems with gait and mobility.

I. POSTURAL HYPOTENSION

Sudden and significant drops in standing blood pressure can lead to decreased perfusion of the brain with subsequent impairment of balance control and consciousness. Most patients do not experience syncope but commonly complain of lightheadedness. Postural hypotension, a drop in systolic blood pressure of 20 mm Hg or more as determined 1 min after standing, is a common finding in the elderly with a prevalence ranging from 6–33% (7). The lowest prevalence is found in healthy, normotensive, community-dwelling elderly, whereas much higher prevalences are seen in patients with polymorbidities who take several medications, both of which may perturb standing blood pressure. An age-related impairment of baroreflex responses primarily accounts for these findings in healthy elderly individuals (8).

Hypertension, a problem common in the elderly, appears to interact with the aging process and results in a further decrement in baroreflex function (8). In the elderly hypertensive, cerebral autoregulation may also be less efficient, such that even a modest fall in standing blood pressure may inordinately decrease cerebral blood flow. Patients with an underlying brain disorder (i.e., prior stroke) are also probably more likely to manifest symptomatic postural hypotension.

Arterial blood pressure is dependent upon the product of cardiac output and peripheral vascular resistance. Symptomatic postural hypotension can occur with sudden drops in cardiac output or peripheral vascular resistance, or both. Specifically, cardiac output may be reduced by decreases in heart rate or stroke volume, the latter governed by venous return and contractile force. Since 70–80% of the blood volume is contained on the venous side, rapid changes in its capacitance will significantly influence the volume of blood returning to the heart. Blood volume is also an important determinant of venous return and is significantly influenced by the hydration status of the patient. In assuming an upright position, gravitational forces lower blood pressure, primarily by pooling blood in the peripheral venous system. Baroreflex mechanisms are quickly activated with standing to increase arterial and venous tone, heart rate, and contractility.

Medications can act detrimentally at every locus involved in the regulatory mechanisms that maintain upright blood pressure. It is easy to imagine an elderly patient receiving a certain combination of drugs wherein each medication mildly interferes with blood pressure regulation at a particular locus, and the sum of these small actions results in a major episode of symptomatic postural hypotension.

Furthermore, numerous studies in healthy or institutionalized elderly have shown significant postprandial reductions in blood pressure (9). In patients with documented postprandial hypotension, it seems reasonable to avoid administering medications that tend to abruptly lower blood pressure on a schedule that is close to meal times.

A. Tricyclic Antidepressants

The most common and serious complication of tricyclic antidepressant therapy is orthostatic hypotension. This hypotensive effect is thought to be principally mediated by competitive inhibition of peripheral α_1 receptors leading to inefficient reflex vasoconstriction of arterioles and capacitance vessels (10). Drops in standing blood pressure usually occur early in treatment, at subtherapeutic doses or plasma levels, and often persist for the duration of treatment. This adverse effect has been noted in several clinical investigations to significantly limit the therapeutic potential of this class of antidepressants. The dual effects of tricyclic antidepressant-induced orthostasis and excess sedation probably accounts for the recently discovered finding that persons 65 years of age and older have a 60% increased risk of hip fracture while receiving tricyclic antidepressants (11). In another study, four fractures occurred in 20% of patients who experienced prolonged dizziness, ataxia, and falls while on imipramine (12).

The incidence of clinically significant postural hypotension varies according to the specific drug and the presence of underlying cardiovascular disease. Imipramine was stopped because of symptomatic hypotension in 7% of patients with normal pretreatment electrocardiograms compared to 32% of patients with cardiac conduction defects (13). In the same study, nortriptyline caused no serious problems with hypotension in patients with a normal pretreatment electrocardiogram while in those individuals with abnormalities only 5% required discontinuation of therapy. For the tricyclic class of antidepressants the tertiary amines (imipramine, amitriptyline, doxepin) produce the highest incidence of orthostatic hypotension while their demethylated derivatives (such secondary amines as desipramine and, especially, nortriptyline) produce considerably less. Dramatic orthostatic drops in blood pressure in the elderly may occur if treatment with a tricyclic antidepressant is initiated with a large dose (i.e., imipramine at 100 mg) instead of using a gradual incremental approach. Host factors that predispose to severe postural drops in blood pressure during treatment with tricyclic antidepressants include (1) the presence of cardiovascular disease; (2) concomitant treatment with other potentially hypotensive medications; and (3) the presence of pretreatment orthostatic falls in blood pressure. Age per se does not appear to be an independent risk factor for antidepressant-induced orthostasis, but certainly in the elderly all of the above host factors are more common.

The newer monocyclic (bupropion) and bicyclic (fluoxetine) antidepressants appear to be nearly devoid of any significant adverse effect on standing blood pressure, making these agents very useful in those elderly patients experiencing antidepressant-induced symptomatic postural hypotension or possessing host factors predisposing to such adverse events (14–16).

B. Antipsychotic Medications

As with the tricyclic antidepressants, postural hypotension is the most troublesome cardiovascular side effect of antipsychotic drugs. Certain of these medications can block peripheral α_1 receptors and this activity may, in part, account for their hypotensive action. This side effect has been more frequently observed with the low-potency antipsychotic drugs (chlorpromazine, thioridazine, mesoridazine) as compared to high-potency agents (e.g., haloperidol, fluphenazine). Despite the widespread use of antipsychotic drugs and their early introduction into clinical medicine (the first clinical trial of chlorpromazine in the U.S. was in 1954!), very few studies have systematically investigated drug and host factors predisposing patients to clinically significant postural hypotension. One investigation in the elderly did demonstrate the occurrence of much greater orthostatic responses during treatment with thioridazine compared to the small blood pressure changes noted with fluphenazine (17). If the occurrence of postural hypotension is a worrisome consideration in a particular patient, a high-potency agent should be prescribed. Until more information becomes available it would be prudent to consider host factors that predispose to tricyclic antidepressant-induced orthostatic hypotension to be applicable to the low-potency antipsychotic drugs.

C. Levodopa and Bromocriptine

Early in its conception as a therapeutic agent, there was concern that the dopamine produced from the peripheral decarboxylation of large oral doses of levodopa would abruptly shock the cardiovascular system into episodes of hypertension and arrhythmias. To the contrary, levopoda did not cause or worsen arrhythmias and *hypo*tensive responses (including syncope) were observed.

Approximately 20–30% of patients experience a 20–30 mm Hg fall in systolic blood pressure during the initiation of levodopa therapy (18,19). In a study that followed 101 patients with Parkinson's disease for over 11 years, 22% experienced postural drops in blood pressure greater than 25 mm Hg (20). In many patients, tolerance to the hypotensive effects of levodopa appears to develop slowly over time with continuous treatment and, in some patients, symptomatic improvement without an objective improvement in standing blood pressures may also be observed.

The addition of a decarboxylase inhibitor does not appear to significantly alter the effects of levodopa on standing blood pressure (21). These findings may be interpreted in two ways. The central action of levodopa may be more critical than its peripheral effects or the threshold concentration for inducing postural hypotension via peripheral mechanisms may be quite low for dopamine. Despite the uncertainty of site of action, recent studies have shown that both levodopa and bromocriptine can attenuate the sympathetic response (i.e., norepinephrine release) to standing, such an effect being intimately linked with orthostatic blood pressure control (22). The direct-acting agonist, bromocriptine, can also provoke serious drops in standing blood pressure.

Postural hypotension occurs in untreated Parkinson's disease and recent studies in such patients have discovered a subset with autonomic dysfunction of the cardiovascular system (23). It is not known if this subset of patients is more vulnerable to the development of severe and symptomatic orthostatic hypotension with levodopa or direct-acting dopaminergic drugs.

D. Antihypertensive Medications

All antihypertensive drugs have the potential for inducing orthostatic hypotension. Fortunately, there are considerable differences between and within classes of antihypertensive agents in their propensity for causing this undesirable effect (these are listed in Table 1). Obviously, those agents with the highest risk should never be considered first-line treatment in elderly hypertensives. Furthermore, particular combinations of cardiovascular medications may predispose certain individuals to severe drops in blood pressure far beyond those expected assuming an

Table 1 Relative Risk of Serious Orthostatic Hypotension from
Antihypertensive Medications

Low	Moderate	High
Ace inhibitors	Alpha-adrenergic	Peripheral adrenergic
Beta blockers	receptor blockers	inhibitors
Calcium entry blockers[a]	Labetalol	Phenoxybenzamine[b]
Central alpha agonists		
Diuretics		
Hydralazine		

[a]Calcium entry blockers of the dihydropyridine type (nifedipine, nicardipine) are potent vasodilators and have been shown to provoke more orthostatic drops in blood pressure than other members in this class.
[b]This agent blocks α_1 receptors irreversibly and is rarely used as an antihypertensive agent; it is being used for the management of benign prostatic hyperplasia and external urinary sphincter disorders.

additive antihypertensive response. The administration of angiotensin-converting enzyme inhibitors to patients pretreated with a vigorous diuretic regimen has been associated with large drops in blood pressure (24). Bradycardia with hypotension has been observed with the combination of a calcium channel blocker and a beta blocker (25,26).

E. Diuretics

Diuretics act on the kidney to promote salt and water loss and there is no doubt that extracellular fluid depletion by these drugs is a common problem in the elderly that can result in the provocation of orthostatic symptoms. Volume depletion results in reduced left ventricular filling pressure and a fall in cardiac output. Studies in healthy elderly subjects have shown that sodium and volume depletion induced by short-term, large-dose (100 mg hydrochorothiazide), diuretic administration resulted in a significant drop in upright systolic blood pressure and an inadequate cardioacceleratory response (27). Several age-related factors increase the risk for diuretic-induced volume depletion and must be taken into account when these agents are prescribed for the elderly. Aging per se is associated with a reduced thirst sensation, a sluggish and suboptimal renin-angiotensin-aldosterone axis that functions as an antinatriuretic force, and a decreased urinary concentrating ability. Added to this risk-enhancing profile are common medical conditions that can result in volume depletion such as fever, vomiting, and diarrhea. Chronic and mild degrees of diuretic-induced volume depletion rarely produce orthostatic hypotension, but in the presence of other modest insults to blood pressure control, its contribution to postural symptoms can be critical. Mild and asymptomatic volume depletion by diuretics may be evidenced by disproportionate elevations in serum urea nitrogen relative to serum creatinine levels, increased serum uric acid concentrations, and a tendency toward water retention.

F. Nitrates

Organic nitrates are a well-recognized cause of postural hypotension. In a large study involving institutionalized elderly patients, nitrate medications were implicated in the majority (73%) of drug-induced cases of postural hypotension with syncope (28). Low doses of nitrates cause pronounced venodilatation, thus reducing venous return. Even with low doses, some arterial vasodilation is seen. Larger doses can cause drops in systolic blood pressure. In fact, a prolonged-release preparation of isosorbide dinitrate (20–40 mg twice daily) produced a selective and sustained decrease in systolic blood pressure in elderly patients with isolated systolic hypertension (29). No tolerance to the nitrate-induced drops in systolic pressure were noted to occur during this 12-week study.

The use of sublingual nitrates in patients who are immobile and upright at the time of administration may be particularly associated with an orthostatic hypotensive effect. All patients beginning nitrate treatment should be told to assume a supine position when the preparation is taken in order determine their susceptibility to its orthostatic effects. The risk of nitrate-induced hypotension may be increased by the concomitant use of other drugs, including (1) beta blockers, which depress sinus node function and may blunt or abolish reflex increases in heart rate that often accompany nitrate-induced vasodilation; (2) aggressive diuretic therapy, which can decrease circulating blood volume and hence potentiate nitrate-induced venous pooling; and (3) alcohol ingestion, which in moderate amounts has a direct vasodilating effect.

II. MYOPATHIES

Drug-induced myopathies are an uncommon cause of gait difficulties in the elderly. Drugs that have been implicated include chloroquine, clofibrate, gemfibrozil, glucocorticoids, kaliuretic diuretics (via their ability to induce significant hypokalemia), lithium, lovastatin, penicillamine, procainamide, and vincristine. Of this medley of medications, two deserve further comment. The highest incidence of drug-induced myopathies is seen with long-term glucocorticoid use. It is estimated to occur in about 7% of recipients (30). Steroid myopathy evolves slowly and often painlessly over time, is usually associated with muscle wasting, and commonly manifests as weakness of all extremities with the lower proximal regions being most affected. Although the risk of myopathy is considered greatest with fluorinated glucocorticoids, use of any steroid of this class should be suspect. Existing myopathies may be treated by tapering and discontinuing the glucocorticoid. Recovery of muscle function is usually seen within a month and can be helped by physical therapy. The propensity for steroid myopathy may be decreased by maintaining the patient on the lowest possible dose, instituting an alternate-day regimen, and participating in a program of daily exercises.

Lovastatin is probably the second most important drug to cause myopathy, with an estimated incidence of about 0.2% with monotherapy (31). Patients complain of muscle aches, tenderness, and weakness. Serum creatinine kinase levels are elevated, but without evidence of inflammation. An apparent synergistic interaction between lovastatin and gemfibrozil has been observed resulting in a nearly 25-fold increase in the incidence of myopathy when compared to lovastatin alone (32). With this combination, there are also numerous case reports of a diffuse, severe myopathy with rhabdomyolysis and, in some individuals, renal failure (33–36). In one study, 8 of 12 such cases were elderly women, which raises questions concerning the benefit versus risk in this age group of pharmacological interventions for lipid abnormalities (33, 36). Furthermore, the risk of lovastatin-induced myopathy appears to be increased with concomitant use of cyclosporin, erythromycin, or nicotinic acid (31, 37).

III. PERIPHERAL NEUROPATHIES

Drug-induced peripheral neuropathies as a cause of gait dysfunction in the elderly are rare. Numerous drugs have been shown to cause neuropathies, including amiodarone, cisplatin, dapsone, disulfiram, ethambutol, hydralazine, isoniazid, metronidazole, nitrofurantoin, phenytoin, procarbazine, and the vinca alkloids.

IV. DRUG-INDUCED PARKINSONISM

Many of the cardinal features of Parkinson's disease, i.e., rigidity, brady-kinesia, and postural instability, are well-recognized for their detrimental impact on gait and mobility. Drug-induced parkinsonism (DIP) can have a similar impact. Besides inducing a parkinsonian state, certain medications may also aggravate preexisting Parkinson's disease. It is important to note that DIP is clinically indistinguishable from idiopathic Parkinson's disease. Because parkinsonism-provoking drugs distribute symmetrically to the brain, the distribution of symptomatology with DIP is nearly always symmetrical in appearance.

Any drug that can interfere with dopamine neuronal uptake, storage, release, and receptor activation can produce DIP. Medications that enhance central acetylcholine activity usually do not induce DIP, but can exacerbate preexisting Parkinson's disease. Table 2 lists important medications known to cause parkinsonism or aggravate Parkinson's disease.

Antipsychotic drugs rank as the most important cause of DIP. The time interval between drug administration and the development of DIP is about 4 weeks, although much longer or shorter intervals may be observed. These medications block striatal dopamine receptors and their propensity to induce parkinsonism seems to be directly correlated to their potency as antipsychotic agents. Clinical reports have emphasized the importance of these drugs as a significant cause of parkin-

Table 2   Drugs That Can Induce Parkinsonism or Aggravate Parkinson's Disease and Their Mechanism of Effect

Drug	Mechanism of Effect
Amoxapine[a]	Blockade of dopamine receptors
Antipyschotics	Blockade of dopamine receptors
Alpha-Methyldopa	Inhibits dopamine synthesis
Metoclopramide[b]	Blockade of dopamine receptors
Papaverine	? Blockade of dopamine receptors
Prochlorperazine[c]	Blockade of dopamine receptors
Reserpine	Inhibits dopamine storage

[a]An active metabolite, 7-hydroxy-amoxapine, is responsible for this effect.
[b]The risk of DIP may be increased in patients with kidney dysfunction since a substantial component of its clearance is renal.
[c]A phenothiazine drug used primarily as an antiemetic and is reported to be a common cause of DIP in the elderly.

sonism in the elderly and indicate a predisposition in this age group to this adverse effect as well (38–40). The much greater frequency of DIP in the elderly may be attributed to an age-related decline in nigral cell counts, tyrosine hydroxylase activity, dopamine levels, and its D_2 receptor (41, 42), thus facilitating the ability of certain medications to disrupt an already compromised system to the threshold for symptom appearance.

Optimal treatment of DIP usually requires discontinuation of the antipsychotic medication. Recovery from symptoms, however, may not occur quickly and a protacted course of recovery may be observed. In a large study of 48 elderly patients with DIP, Stephen and Williamson (39) found that with remedial measures (i.e., usually stopping the offending drug) only 66% of these cases resolved and required on average 7 weeks for symptom abatement. Eleven percent of their patients still had symptoms despite stopping the medication, and an equal number later developed idiopathic Parkinson's disease despite a good initial response to drug discontinuation. The latter two findings suggest that subclinical Parkinson's disease may have been present in these patients prior to antipsychotic drug therapy. The prolonged recovery phase seen in the majority of elderly patients with DIP may be due to the high affinity of antipsychotic agents for dopamine receptors in the brain, such that a disequilibrium exists between brain and blood drug concentrations, with brain drug levels persisting far longer than those in blood.

Because DIP is a serious threat to mobility and to safety of gait, the indications for continued use of the offending medication must be thoroughly reevaluated and alternative therapies considered. When parkinsonian symptoms emerge during antipsychotic drug therapy, several measures can be taken to reduce or eliminate these potentially debilitating drug effects. If symptoms are mild, they may disappear within a few months despite continued treatment. Often the dose of antipsychotic drug is reduced with a consequent reduction in parkinsonian symptoms. Alternatively, a low-potency antipsychotic medication (thioridazine) may be substituted for a high-potency agent (i.e., haloperidol, perphenazine, fluphenazine, thiothixine). Although studies in the elderly have shown that low-potency agents induce significantly less rigidity than high-potency drugs (17), there are still numerous reports of thioridazine causing severe parkinsonian reactions in this age group (39,40). Centrally acting anticholinergic drugs may be used if dosage reduction or changing to a lower potency agent fails to relieve troublesome parkinsonian symptoms. Agents such as benzotropine or trihexyphenydyl are remarkably effective for treating antipsychotic drug-induced parkinsonism. Prescribing anticholinergic drugs as routine prophylaxis of anticipated DIP in the elderly is not recommended since this side effect does not occur in all patients who receive antipsychotic agents. Furthermore, because prolonged administration of anticholinergic drugs may increase the risk of developing tardive dyskinesias, they should be gradually withdrawn after 3 months of use in order to determine if drug-induced parkinsonism has subsided spontaneously.

Unfortunately, the elderly are more prone to developing serious side effects from anticholinergic drug therapy; these include confusion, delirium, urinary retention, obstipation, and esophagitis (43). If an elderly patient cannot tolerate an anticholinergic drug or has a preexisting medical condition that may be exacerbated by cholinergic blockade, then a trial with amantadine should be considered. This drug is thought to facilitate the release of striatial dopamine and has little or no anticholinergic activity. Amantadine is, however, excreted solely by renal routes (glomerular filtration and tubular secretion) and its dosage must be adjusted downward in the elderly. Most recently, clozapine, an "atypical" antipsychotic drug (i.e., lacking extrapyramidal side effects), has proved to be an effective medication in treating psychosis in Parkinson's disease without exacerbating motor function or requiring an adjustment in antiparkinsonian therapy (44).

V. ATAXIA

Problems with balance and gait may result from drug-induced ataxia. Such a reaction may be ascribed to toxic drug effects on the cerebellum, vestibulosensory, or proprioceptive control systems. High degrees of drug-induced sedation may also produce an ataxic syndrome due to decreased cortical awareness of head and body motion and position. Numerous drugs have been implicated as causes of ataxia, including alcohol, aminoglycoside antibiotics, anticonvulsants, benzodiazepines, minocycline, nonsteroidal anti-inflammatory drugs, and quinidine. From this list benzodiazepines and anticonvulsants need further elaboration because of their high use in the elderly and their large propensity for producing ataxic reactions.

Ataxia is a side effect that occurs commonly with the administration of therapeutic doses of benzodiazepines. Several carefully performed studies have shown that benzodiazepine administration is associated with increases in body sway and in the rate of loss of balance (45–48). Although benzodiazepine-induced ataxia may be partly attributed to a sedative effect, a direct action on cerebellar function is likely. Benzodiazepine receptors have been discovered in the cerebellum (in addition to the frontal cortex) and animal studies have shown that benzodiazepines have a direct effect on Purkinje cell activity in the cerebellum (49, 50).

Several dynamic studies of benzodiazepine response have shown their effects on postural sway to be significantly accentuated in the elderly (45–48). These studies point out that the observed sensitivity to benzodiazepines in the elderly still persists even when potential pharmacokinetic differences between age groups is accounted for. Thus the aging brain appears to be uniquely susceptible to benzodiazepine-induced ataxia. Failure to consider a downward dosage adjustment of those benzodiazepines that are not as efficiently metabolized in the elderly as compared to younger subjects further enhances the risk for inducing ataxia. Additionally, studies have shown that in the elderly use of benzodiazepines with long elimination half-lives is more likely to be associated with falls and hip fractures than shorter half-life entities (51). Although the mechanisms responsible for falls and fractures are not known, it seems reasonable to assume that they are related to drug-induced perturbations in sway, balance, and level of alertness. Clinicians wishing to avoid the use of long half-life benzodiazepines in the elderly can consult Table 3, which categorizes this drug class according to elimination half-life.

Table 3 Classification of Benzodiazepines by Elimination Half-Life

Short	Intermediate	Long
Triazolam	Alprazolam	Chlordiazepoxide[a]
	Estazolam	Clonazepam
	Lorazepam	Clorazepate[a]
	Oxazepam	Diazepam
	Temazepam	Flurazepam[a]
		Halazepam[a]
		Prazepam[a]
		Quazepam

[a]These drugs by themselves have short or intermediate half-lives, but are converted to active metabolites with long elimination half-lives.

All of the commonly prescribed anticonvulsant medications have been shown to produce ataxic reactions. A direct effect of these drugs on cerebellar function has been demonstrated and probably accounts for these reactions (52). Ataxia is most commonly observed with initiation of anticonvulsant therapy or upon dosage increases, and it improves or disappears over time. The development of ataxia during chronic treatment is usually due to excessive serum levels of anticonvulsant drug. Polytherapy with anticonvulsants would be expected to increase the risk for ataxia. There have been anecdotal indications that the elderly have an increased propensity for neurotoxic reactions from phenytoin or carbamazepine therapy but, despite their widespread use in this age group, little or no effort has been made to verify these impressions (53, 54).

The development of ataxia in any patient on chronic anticonvulsant therapy should always raise a strong suspicion that it is drug related. Serum drug levels should be determined. However, since certain anticonvulsant drugs are highly bound to serum albumin (i.e., phenytoin, valproic acid, carbamazepine), interpretation can be difficult in situations where hypoalbuminemia is present (55). This situation is analogous to interpreting serum calcium or thyroxine concentrations in states of altered protein binding. Just as these endogenous substances can be more accurately interpreted by measuring their ionized or unbound levels, respectively, so can unbound anticonvulsant levels provide a more sensitive index for their clinical interpretation.

Two common causes of elevated anticonvulsant blood levels are excessively rapid dose escalations and inhibitory drug–drug interactions. Serum phenytoin levels increase disproportionately to increases in dose, often resulting in unexpectedly high serum drug concentrations with just modest dose escalations (56). This clinical problem is due to saturation of hepatic drug metabolizing enzymes, which biotransform phenytoin into inactive metabolites. Daily maintenance doses should be escalated in increments of 30–100 mg. If serum phenytoin levels are already 10 μg/ml, then the daily maintenance dose should be adjusted by only 30–50 mg. Furthermore, dose–serum drug concentration responses can only be evaluated under steady-state conditions. Thus dose escalations with any anticonvulsant medication should be based on steady-state drug concentrations, which may not be achieved if such escalations occur so frequently that not enough time is allowed for a plateau concentration to be reached. Finally, many coadministered medications can inhibit the hepatic metabolism of anticonvulsants, resulting in elevated serum concentrations and potentially toxic effects (see Table 4).

Table 4 Selected Drugs That Can Elevate Anticonvulsant Serum Levels by Inhibiting Their Metabolism

Anticonvulsant			
Carbamazepine	Phenytoin	Phenobarbital	Valproic Acid
Cimetidine	Amiodarone	Valproic acid	Salicylates
Danazol	Chloramphenicol	Propoxyphene	
Erythromycin	Cimetidine		
Fluoxetine	Disulfiram		
Isoniazid	Fluconazole		
Propoxyphene	Isoniazid		
Valproic acid	Valproic acid		
Verapamil			

Of all the available anticonvulsants, phenytoin has been the best studied for its ability to produce ataxia. Kutt et al. characterized phenytoin-induced ataxia (observed with tandem walking) as being reversible with dosage reduction or discontinuation, manifesting in some patients at serum concentrations in excess of 20 μg/ml, and becoming common at levels of 30 μg/ml and above (53). In this classic report, a step-wise progression of side effects is apparent, beginning with nystagmus, followed by ataxia, and culminating in mental changes (problems with cognition and memory). This catenation of adverse central effects, however, is not always seen and one or more may be absent. Although ataxia often occurs as an acute reaction to excessive blood phenytoin levels, studies have shown that it may be delayed in appearance, occurring insidiously over several months (57). Its occult development has sometimes been mistaken as a recurrence of an intracranial tumor or as progression of a traumatic head injury. Irreversible cerebellar damage from chronic phenytoin use has also been described in several isolated case reports (58,59). Although there is no uniform agreement that this relatively rare effect is indeed phenytoin-induced (60), it seems prudent to monitor serum phenytoin levels in order to prevent sustained exposure of the cerebellum to excessive concentrations and to examine patients receiving phenytoin periodically for cerebellar dysfunction.

Less well characterized are the serum concentration thresholds for ataxic reactions to carbamazepine, phenobarbital, or valproic acid. The therapeutic range for carbamazepine is 4–12 μg/ml (61) and the threshold serum concentration for the development of ataxia and other common neurological effects is considered above 6.0 μg/ml (62,63). During chronic treatment with phenobarbital, ataxia can occur with serum concentrations above 35 μg/ml, the therapeutic range of serum levels being 15–40 μg/ml/ (62). Valproic acid rarely causes ataxia when used as monotherapy (62). The appearance of ataxia or other neurological side effects with initiation of valproic acid therapy is usually due to its inhibitory effects on the hepatic metabolism of other concurrently administered anticonvulsant medications (see Table 4).

It cannot be overemphasized that prescribed medications can cause or aggravate gait and balance disturbances in the elderly. A careful evaluation of medications including over-the-counter preparations and alcohol must be performed in any patient requiring an examination for abnormalities in gait or balance. Focusing attention on a single drug etiology may cause one to miss the possibilities of an additive detrimental effect of two or more medications. Appropriate laboratory tests should be ordered (BUN, electrolytes, serum drug concentrations, etc.), since they may be very helpful in identifying a drug etiology in certain situations. Harold Kaminetzky's comment of nearly 30 years ago, "There are no really safe biologically active drugs, there are only safe physicians, " should remind us of our responsibility to fully understand the polypharmacological effects of medications and the population to whom they are given (64).

REFERENCES

1. Sudarsky L. Geriatrics: Gait disorders in the elderly. N Engl J Med 1990; 322: 1441.
2. Lamy P. Clinical pharmacology. Ger Clin North Am 1990; 6: 229–457.
3. Swift CG (ed.). Clinical Pharmacology in the Elderly. New York: Marcel Dekker, Inc., 1987.
4. Tinetti ME, Speechley M, Ginter SF. Risk factors for falls among elderly persons living in the community. N Engl J Med 1988; 319: 1701.
5. Rubenstein L, Robbins A, Josephson K et al. Predictors of fall in an institutional elderly population: results of a case-control study. J Am Geriatr Soc 1988; 36: 578.
6. Campbell AJ, Borrie MJ, Spears GF. Risk factors for falls in a community-based prospective study of people 70 years and older. J Gerontol 1989; 44: M112.
7. Mader SL. Aging and postural hypotension: an update. J Am Geriatr Soc 1989; 37:129.

8. Lipsitz L. Orthostatic hypotenion in the elderly. N Engl J Med 1989; 321: 952.

9. Jansen RW, Hoefnagels MM. Hormonal mechanisms of postprandial hypotension. J Am Geriatr Soc 1991; 39: 1201.

10. Middleton HC, Maisey DN, Mills IH. Do antidepressants cause postural hypotension by blocking cardiovascular reflexes? Eur J Clin Pharmacol 1987; 31: 647.

11. Ray WA, Griffin MR, Malcolm E. Cyclic antidepressants and the risk of hip fractures. Arch Int Med 1991; 151: 754.

12. Glassman AH, Bigger JT, Giardina EV, et al. Clinical characteristics of imipramine-induced orthostatic hypotension. Lancet 1979; 1: 468.

13. Roose SP, Glassman AH, Giardina EGV, et al. Tricyclic antidepressants in depressed patients with cardiac conduction disease. Arch Gen Psychiatry 1987; 44: 273.

14. Roose SP, Glassman AH, Giardina EGV, et al. Cardiovascular effects of imipramine and bupropion in depressed patients with congestive heart failure. J Clin Psychopharmacol 1987; 7: 247.

15. Roose SP, Dalack GW, Glassman AH, et al. Cardiovascular effects of bupropion in depressed patients with heart disease. Am J Psychiatry 1991; 148: 512.

16. Chouinard G. A double-blind controlled clinical trial of fluoxetine and amitriptyline in the treatment of outpatients with major depressive disorder. J Clin Psychiatry 1985; 46 (Ser 2): 32.

17. Branchey MH, Lee JH, Amin R, et al. High- and low-potency neuroleptics in elderly psychiatric patients. JAMA 1978; 239: 1860.

18. Yahr MD, Duvoisin RC, Schear MJH, et al. Treatment of parkinsonism with levodopa. Arch Neurol 1969; 21: 343.

19. McDowell F, Lee JE, Swift T, et al. Treatment of Parkinson's syndrome with L-dihyroxyphenylalanine (levodopa). Ann Intern Med 1970; 72: 29.

20. Selby G. The long-term prognosis of Parkinson's disease. Clin Exp Neurol 1984; 20: 1.

21. Liebowitz M, Lieberman A. Comparison of dopa decarboxylase inhibitor (carbidopa) combined with levodopa and levodopa alone on the cardiovascular system of patients with Parkinson's disease. Neurology 1975; 23: 917.

22. Durrieu G, Senard JM, Tran MA et al. Effects of levodopa and bromocriptine on blood pressure and plasma catecholamines in parkinsonians. Clin Neuropharmacol 1991; 14: 84.

23. Micieli G, Martignoni E, Cavallini A, et al. Postprandial and orthostatic hypotension in Parkinson's disease. Neurology 1987; 37: 386.

24. Kamper AL. Angiotensin converting enzyme (ACE) inhibitors and renal function. Drug Safety 1991; 6: 361.

25. Winniford MD, Fulton KL, Hillis LD. Symptomatic sinus bradycardia

during concomitant propranolol-verapamil administration. Am Heart J 1985; 110: 498.

26. Sagie A, Strasberg B, Kusnieck J, et al. Symptomatic bradycardia induced by the combination of oral diltiazem and beta blockers. Clin Cardiol 1991; 14: 314.

27. Shannon RP, Wei JY, Rosa RM, et al. The effect of age and sodium depletion on cardiovascular response to orthostasis. Hypertension 1986; 8: 438.

28. Lipsitz LA, Pluchino FC, Wei JY, et al. Syncope in institutionalized elderly: the impact of multiple pathological conditions and situational stress. J Chron Dis 1986; 39: 619.

29. Ducher J, Iannascoli F, Safar M. Antihypertenisve effect of sustained-release isosorbide dinitrate for isolated systolic systemic hypertension in the elderly. Am J Cardiol 1987; 60: 99.

30. Lacomis D, Samuels MA. Adverse neurological effects of glucocorticoids. J Gen Intern Med 1991; 6: 367.

31. Tobert JA. Efficacy and long-term adverse effect pattern of lovastatin. Am J Cardiol 1988; 62: 28J.

32. Tobert JA. Reply (letter). N Engl J Med 1988; 318: 48.

33. Pierce LR, Wysowski DK, Gross TP. Myopathy and rhabdomyolysis associated with lovastatin-gemfibrozil combination therapy. JAMA 1991; 264: 71.

34. Marais GE, Larsom KK. Rhabdomyolysis and acute renal failure induced by combination lovastatin and gemfibrozil therapy. Ann Intern Med 1990; 112: 228.

35. Manoukian AA, Bhagavan NV, Hasashi T, et al. Rhabdomyolysis secondary to lovastatin therapy. Clin Chem 1990; 36: 2145.

36. Goldstein MR. Myopathy and rhabdomyolysis with lovastatin taken with gemfibrozil. JAMA 1990; 264: 2991.

37. Spach DH, Bauwens JE, Clark CD, et al. Rhabdomyolysis associated with lovastatin and erythromycin use. West J Med; 154: 213.

38. Ayd FJ. A summary of drug-induced extrapyramidal reactions. JAMA 1961; 175: 1054.

39. Stephen PJ, Williamson J. Drug-induced parkinsonism in the elderly. Lancet 1984; 2: 1082.

40. Murdoch PS, Williamson J. A danger in making the diagnosis of Parkinson's disease. Lancet 1982; 1: 1212.

41. McGeer PL, McGeer EG, Suzuki JS. Aging and extrapyramidal function. Arch Neurol 1977; 34: 33.

42. Wong DF, Wagner HN, Dannals RF, et al. Effect of age on dopamine and serotonin receptors measured by positron tomography in the living human brain. Science 1984; 226: 1393.

43. Peters N. Snipping the thread of life: Antimuscarinic side effects of medications in the elderly. Arch Intern Med 1989; 149: 2414.

44. Friedman JH. The management of levodopa psychosis. Clin Neuropharmacol 1991; 14: 283.
45. Swift CG, Haythorne JM, Clarke P, et al. The effect of ageing on measured responses to single doses or oral temazepam. Br J Clin Pharmacol 1981; 11: 413P.
46. Swift CG, Ewen JM, Clarke P, et al. Responsiveness to oral diazepam in the elderly:relationship to total and free plasma concentrations. Br J Clin Pharmacol 1985; 20: 111.
47. Swift CG, Swift MR, Ankier SI, et al. Single dose pharmacokinetics and pharmacodynamics of oral loprazolam in the elderly. Br J Clin Pharmacol 1985; 20: 119.
48. Robin DW, Hasan SS, Lichtenstein MJ, et al. Dose-related effect of triazolam on postural sway. Clin Pharmacol Ther 1991; 49: 581.
49. Braestrup C, Albrechsten R, Squires RF. High densities of benzodiazepine receptors in human cortical areas. Nature 1977; 269: 702.
50. Haefely W, Pieri L, Polc P, et al. General pharmacology and neuropharmacology of benzodiazepine derivatives. In Hoffmeister F, Stille G, eds., Handbook of Experimental Pharmacology. Berlin: Springer-Verlag, 1981: 13.
51. Ray WA, Griffin MR, Downey W. Benzodiazepines of long and short half-life and the risk of hip fracture. JAMA 1989; 262: 3303.
52. Halperin MH, Julien RM. Augmentation of cerebellar purkinje cell discharge rate after diphenylhydantoin. Epilepsia 1972; 13: 377.
53. Kutt H, Winters W, Kokenge R, et al. Diphenylhydantoin metabolism, blood levels, and toxicity. Arch Neurol 1964; 11: 642.
54. Gram L, Jensen PK. Carbamazepine: Toxicity. In: Levy R, Mattson R, Meldrum B, eds, Antiepileptic Drugs. New York: Raven Press, 1989: 555.
55. Gugler R, Azarnoff DL. Drug protein binding and the nephrotic syndrome. Clin Pharmacokin 1976; 1: 25.
56. Richens D, Dunlop A. Serum phenytoin levels in the management of epilepsy. Lancet 1975; 2: 247.
57. Husby J. Delayed toxicity and serum concentrations of phenytoin. Danish Med Bull 1963; 10: 236.
58. Reynolds EH. Chronic antiepileptic toxicity: a review. Epilepsia 1975; 16: 319.
59. McLain LW, Martin JT, Allen JH. Cerebellar degeneration due to chronic phenytoin therapy. Ann Neurol 1980; 7: 18.
60. Dam M. Chronic toxicity of antiepileptic drugs with respect to cerebellar and motor function. Antiepileptic Therapy: In: Oxley J, Janz D, Meinardi H, eds, Chronic Toxicity of Antiepileptic Drugs. New York: Raven Press, 1983: 223.
61. Levy RH, Wilensky AJ, Friel PN. Other antiepileptic drugs. In Evans WE, Schentag JJ, Jusko WJ, eds), Applied Pharmacokinetics: Principles of

Therapeutic Drug Monitoring. Spokane, WA: Applied Therapeutics, Inc., 1986: 540.

62. Penry JK, Newmark ME. The use of antiepileptic drugs. Ann Intern Med 1979; 90: 207.

63. Reynolds EH. Neurotoxicity of carbamazepine. Adv. Neurol. 1975; 11: 345.

64. Kaminetzky H. A drug on the market. Obstet Gynecol 1963; 21: 512.

11

Falls in Older Persons

REIN TIDEIKSAAR

Mount Sinai Medical Center, New York, New York

I. INTRODUCTION

Falls are a common problem for persons aged 65 and older. About one-third of community-dwelling older persons fall each year (1). Of these individuals, one-half suffer multiple falling episodes (1). Among older persons residing in institutional settings, the incidence of falls is equally alarming. Falls represent a leading cause of adverse events in acute care hospitals, accounting for up to 40% of incidents (2). Older patients experience an overwhelming majority of fall-related incidents. Up to 10% of older hospital patients fall repeatedly (3). In the nursing home, about 50% of residents fall annually (4). Over 40% of persons have recurrent falling episodes. In all clinical settings the risk of falling increases with advancing age, with the highest incidence occurring in the 80- to 89-year age group (5).

Historically, falls in older persons have for the most part been considered as either accidental, random events, or as "normal" consequences of the aging process. Similarly, falling has been attributed solely to the carelessness of the older person involved. However, contrary to popular myth, falls are neither "accidental" nor strictly age-related events but, to a large degree, are predictable occurrences that stem from a multitude of host-related and environmental factors. Many of these factors are potentially amenable to interventions. The purpose of this chapter is to acquaint clinicians with the consequences of falls, the conditions under which falls occur, and the factors associated with fall risk. An approach to clinical assessment procedures and intervention strategies to reduce the risk of falls is presented as well.

II. CONSEQUENCES

Falls are a major health problem, not only because they occur with increasing frequency in the older population, but because of their associated mortality and morbidity. Falls are a leading cause of unintentional injury-related deaths in the United States, accounting for about 9500 fatalities per year (6). An estimated 5% of falls in both community- and institution-residing older persons result in a fracture (6). The most common fall-related fractures are those of hip, pelvis, distal forearm, and ankle (6). An additional 10% of falls lead to head injuries, soft tissue trauma, joint dislocations, and muscle sprains (6,7).

A fracture of the femoral neck is the most devastating injury. It has been estimated that each year in the United States alone almost 200,000 persons over the age of 65 suffer hip fractures from falls (8). The cost of hip fractures is approximately 7 billion dollars a year (9). Up to 27% of older persons with hip fracture die within 1 year following the injury (10). A high incidence of coexisting chronic diseases in persons with hip fracture contributes to the increased mortality rate (6,7). In those persons who survive a hip fracture, many never regain their premorbid level of ambulation. Approximately 60% of persons experience mobility limitations, and another 25% become functionally dependent in walking, requiring either mechanical or human assistance (11). Many persons who become dependent in ambulation require long-term care placement. Hip fractures represent the second most common cause of nursing home admission, accounting for about 60,000 admissions annually (9). A multitude of interacting circumstances consisting of both host-related factors (i.e., osteoporosis, reduced fat around the hip, neuromuscular dysfunction affecting the lower extremities) and environmental conditions (i.e., nonabsorptive ground surfaces) increase the risk of hip fracture (12). The presence of a gait disorder can result in a backward displacement of balance (i.e., a slip) and, when occurring in combination with a fall that strikes the hip, impacts against osteoporotic bone and a hard ground surface, with the likelihood of a fracture increased.

In the absence of physical injury, falls are commonly associated with a restriction of activities and loss of mobility. Falls can lead elderly persons to lose confidence in their ability to function safely and result in a fear of further falls. Up to 50% of older persons who have suffered multiple falling episodes admit to avoiding everyday activities because they fear additional falls and subsequent injury (13). In those persons who continue to perform activities despite a fear of falling, ordinary tasks can provoke a great deal of anxiety and are often achieved by clutching or grabbing environmental structures (i.e., furnishings, walls, sink edges) for support. Developing a fear of falling is increased in those persons who live alone, have an underlying gait and balance impairment, and experience recurrent falls over a short time period. In those falls associated with injury or prolonged postfall times (i.e., persons are unable to get up from the floor by themselves), the fear becomes intensified.

Either an injury or a fear of falling can lead to episodes of immobility. Prolonged immobility places persons at risk for a host of physical and psychological complications. Some of the most significant include osteoporosis, muscle weakness, pressure sores, social isolation, and depression. The risk of complications increases with the duration of immobility. In turn, any resulting loss of functional status places persons at further fall risk and, possibly, long-term institutional placement. Falls and immobility are a contributing factor in up to 40% of nursing home admissions (6).

III. CAUSES OF FALLING

The risk of falling is intensified when a person engages in an activity that results in a loss of balance and the body mechanisms responsible for compensation fail. Those activities most often associated with balance loss consist of everyday tasks such as walking, descending and climbing steps, transferring on and off chairs, beds, and toilets, getting in and out of bathtubs, and reaching or bending to retrieve and place objects. Any consequent fall is typically a sign or symptom of an underlying problem indicative of intrinsic factors (e.g., age-related changes, pathological diseases, medication effects) and/or extrinsic factors (i.e., environmental hazards and obstacles). In general, the etiology of falls in older persons is multifactorial, due to a combination of both intrinsic and extrinsic factors.

A. Age-Related Changes

With advancing age, several physiological changes contribute to the risk of falling. The most significant occur in the visual and neuromuscular systems and exert an influence on gait and balance.

1. Vision

The ability of the eye to adjust to various environmental stimuli diminishes with age. The response to varying levels of light and darkness is reduced (14). As a result, persons require more time to adapt to lighting changes. Dark adaptation, the capability of the eye to adjust to low levels of illumination, is particularly affected by age (14) and is associated with the risk of falling. This change may compromise an individual's capacity to view environmental surroundings and potential hazards under conditions of low illumination. Bright lighting produces similar effects. With age, pupillary response and accommodation decline (15). As a consequence, excessive illumination may lead to blindness until the eyes are able to adjust.

Also, a greater sensitivity of the aging eye to glare (e.g., a dazzling effect associated with a source of intense illumination) can interfere with vision (14). Common sources of glare include sunlight and unshielded light bulbs, either isolated or combined with reflected glare from window panes or polished floors. As a consequence, potential ground hazards that can lead to trips and slips are hidden from view. As well, persons may perceive glare-producing surfaces as slippery. In an effort to compensate, they may alter their gait in an attempt to maintain a safe level of ambulation. Similar to walking on ice, the gait tends to be slower and flat-footed, with a wide base of support. The gait change can be hazardous, leading to unsteady balance and falls.

A decline in depth perception also occurs with age (14). This change can interfere with the visual detection and interpretation of environmental surroundings. Environmental objects of low visual contrast such as carpet, step edges, and door thresholds that are indistinguishable from their background may not be easily visualized. Linoleum and carpet designs that are patterned, checkered, or floral may appear to the aging eye as either ground elevations or depressions, and can lead to hazardous gaits.

2. Balance

Balance is a complex function. The ability to maintain upright stability is dependent on the operation of the neurological and musculoskeletal systems and the capability of their individual components, consisting of vision, vestibular input, proprioceptive feedback, muscular strength, and joint flexibility. Working in unison, these components culminate in postural sway, an anterioposterior and lateral motion or movement of the body that counters the effects of gravity and controls stability. In the standing position, balance is achieved by constantly positioning the body's center of gravity (COG) over a base of support (BOS), the area surrounding the borders of the feet (Fig. 1). During ambulation, the COG extends beyond the BOS and stretches the limits of stability (Fig. 2). Imbalance is detected by the visual, proprioceptive, and vestibular components of the central nervous system. Signals are sent to stretch receptors located in the joints and muscles of the lower extremities. In turn, these messages initiate a set of coordinated movements that read-justs the body's COG in alignment with the BOS. The protective move-ments most commonly employed to maintain balance consist of an an-kle, hip, and stepping strategy. An ankle strategy shifts the body's COG by rotating the body about the ankle joints. A hip strategy repositions the COG by flexing or extending the body at the hips. A stepping strategy realigns the BOS with the COG with rapid forward or backward shifting of the feet. The use of a particular strategy depends on the configuration of the ground or support surface and the size or extent of the balance displacement. An inability to initiate or complete these strategies successfully results in balance loss and fall risk.

The proprioceptive system, which arises from joint mechano-receptors located in the spine and extremities, supplies the body with kinesthetic information or feedback on the surrounding environment. With respect to ambulation, proprioception provides a person with proper orientation to ground conditions. With advanced age, proprio-ceptive feedback declines (16); malfunction is associated with increased postural sway or instability that can place persons at risk for balance loss and falls. Vision can augment proprioceptive function or provide a sub-stitute for its loss. This is demonstrated by older people with proprio-ceptive loss who ambulate by viewing the location of their feet on the ground to ensure proper placement. When visual input is decreased, maintaining balance becomes difficult (e.g., when asked to stand with their eyes closed, persons often demonstrate unsteady balance).

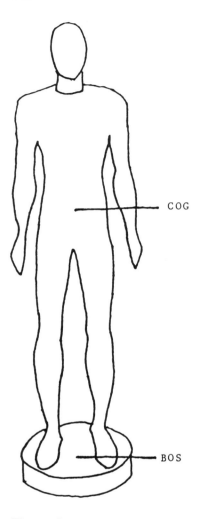

Figure 1 The center of gravity (COG) in relationship to the base of support (BOS).

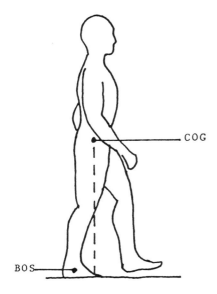

Figure 2 The center of gravity (COG) in relationship to the base of support (BOS) during ambulation.

The vestibular system achieves balance by helping to maintain visual perception and body orientation in moving about the environment. During episodes of body displacement, vestibular receptors located in the semicircular canals and otoliths initiate a series of compensatory limb, trunk, and head movements which serve to control postural sway and stability. This body-orientating response or righting reflex diminishes with age (17). As a result, if a person trips or slips (i.e., balance displacement) the chances of regaining stability and avoiding a fall declines.

Normally there is some redundancy in the sensory information needed to maintain balance; the failure of one source of input can be compensated for by feedback from another system. For example, intact proprioceptive and vestibular feedback can compensate for a decline in vision. However, dysfunction in more than one system is likely to result in a lowered balance threshold and increase the risk of falls. Older persons who fall demonstrate greater sway or unsteadiness than non-fallers and those persons with recurrent falls have appreciably more sway than single fallers (18).

3. Gait

Gait, simply defined as the manner or style of walking, consists of two phases: stance and swing. The stance phase occurs when one leg is in contact with the ground and the swing phase occurs when the other leg advances forward to take the next step. Walking is accomplished by a series of reciprocal leg movements alternating between stance and swing (Fig. 3): pushing off on the leg in stance swing, while at the same time swinging the other leg forward. To allow for adequate ground clearance during the swing phase, the leg is flexed at the knee and dorsiflexed at the ankle. When the heel of the swing leg strikes the ground (a return to the stance phase), the knee extends and the foot plantar flexes to provide sufficient ground support.

Changes in gait are one of the most frequent concomitants of aging. Compared to younger persons, older individuals experience a number of alterations in gait. The velocity or speed of walking, stride length (the distance the foot travels during the swing phase), heel lift (i.e., the level of ground clearance by the foot during swing phase), and ankle plantar and dorsiflexion declines (18,19). During ambulation, older persons also display a slight anteroflexion or kyphosis of the

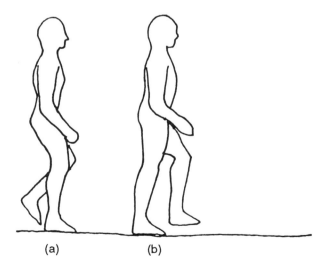

(a)   (b)

Figure 3   The (a) stance and (b) swing phase of gait.

upper torso with flexion of the arms and knees, and diminished arm swing. In response, this forward or stooped posture may alter the person's balance threshold. The COG is shifted forward, beyond the BOS or critical point of stability. Subsequently, it becomes more difficult to thrust the foot forward (i.e., stepping strategy) fast enough to preserve stability during balance displacements. In addition, an age-associated decline in ankle muscle strength complicates the execution of this movement, making it difficult to adjust the COG in line with the BOS rapidly enough to avoid a fall. Despite the preceding discussion, it remains speculative as to whether age-related gait changes contribute to falls. However, impaired gait is more often present than absent in persons with a history of falls (20).

B. Pathological Diseases

Disease states and their associated impairments are more decisive as factors in falls than are age-related physiological changes that occur in isolation. Evidence indicates that persons who fall have more medical diagnoses than nonfallers (1). Both acute and chronic conditions play a role.

A fall may be premonitory, in that the event represents the initial presentation of an underlying acute illness. Acute disease processes most often identified as contributing to falls are those that interfere with postural stability. These include syncope; hypovolemia (e.g., dehydration, blood loss): cardiac arrhythmias; electrolyte disturbances; seizures; stroke; febrile conditions (e.g., urinary tract infections, pneumonias, etc.); and acute exacerbations of chronic diseases such as congestive heart failure and obstructive pulmonary disease.

Chronic disease processes that predispose to falling include any persistent conditions that interfere with mobility. The most common originate in the sensory and neuromuscular systems. For example, diseases of the eye (e.g., cataracts, macular degeneration, and glaucoma) adversely affect visual perception, acuity, and dark adaption. When combined with low illumination, these alterations in visual function can result in poor recognition of ground hazards (e.g., upended floor tiles and carpet edges, low-lying furnishings, etc.) and predispose to tripping. Parkinsonism affects postural control; and disease is associated with a loss of autonomic postural reflexes; propulsion (i.e., an uncontrolled forward motion); retropulsion (i.e., loss of balance backwards); and gait changes (i.e., short-stepped and shuffling, barely clearing the ground;

poor initiation and freezing of gait). Abnormalities such as these can lead to a displaced center of gravity during ambulation, balance loss, and fall risk.

Proximal muscle weakness of the lower extremities, concomitant with conditions such as osteomalacia, thyroid disease, polymyalgia rheumatica, or deconditioning can lead to a waddling ("penguin's") gait and balance loss (i.e., gluteal muscle weakness results in exaggerated lateral trunk movements). Lower extremity hemiplegia or paresis results in decreased ankle dorsiflexion on foot clearance when walking and places the person at risk for tripping. Osteoarthritis of the hips and knees can lead to a decrease in single limb support (i.e., the result of pain when weight bearing on the joint) and instability during ambulation. Foot disorders (e.g., uncut nails, bunions, and calluses, etc.) can lead to mechanical gait disorders. Chapter 9 provides a review of common foot disorders.

C. Medications

Any drug that interferes with postural control and cognitive function may influence gait and balance and place persons at fall risk. Common offenders include sedatives, antipsychotics, antihypertensives, and antidepressants (13). The risk of drug-related falls is increased with medications that have extended half-lives (i.e., greater than 24 h) and with the numbers of medications taken simultaneously (1). Chapter 10 discusses this issue more fully.

D. Environmental Factors

The overwhelming majority of falls experienced by community-residing older persons take place in the home setting (5). Falls in the hospital and nursing home occur most often in the bedroom and bathroom, a reflection of the increased time persons spend in these locations (3,5). Several environmental obstacles and design features in conjunction with host-initiated activities are associated with falling. These consist of transferring from inappropriately low or elevated bed heights or climbing over side rails; rising from and sitting down on unstable, low-seated, and armless chairs, or low-seated toilets that lack grab bar support; walking in poorly illuminated areas and tripping over low-lying objects or floor coverings such as thick pile carpets, and unsecured rug edges; slipping on polished or wet ground surfaces and sliding rugs; climbing and descending stairs that lack handrail support and sufficient lighting; and reaching up to place or retrieve objects from inappropriately high shelves (5). The likelihood of the environment contributing to the risk of falls is greatest for those persons with mobility problems since the physical demands of activities or tasks can exceed the competence level of these individuals.

Assistive devices (i.e., canes, walkers) that support mobility can contribute to falls, particularly if they are utilized improperly or are in poor repair (i.e., worn rubber tips, structural deterioration). As well, improper footwear can alter gait and balance. High-heeled shoes can lead to instability. They narrow the standing and walking BOS, decrease stride length, and cause the person to assume a forward-leaning posture. Poorly fitting shoes, particularly when loose, can also alter a person's gait patterns. In an effort to keep their feet in the shoes, persons assume a shuffling type of gait, which can lead to tripping. Wearing leather-soled shoes or plain socks promotes slipping. The use of rubber crepe soles, promoted as slip resistant, may stick to linoleum floor surfaces. In those persons with decreased foot-ground clearance, rubber soles can cause an immediate halting gait, producing balance loss and falls. Thick-soled footwear (e.g., running shoes, tennis sneakers) may decrease proprioceptive feedback (gained from the foot striking on the ground) and contribute to balance loss.

E. Fall Risk Factors

A host of intrinsic and extrinsic (environmental) factors are associated with falling. Effective preventive measures are dependent upon identifying specific fall risk factors. Several host-related or intrinsic factors have been repeatedly found to correlate with the risk of falls: reduced lower extremity strength and sensory impairment; decreased vision; altered cognition; urinary dysfunction (e.g., incontinence, nocturia); and polypharmacy (i.e., taking more than four drugs simultaneously) (1,4,13). The risk of falling increases with the number of factors present. When these intrinsic risk factors are combined with undesirable environmental conditions, the risk of falling increases further.

IV. CLINICAL ASSESSMENT

The primary aim of the clinical assessment is to identify persons at fall risk and discover the causative factors in those with a history of falls.

A. The Fall History

Following an episode of falling, one should first evaluate and treat for the presence of physical injury and/or any life-threatening acute medical condition that might have precipitated the event. Once the person is medically stable, the circumstances surrounding the fall should be ascertained with a fall history. Fall histories include: asking the person about the presence of symptoms, the location of the fall, the activity they were engaged in at the time, the time of the fall (i.e., hour of the day); and the consequences of the fall (i.e., injury, prolonged postfall lie time, fear of falling). While some persons give a clear account of their fall, others, because of memory problems stemming from depression or dementia, may not be able to recall the circumstances. Still other persons, out of embarrassment or a fear of being viewed as frail and dependent, underreport or fail to fully disclose the true extent of their falls. In this case, a history should be obtained from family members and significant others.

Information acquired from fall histories usually provides important clues to the diagnosis of falling and its effect on the person. For example, tripping suggests lower extremity dysfunction (e.g., decreased ankle dorsiflexion, shuffling gait) and/or failing to clear an environmental ground hazard. A loss of balance and falling in the dark may indicate a problem with proprioception. Associated dizziness may signify a cardiovascular or vestibular etiology. Prolonged fall lie time and/or fear of falling in a person living alone indicates a potential need for human assistance at home.

Also, inquiring about previous falls and their circumstances helps to determine if there is a pattern. For example, falls occurring over a short time period may be due to a solitary cause. If a person has a total of five previous falls, all occurring in the bedroom while getting out of bed in the morning, accompanied by symptoms of dizziness, the possibility of orthostatic hypotension must be considered. A convenient acronym to help remember and record the components of the fall history is SPLATT; Symptoms, Previous falls, Location, Activity, Time, and Trauma (i.e., the physical and psychological consequences).

Once the fall history is obtained, past medical problems, current complaints, and medications should be reviewed. The latter is particularly important as recent prescription drug or dosage changes, or the use of over-the-counter medications may provide a clue to the cause of the fall.

B. The Assessment of Gait and Balance

The next step is to examine the person. In the absence of an identifiable medical cause of falling, an assessment should begin with a performance-oriented mobility screen (POMS) that appraises the person's gait and balance. The components include observing the person perform a number of mobility tasks and noticing the manner in which each is accomplished. Ask the person to rise from a chair (not using the armrests for assistive support); stand without assistive support; walk in a straight line and turn around (with assistive devices if used); bend down and pick up an object from the ground; return to the chair and sit down. Last, place the person on the ground and ask him or her to get up unassisted (assess the risk of prolonged postfall lie times). Normal performance is demonstrated by the person being able to accomplish each task (i.e., chair transfers, immediate standing, bending down, floor rising) in a smooth and controlled manner, without a loss of balance. The gait pattern is continuous, without hesitation or sway (i.e., excessive deviation from path), and both feet clear the floor. The steps taken during turning movements are continuous, without staggering or balance loss.

At this point, a Romberg maneuver (to assess proprioception) and sternal nudge test (to assess postural competence) should be performed. The latter is accomplished with the person in the standing position, with the examiner tapping the person's sternum with enough pressure to elicit a displacement of balance backwards. A normal response is a rapid step backward, often associated with a brisk forward movement of both arms (i.e., the righting reflex or response). An abnormal response consists of the person falling into the examiner's arms because of an ineffective stepping strategy (to preserve balance), or a complete absence of the righting reflex. An alternative method to invoke a postural response is to stand behind the person and pull sharply backward on the hips or shoulders.

An abnormal POMS provides clues as to the cause of falling, particularly in those persons with chronic disease. It helps to localize the organ systems involved and isolate potential environmental problems (Table 1).

C. The Assessment of Fall Risk

Older persons at fall risk can be identified first by reviewing the medical history for conditions and medications that place individuals at risk (Table 2). Next, complete the POMS (as described above) to assess the person's mobility. In the absence of identifiable risk factors and a nor-

Table 1 Differential Diagnoses of Abnormal Performance-Oriented Mobility Screen (POMS) Maneuvers

Impaired maneuver	Intrinsic factor	Extrinsic factor
Chair transfer (possibly impaired bed, toilet, and bathtub transfers)	Parkinsonism Arthritis Deconditioning	Poor chair design (possibly faulty bed, toilet, and bathtub design)
Standing balance	Postural hypotension Vestibular dysfunction Adverse drug effects	
Romberg test	Proprioceptive dysfunction Adverse drug effects	Poor illumination Overly absorptive footwear and/or carpeting
Sternal nudge test	Parkinsonism Normal pressure hydrocephalus Adverse drug effects	
Bending down	Neuromuscular dysfunction Adverse drug effects	
Walking/turning	Gait disorders (Parkinsonism, hemiparesis, or foot problem) Sensory dysfunction Adverse drug effects	Improper footwear Improper size, utilization of ambulation devices Hazardous ground surfaces (slippery, uneven)
Rising up from floor	Neuromuscular dysfunction	

mal POMS, the person is at low fall risk. However, the presence of one or more risk factors and/or any abnormalities discovered on the POMS indicate fall risk and should trigger further investigations to search for modifiable factors.

D. The Physical Assessment and Diagnostic Evaluation

The last steps in the evaluation process of both falls and fall risk consist of performing a physical examination and obtaining diagnostic and laboratory studies. The extent of the physical examination is dictated by the

Table 2 Fall Risk Factors

Previous falls
Lower extremity weakness
Arthritis (hips, knees)
Gait disorders
Balance disorders
Cognitive disorders (depression, dementia, poor judgment)
Visual disorders
Postural hypotension
Bladder dysfunction (frequency, urgency, nocturia, incontinence)
Medications (psychotropics, sedatives, hypnotics, antihypertensives)

information gathered from the fall history, risk factor assessment, and POMS. In the absence of historical information, the physical exam should focus on detecting diseases that affect gait and balance. The neuromuscular exam is performed to identify conditions leading to lower extremity dysfunction (i.e., Parkinson's disease, previous strokes, peripheral neuropathy, arthritis, muscular weakness) and postural instability (i.e., vestibular and proprioceptive disorders). The cardiovascular system is evaluated to rule out arrhythmias, postural hypotension, and carotid hypersensitivity. Visual testing should be performed to examine acuity, visual fields, and depth perception. Last, cognitive function is assessed to identify dementia and depression, conditions associated with poor judgment, hazardous mobility, and fall risk.

Diagnostic tests and laboratory studies used to investigate falls and risk should be selective, based upon clinical suspicions derived from all previous evaluations. Obtaining routine laboratory studies (e.g., chemistries, hematology) is rarely beneficial in the absence of symptoms or demonstrated physical findings. In addition, diagnostic testing (i.e., Holter monitoring, brain imaging, EMG) should be pursued only when focal findings are present.

V. INTERVENTIONS

Interventions aimed at minimizing fall risk by ameliorating or eliminating the contributing factors are the goal of all fall prevention programs. At the same time, the person's autonomy and mobility should be maintained or improved. Based on accepted risk factors and postulated causes of falls, potential intervention strategies are classified as medical, rehabilitative, and environmental. In most cases, the management approach includes components of each. While there is little direct evidence on the effectiveness of these approaches, common sense suggests that many are promising and should be attempted.

A. Medical

The importance of identifying persons at fall risk and those with falls, and following through with a clinical assessment to search for modifiable factors cannot be overemphasized. A fall or the presence of risk factors may represent a sign of an underlying disease or medication effect that demands the clinician's attention first, to rule out contributing acute and chronic medical conditions and medications and second, to treat each accordingly. This point is illustrated by the following case.

CW is an 89-year-old female who presented to the clinic with multiple falling episodes. She stated that her falls occurred at night after arising from bed to walk to the bathroom. At the time of falling, the patient complained of "balance loss." Her medical history was remarkable for hypothyroidism, moderate obesity, degenerative arthritis of the knees (treated with a nonsteroidal anti-inflammatory drug), and nocturia. Her urinary problem coincided with the start of her falls. After an evaluation, it was determined that CW's nocturia was due to the onset of congestive heart failure, which resolved with treatment. Her loss of balance was the result of several conditions: proprioceptive loss (due to pernicious anemia), environmental exposure (walking about in the dark), decreased visual input (low illumination), and mild orthostatic hypotension (secondary to iron deficiency anemia caused by NSAIDs). Following treatment of the anemia (B-12 and iron supplementation, and discontinuing the NSAID) and the addition of night lights in the bedroom and bathroom, CW's falls stopped.

This patient had several chronic diseases (e.g., hypothyroidism, arthritis) that affected her gait and balance, and placed her at fall risk. Despite these conditions, she was able to compensate and avoid falls. However, with the onset of acute problems (i.e., nocturia, proprioceptive loss, orthostatic hypotension) and unfavorable environmental conditions (i.e., poor lighting), which adversely influenced her ability to compensate for proprioceptive loss, her balance was compromised. Once CW's falls were recognized as being caused by the onset of numerous acute conditions, her risk of sustaining further falls was reduced by the evaluation and treatment of each problem.

B. Rehabilitative

Those persons who fail to improve with conventional medical treatment and remain at fall risk, particularly those with chronic neuromuscular disorders that affect mobility, may respond to a number of rehabilitative strategies. These consist of exercises to improve mobility, attention toward wearing proper footwear, and utilizing ambulation devices (see Chap. 13 for further details).

A growing body of evidence suggests that older persons respond to and dervie benefit from exercise training in exactly the same way as younger persons do (21). This response extends to persons of extreme age and frailty, and may be of benefit in reducing the risk of falls and injury. Exercises that focus on improving flexibility, muscle strength, and endurance may produce improvements in gait and balance. Exercises that concentrate on improving the function of antigravity muscles (i.e., hip and knee extensors, muscles surrounding the ankles) are the most beneficial. These muscle groups are particularly susceptible to the effects of immobility and the most important in maintaining effective walking and transferring activities. Also, exercise programs may help to reduce the fear of falling or instability. Older persons who exercise on a regular basis build self-confidence in performing activities. As well, providing persons with weight-bearing exercises (e.g., walking, stair climbing) improves bone strength and reduces the risk of injury (i.e., hip fracture) in the event of a fall. Because older persons have a host of medical problems and take numerous medications, exercise regimens should be individually designed to avoid the risk of injury. In this sense, the prescription of exercises demands the same consideration used in prescribing medications. There are several publications available that provide exercises and guidelines on methods to ensure their success and avoid adverse effects (22,23). Chapter 14 reviews exercise in older adults in greater detail.

Paying attention to the type and fit of footwear often supports safe gait patterns. In a study of older persons with multiple falls and gait disorders, correcting improper footwear resulted in improved mobility and reduction of falls (24). Shoes and slippers should fit properly (i.e., not too tight or loose) and their soles should be slip resistant. Persons with foot problems (e.g., hammer toes, bunions, nail disorders) that interfere with wearing properly fitting footwear should be referred for podiatric care. Footwear with rubber or crepe soles will provide adequate slip resistancy on most ground surfaces. Socks with nonskid tread design on the soles are a good choice for persons who are accustomed to walking about without shoes or slippers.

For those persons with a shuffling gait or poor stepping height (i.e., not picking the feet up from the floor), slip-resistant soles may stick to ground surfaces and interfere with safe ambulation. Footwear with leather soles that promote gliding on linoleum and carpeted floor surfaces may constitute a better choice. The best way to ensure that sole surfaces are adequate is to observe the person walk over different floor surfaces in their environment.

Wearing high-heeled shoes should be discouraged, as they tend to adversely affect gait and balance. Footwear with low and broad surface heels are better suited for safe ambulation. Some persons will insist on wearing high heels, either for reasons of style or because of a life-long use of high-heeled footwear leads to a shortening of the achilles tendon and necessitates their use. For these persons, shoes with wedge heels should be suggested. They provide a better base of support than high heels. Wedge heels are also less likely to get caught on uneven floor surfaces (e.g., upended carpets or tiles, door thresholds). To ensure that older persons wear suitable footwear, information on their selection should be provided. Table 3 provides guidelines for purchasing footwear and can be used by older persons to help them select appropriate shoes.

Ambulation devices (e.g., canes, walkers) are designed to improve mobility in persons with gait and balance disorders. They function by increasing the person's standing and walking BOS (i.e., they provide an additional point(s) of ground contact), increasing stability by supplying proprioceptive feedback through the handle(s), and reducing the load on weight-bearing joints (e.g., hips and knees). Also, walking devices provide the person with visual support during ambulation. This affords the person a sense of confidence and helps reduce the fear of instability and falling.

The type of cane or walker selected must be individualized, as the choice of a particular device is based on the person's mobility needs and environmental situation. As a result, the purchase of a device should never be left to the person's whim, as they will unintentionally often select the wrong device and increase their risk of falling. Rather, devices need to be "prescribed" items, specific to correct the underlying gait and balance problem and tailored to fit the person (i.e., properly sized) and the individual's environment. As well, persons need to be instructed on the proper use of the device for walking and transferring activities. This is best accomplished by referring persons to a physiatrist or physical therapist, as reviewed in Chapter 13.

Table 3   Guidelines for Purchasing Footwear

Buy shoes in the late afternoon, as the feet swell during the day.
Never buy shoes without trying them both on, as the feet may be of different
   sizes. Buy the pair that fits the longer, wider foot. Shoe inserts can be used
   to make the larger shoe fit the smaller foot.
Choose shoes with slip-resistant soles to guard against slipping on wet surfaces.
Choose shoes with heels that are no more than 3.5 cm in height, and at least
   5.5 cm in width. These dimensions provide maximum balance support.
Choose shoes with ample room in the toe box (the space between the tip of the
   longest toe and front of the shoe). This space should be at least ¼ of an inch
   in length (the size of a thumb nail) and wide enough to avoid rubbing the
   large and/or small toe against the sides of the shoe. These dimensions allow
   free movement of the toes when walking and help to prevent injuries.
Choose shoes with inner soles that cushion the feet. A cushioned sole absorbs
   pressure on the feet and protects the feet from impact injuries that may
   occur when walking on hard surfaces.
Choose shoes that have firm heel support. When walking, the heel of the shoe
   should remain stable on the foot (not sway from side to side) and fit the foot
   snugly (not ride up and down).
Shoes that fit well are comfortable and appropriate for walking, cause neither
   rubbing, friction, or pressure on the feet.

Despite the best efforts to prescribe the right device, many persons still have ill-fitting canes and walkers. Walking devices that are
too short in height (i.e., the distance from stem tip to handle), often
lead to kyphotic postures and the risk of balance loss. The person has
to bend over in order to place the hand(s) on the handle(s). Similarly,
devices that are too long can lead to elbow and shoulder discomfort.
The person is forced to hold the device's handle(s) with their arm(s) in
an elevated position. Measurement of canes and walkers is similar
regardless of type. Have the person stand erect (wearing everyday
footwear) and place the cane tip (6 in to the front and side of the
person's shoe) or front legs of walker (10 to 12 in. in front of the
person's feet). In this position, the handle(s) should come to approximately the level of the greater trochanter, and the elbow(s) should be
flexed at 20 to 30 degrees. Elbow flexion is the most important indicator of correct height, as it allows the arm to shorten and lengthen
during different phases of gait.
   Physicians and other health-care professionals, as part of the evaluation process, should always assess a person's walking device. This is
achieved by checking first that the device is of the proper size and second,

Table 4   Environmental Hazard Checklist

Illumination
   Are lights bright enough to support vision and mobility?
   Are lights and lighting conditions glare free?
   Are light switch plates and lamp pull cords/switches in all rooms and stair-
      ways both visually and physically accessible?
   Are light switch plates located by the entry way of all rooms and at the top
      and bottom of stairs (to avoid ambulation in the dark)?
   Are night lights available in the bedroom and bathroom?
Floor Surfaces
   Are floor surfaces slip resistant?
   Are carpet edges tacked or taped down?
   Are throw rugs nonslip?
   Are pathways free of low-lying and difficult-to-visualize objects?
Stairways
   Are step surfaces in good repair and slip resistant?
   Are handrails present to support mobility?
Furnishings
   Are beds low in height and stable to support transfers?
   Are chairs outfitted with armrests and stable to support transfers
   Are bedside and dining room tables stable to support seating and walking
      mobility (if leaned upon)?
Bathroom
   Are toilet grab rails available to support transfers?
   Are bathtub grab rails available to support transfers?
   Are bathroom grab rails securely fastened to toilets and bathtub or mounted
      on walls?
   Are bathtub surfaces slip resistant?

---

that the device is in good repair. As if the person uses the cane or walker, and whether the device helps or interferes with mobility. As well, instruct the person to walk and transfer (on and off a chair) with the device and observe whether the tasks are being accomplished properly.

C. Environmental

The goal of environmental interventions to reduce fall risk is twofold: first, to identify and eliminate hazardous conditions that may interfere with safe mobility (Table 4 includes an environmental hazard checklist that community-residing older persons, their family members, and institutional staff can use); second, to simplify or maximize mobility tasks

Table 5 Environmental Modifications

Lighting

Low illumination: Lighting levels can be increased by using 100–200-W bulbs. Light-colored wall coverings increase the reflection of available light. Rheostatic light switches and three-way light bulbs allow persons to increase and decrease illumination levels as desired. (Control of lighting levels should rest in the hands of the person.)

Lighting glare: Glare from unshielded light sources is eliminated by placing translucent shades or coverings on exposed bulbs or using glare-free frosted light bulbs. Window glare is controlled with sheer drapery or tinted mylar shades that diffuses glare without reducing the amount of available light. Floor glare is reduced by using carpets or floor finishes that diffuse rather than reflect light.

Lighting is unavailable: Provide extra lighting (i.e., night lights that turn on automatically when lighting levels are low) in high-risk fall locations such as the top and bottom of stairways, bedrooms, and bathrooms.

Ground Surfaces

Patterned carpet designs: Avoid using carpets and rugs that have checkered or floral designs. These patterns can lead to a loss of depth perception and balance instability. If possible, replace with carpeting that is solid in color.

Sliding throw rugs: Replace rugs or apply double-sided slip-resistant adhesive backings to prevent sliding.

Carpet edges are up-ended: Either tack or tape down all carpet edges that are prone to buckling or curling.

Slippery linoleum and tiled floors: Apply nonskid finishes to linoleum floors. Bathroom tiles can be rendered slip resistant by applying nonskid strips or decorative decals on the floor next to the toilet, sink, and bathtub. Indoor–outdoor carpet has similar benefits and also provides cushioning in the event of a fall.

Chairs

Seating height is low: A cushion can increase seating height. The cushion's width or thickness is determined by the amount of height needed to support independent transfers.

Lack of arm rests: All chairs used by older persons should have arm rests. Arm rests provide leverage during rising and gradual deceleration when sitting. As well, arm rests can compensate for low seat heights. To provide maximum support, arm rests should be located approximately 7 in above the seat and extend beyond seat edges by 1 or 2 in.

Stairs

Lack of handrails: Stairway handrails are essential to support mobility. The best handrails are round in shape, extend approximately 30 in higher than the stairs, and are positioned at least 2 in from the wall. These dimensions provide effective grasp. Handrails should color contrast with the background of the wall to be noticeable.

Table 5   (Continued)

Steps are slippery: Apply nonskid treads to all steps or place nonskid adhesive
  strips that run parallel to step edges. Use color-contrasting treads and strips
  to help persons with visual impairment.

Bathrooms

Low toilet seats: The addition of a height adjustable double arm rest grab rail
  (that attached to the toilet) provides assistance with transfers. These devices
  offer better support and leverage then wall-attached grab rails.

Towel bars/sink edges are used for mobility support. Replace towel bars with
  grab rails, which provide better support. Grab rails should be securely fixed
  to the studs of the wall, constructed of a nonslip material, and color contrasted from the wall for visibility. Nonslip adhesive strips can be placed on
  the top of sink edges to guard against hand slippage.

Slippery bathtub floor: A rubber mat or nonslip adhesive strips applied on the
  tub floor surface will provide stable footing. Wall-mounted grab rails in the
  bathtub provide support during tub transfers. An adjustable grab rail that
  attaches onto the edge of the bathtub can be used as an alternative.

Shelves

Shelf heights are too high/low: To remedy this situation, frequently used items
  should be placed at levels that avoid excessive bending and reaching (i.e.,
  between the person's eye and hip level). A hand-held reacher device can be
  employed as an alternative.

through the modification of the environment and existing furnishings.
(Table 5 outlines the most common environmental features that can
interfere with mobility and recommendations for their correction.)

While this information is useful in helping to reduce fall risk, the
best approach to ensuring a safe environment is to observe the older
person functioning in the environment. This approach will determine
whether a particular environmental area of furnishing is safe or hazardous, relative to the person's functional capacity. Ask the person to walk
through every room; over present floor surfaces (e.g., carpets, linoleum
tiles, door thresholds); transfer on and off the bed, chairs, and toilet; get
in and out of the bathtub or shower; climb and descend stairs; reach up
to obtain objects from kitchen and closet shelves; and bend down to
retrieve objects from cabinets. Note which environmental features interfere with mobility and recommend adaptive modifications. The institutional assessment of the environment is similar to the home evaluation,
with the exclusion of tasks that are performed only with human assistance (i.e., bathing). To maintain safe conditions, the environmental

assessment needs to be completed on a regular basis or whenever the person's mobility needs change. Referral to allied health professionals (e.g., nurses, occupational and physical therapists), for the purpose of completing the environmental evaluation and instituting modifications, can be an effective approach.

VI. SUMMARY

Falls are an significant problem for older persons and result in significant mortality and morbidity. Most falls result from the presence of multiple intrinsic and extrinsic factors and their cumulative affects on mobility. Prevention requires a multifaceted approach aimed at: first identifying and assessing persons who have sustained falls or are at fall risk, and second, attempting interventions focused on reducing their contributing factors and supporting mobility in those who remain at fall risk.

REFERENCES

1. Tinetti ML, Speechley M, Ginter SF. Risk factors for falls among elderly persons living in the community. N Engl J Med 319: 1701.
2. Jones W J, Smith A. Preventing hospital incidents: What can we do. Nurs Manage 1989; 20 (9):58.
3. Morgan V R, Mathison J H, Rice J C, et al. Hospital falls: A persistent problem. Am J Pub Health 1985; 75: 775.
4. Rubenstein L Z, Robbins A S, Schulman B L., et al. Falls and instability in the elderly. J Am Geriatr Soc 1988; 36: 266.
5. Tideiksaar R. Falling in old age: Its prevention and treatment. New York: Springer Publishing Company, 1989.
6. Tinetti M E, Speechley M. Prevention of falls among the elderly. N Engl J Med 1989; 320: 1055.
7. Tinetti M E. Factors associated with serious injury during falls by ambulatory nursing home residents. J Am Geriatr Soc 1987; 35: 644.
8. Felson D T, Anderson J J, Hannan M T, et al. Impaired vision and hip fracture. J Am Geriatr Soc 1989; 37: 495.
9. Lindsay R. Osteoporosis. Clin Geriatr Med 1988; 4: 411.
10. Melton LJ, Riggs BL. Risk factors for injury after a fall. Clin Geriatr Med 1985; 1: 525.
11. Evans JG, Prudham D, Wandless I. A prospective study of fractured proximal femur: incidence and outcome. Publ Health 1979; 93: 235.
12. Cummings SR, Nevitt MC. A hypothesis: The causes of hip fractures. J Gerontol 1989; 44: M 107.

13. Nevitt MC, Cummings SR, Kidd D, et al. Factors for recurrent non-syncopal falls: A prospective study. JAMA 1989; 261: 2663.

14. Kolanowski AM. The clinical importance of environmental lighting to the elderly. J Gerontol Nurs 1992; 18: 10.

15. Kokeman E, Bossemyer RW, Barney J, et al. Neurologic manifestations of aging. J Gerontol 1977; 32: 411.

16. Skinner HB, Barrack RL, Cook SD. Age-related decline in proprioception. Clin Orthoped 1984; 184: 208.

17. Sloan PD, Baloh RW, Honrubia A. The vestibular system in the elderly: clinical implications. Am J Otolaryngol 1986; 10: 422.

18. Gabell A, Nayak USL. The effect of age on variability of gait. J Gerontol 1984; 39: 662.

19. Sabin T. Biologic aspects of falls and mobility limitations in the elderly. J Am Geriatr Soc 1982; 30: 51.

20. Guimaraes RM, Issacs B. Studies of gait and balance in normal old people and in people who have fallen. Intern Rehab Med 1980; 2: 177.

21. Smith EL, Di Fabio RP, Gilligan C. Exercise intervention and physiologic function in the elderly. Top Geriatr Rehab 1990; 6: 57.

22. Flatten K, Wilhite B, Reyes-Watson E. Exercise activities for the elderly. New York: Springer Publishing Company, 1988.

23. Lewis CB. Improving mobility in older persons: A manual for geriatric specialists. Rockville, MD: Aspen Publishers Inc., 1989.

24. Tideiksaar R. Footwear in the elderly: factors involved in causing and preventing falls. Clin Gerontol, in press.

12

Neuromuscular and Systemic Effects of Immobilization

ROBERT E. WHITE

Rehabilitation Hospital of Lafayette, Lafayette, Louisiana

KEVIN C. O'CONNOR

University of Medicine and Dentistry of New Jersey, Newark, New Jersey

I. INTRODUCTION

Humans are affected by gravity more than any other animal because of their normal erect posture (1). Over time, adaptive changes have allowed the ability to bear weight on the spine and to walk upright. With recumbancy, gravity is still present, but head-to-foot loading of the body along its long axis is minimized and its load is redistributed. Changes occur again as the body rapidly adapts to this new physiological state and the ability to adjust to an upright body position is reduced. Under these conditions, the various physiological systems deteriorate according to different time sequences (2). The objective of this chapter is to review those deleterious effects of bed rest and immobilization upon the human body.

II. CARDIOVASCULAR SYSTEM

In response to gravity, the human body has evolved a system of receptors that sense body position while erect and direct compensatory mechanisms. Normally, 70% of the body's blood volume is in systemic veins, 15% in the heart and lungs, 10% in systemic arteries, and 5% in capillaries. When a person moves from supine to erect, 700 cc of venous blood shifts from the upper to the lower extremities, with 400 cc coming from the heart and lungs. The loss of central blood volume causes a 25% decrease in cardiac output, a 40% decrease in stroke volume, a 25% increase in heart rate, but little change in the blood pressure of a normally active person (3–6).

While erect, the human body can offset these positional changes in three ways. The first compensatory mechanism is the rapid contraction and relaxation of smooth muscle of the venous wall combined with contraction of lower extremity muscles, which enhances blood return to the central circulation (7). The second line of defense occurs when the pre- and postcapillary sphincters act to decrease or increase fluid in the tissues. The third mechanism depends upon stimulation of baroreceptors, which in turn stimulate sympathetic nervous system activity and inhibit the release of hormonal regulators, especially antidiuretic hormone (ADH) (8). Padfield and Morton (9) suggested that ADH may be important in maintaining blood pressure, and in the regulation of plasma volume. In addition, atrial distention may release a natriuretic factor that controls electrolyte loss by the kidneys (10). These last two mechanisms are more important for long-term adjustments and adaptations of the circulation to changes of gravity.

During the first few days of bed rest, a diuresis occurs that is primarily associated with a suppression of ADH secretion (11,12). This diuresis leads to a rapid 8–12% loss of plasma volume, which stabilizes to a 15–20% decrease after 2–4 weeks (13). Studies lasting 100–200 days have shown a 30% loss of plasma volume (13). With the loss of plasma volume, the hematocrit increases and, with bed rest longer than 2 weeks, it leads to a decrease in red cell mass and a slight reticulocytosis (14,15). These changes stabilize but remain suppressed after 60 days of immobilization (14).

Cardiac function also changes with prolonged bed rest. Initially, with the change from upright to supine, body fluids shift toward the head, leading to increased central circulating volume. These changes lead to an increase in stroke volume and cardiac output (16). As bed rest continues, baroreceptors and volume receptors react to restore central volume and stroke volume and cardiac output decreases toward normal levels. Persistent bed rest results in further adaptation, where stroke volume and cardiac output continue to decline, but eventually stabilize at lower levels than normal (17).

End diastolic volume changes are influenced by the state of conditioning, with athletes showing greater bed rest losses. After 2 weeks, end diastolic volume fell 11% in seven athletic males, while in seven nonathletic males, end diastolic volume decreased only 6% (18). A 12% decrease in end diastolic volume has been noted in nonathletic females (19). Resting stroke volume and cardiac output also fell during inactivity secondary to a decrease in heart size, a loss of muscle mass, and decreased metabolic demand. In males, resting stroke volume decreased 3–9% and cardiac output declined 6–13%, while females had 25% and 21% decreases, respectively (19,20).

Resting pulse rate increases one-half beat per minute per day during the first 2 months (21). Studies of heart rate have shown increases in heart rate of 12 to 32 beats per minute after 10 days of bed rest (22,4). This increase appears to level off after 60 days, with heart rate increasing thereafter by one to five beats per minute per week. Other investigators have found little or no change (7), and even a decrease in heart rate following bed rest (23). Resting diastolic and systolic blood pressure during bed rest usually do not change, although diastolic pressure increases (24) and systolic pressure decreases have been reported (4).

Studies on thromboembolic events reveal a direct relationship between the frequency of deep vein thrombosis and the duration of bed rest (25–27). Virchow's triad postulates that the interaction of stasis, increased blood coagulability, and damage to the blood vessel wall cause a vein thrombosis. Although stasis of the blood in the lower extremities has long been proposed as the primary mechanism for the formation of vein thromboses, studies have shown that the blood flow in the lower extremity veins is actually greater in the recumbent position than in standing or sitting (28). More likely, vein thrombosis may be related to the hypercoagulable state induced by plasma volume reduction and dehydration (26). Because 50–80% of pulmonary emboli occur in patients in whom leg vein thromboses were undetected, the emphasis should be on prevention rather than treatment of established phlebothrombosis (2).

With prolonged inactivity and bed rest, the normal compensatory responses on assuming an upright position are significantly altered, lead-

Table 1 Cardiovascular Effects of Immobilization

Parameter	% Change	Comment
A. *Decreased*		
1. Plasma volume	8–30	8–12 initially, 15–20 @ 2–4 weeks, 30% @ 100–200 days
2. Total blood volume		
3. Coronary blood flow		
4. End diagnostic volume	6–12	
5. Stroke volume	3–9 (males) 25 (females)	with exercise 23%
6. Cardiac output	6–13 (males) 21 (females)	
7. Orthostatic tolerance		
8. Red cell mass		
9. Maximal oxygen uptake	17–28	
B. *Increased*		
Heart Rate	12–32 bpm (½ beat/day)	with exercise 19%
C. *No Change*		
Resting or exercising arteriovenous oxygen differences		
Blood pressure		

ing to postural hypotension. Although this has been thought to be in response to increased venous pooling in the lower extremities (29), this hypothesis has not been confirmed (30,29,19). Instead, an increase in the sympathetic nervous system beta-adrenergic activity may be the possible mechanism. Melada (31) and Sandler (18) demonstrated that beta-adrenergic blockade with propranolol improved, but did not completely alleviate, postbed-rest postural hypotension.

Both exercise tolerance and work capacity are significantly reduced following bed rest. Measurements during exercise testing have demonstrated decreases in oxygen uptake, stroke volume, and cardiac output following bed rest. Little to no change has been noted in ventilatory volumes, maximal heart rate, and arteriovenous oxygen differences (32).

Most investigators reported a decrease in maximal oxygen uptake of 17–28% (10, 33–35). It appears that the increased duration of inactivity negatively correlated with changes in the maximal oxygen uptake (VO_2Max) (36). Work capacity is also impaired following bed rest and may result from loss of skeletal muscle strength, decreased muscle me-

Table 2 Other Physiological Effects of Prolonged Bed Rest

Decreased	Increased	No change
Total lung diffusing capacity	Diuresis	Vital capacity
	Nitrogen loss	Maximum voluntary ventilation
Hormones (adrenal, ADH)	Urinary calcium and phosphorus	
Muscle mass and strength	Cholesterol	Total lung capacity
Serum proteins	Growth hormone	
Insulin sensitivity	Deep vein thrombosis risk	
Resistance to infection	Psychosocial dissociation	
Bone calcium, density	Urinary tract infections and calculi	

tabolism, and loss of lower limb skeletal muscle strength (37). At submaximal exercise, bed rest lowers the stroke volume up to 23%, while heart rate increases up to 19% (38–41).

Decreased exercise tolerance has been found to deteriorate equally in both supine and upright exercise (10). Saltin (37) concludes that the most important factor, then, is the decrease in myocardial performance, rather than orthostatic intolerance, that reduces effort tolerance.

Several studies have also shown a poorer orthostatic tolerance and exercise tolerance for athletically conditioned subjects following bed rest, indicating that athletes decondition at a faster rate than nonathletes (42,43). Although definitive studies have not been completed, the most likely explanation is an alteration in baroreceptor function (44). The cardiovascular effects of immobilization are summarized in Table 1; other physiological effects of prolonged bed rest are summarized in Table 2.

III. PULMONARY SYSTEM

The mechanics of air exchange appear to be only minimally affected by immobility. Strict bed rest produced little change in total lung capacity, functional vital capacity, functional expiratory volume, alveolar-arterial oxygen tension difference, and membrane diffusing capacity. When exercise was performed following bed rest, the tidal volume was lower and the respiratory rate was higher than prior to bed rest (1).

The supine position interferes with the normal ciliary mechanism for the clearance of secretions from the bronchioles (2). This predisposes to pneumonia, most frequently in the lower lobes (45). In addition, arteriorvenous shunting of the dependent pulmonary segments has been described. This occurs because the dependent portions of the lung are poorly ventilated, whereas blood perfusion continues at a normal rate. When this unoxygenated blood mixes, a relative arterial hypoxemia is produced (39).

IV. BONE AND CALCIUM METABOLISM

Bone is in a dynamic and constant state of change through accretion and resorption. In each bone, collagen is mineralized in a highly ordered laminated fashion to form two types of bone, trabecular and cortical. The amount of surface in relation to calcified matrix is greater in trabecular than in cortical bones. Therefore, certain bones, e.g., vertebrae, which have a larger amount of trabecular bone, are more vulnerable to the change in surface metabolic activities (46).

Bone functions not only as a mechanical support, but also in the regulation of mineral metabolism (calcium homeostasis). These functions are carried out by osteocytes: osteoblasts (bone-forming cells), and osteoclasts (bone-resorbing cells). Bone remodeling or renewal is initiated by a variety of stimuli including parathyroid hormone (PTH), which activates the osteoclast to resorb calcified matrix. Osteoblasts synthesize new matrix, which is later calcified.

Although the skeleton contains most of the body's calcium, the renal tubule, intestinal mucosa, and bone surfaces all participate in calcium homeostasis. In addition, it is dependent upon the interaction of three hormones: PTH, calcitonin, and vitamin D, along with magnesium, phosphorus, sodium, hydrogen, and calcium (46). Both PTH and 1,25-dihydroxy vitamin D increase extracellular calcium, while calcitonin acts in the opposite direction to maintain a constant serum calcium (47). A useful marker of bone metabolism is hydroxyproline, 25% of which is excreted in urine and can be used as an index of bone resorption in healthy adults (48).

Wolff's law states that bone morphology and density are dependent upon the forces that act on the bone (49,50). With immobilization, the normal forces acting upon bone are disrupted. Animal studies have demonstrated that increased bone resorption during immobilization appears to be the primary factor in bone loss. Bone loss occurs in several stages. The initial stage is a rapid loss of bone with an equally rapid reversal. The second stage begins after about 12 weeks of immobilization and, while slower, is longer lasting. During the final stage, bone volume is maintained at 40–70% of the original volume (51,52). The rate of bone loss is higher in younger individuals and in weight-bearing bones (53). Osteopenia due to immobilization is characterized by the loss of calcium and hydroxyproline from the cancellous bone of long bone epiphyses and metaphyses. Rates of bone loss for healthy bed-rested subjects average 5% per month (54).

Age and bone turnover rate are critical in the response to inactivity. There is a more rapid bone loss in younger individuals, with higher rates of bone turnover than in older individuals, who tend eventually to lose a quantitatively similar amount of bone but do so more slowly (55). Total serum calcium concentration and serum phosphorus generally remain normal, but urinary calcium, phosphorus, and hydroxyproline are all significantly increased resulting in a negative nitrogen balance (56).

Urinary calcium excretion increases above normal levels on the second and third days of recumbency, with maximum loss during the fourth and fifth week. On average, calcium loss is 1.5 g per week. This decrease in total calcium continues even after resumption of physical activity and calcium balance may not be achieved for months or even years (57). The calcium loss probably occurs through suppression of the PTH-1,25-dihydroxy vitamin D axis (58,59). Complications of this altered calcium metabolism include fractures with minimal trauma, especially compression fractures of the vertebrae and ectopic calcification in muscles and other soft tissues (60).

Another consequence related to disordered calcium metabolism is the syndrome of immobilization hypercalcemia, seen particularly in adolescent boys after acute spinal cord injury. Up to 50% of healthy children with single fractures of the lower limb on bed rest will have hypercalcemia (61). Symptomatic hypercalcemia is characterized by anorexia, abdominal pain, nausea, vomiting, constipation, hypertension, and progressive neurological signs including coma (62). Treatment relies on achieving calcium excretion through hydration and furosemide (63,64). The hallmark of both treatment and prevention of the skeletal complications of immobility is the resumption of weight bearing and resistive exercises as early as possible (16).

V. MUSCULAR SYSTEM

Skeletal muscle is adaptable and readily changes with daily activity. Regular exercise, training and physical conditioning result in morphological and metabolic changes that increase muscle mass and strength.

Both an increase in fiber size (hypertrophy) and number (hyperplasia) are thought to occur, although the latter concept is controversial (16).

Lack of mobility leads to loss of muscle mass because of minimal muscle activity and the redistribution of gravitational forces. With immobilization, a muscle will lose 10–15% of its strength per week, or about 1–3% per day, and 50% in 3–5 weeks. After 4 months, a significant number of muscle fibers degenerate, and full recovery is not possible (65). During bed rest, the antigravity muscles of the leg and trunk which are used to resist gravity are more affected. Deitrick (66), using healthy individuals in body casts, found the greatest loss of strength (measured by ergometer) in the gastrocnemius-soleus muscle (20.8%), followed by the anterior tibialis muscle (13.3%), the shoulder girdle (8.7%), and the biceps muscle (6.6%). Strength in hand grip, back extensors, and abdominal muscles did not decline. Type I muscle fibers atrophied predominantly (66).

Physiologically, with prolonged inactivity, oxidative enzymatic activity is reduced, resulting in lower tolerance to oxygen debt and earlier and longer accumulation of lactic acid (67–69). Also, fuel storage by individual muscle cells is impaired, which can contribute to the negative nitrogen balance.

Using submaximal exercise, disuse weakness can be reversed at a rate of 6% per week, significantly slower than seen in the original loss (65). After a few weeks' delay, an increase in muscular size will follow an increase in power, mainly due to enlargement of individual fibers and increased capillary density. Disuse weakness is simple to prevent. Muscle strength can be maintained with a program of daily muscle contractions of 20–30% of maximal tension for several seconds each day. A more vigorous contraction (50% of maximum) performed for 1 s per day will also be effective (65,70,4). In addition, isolated muscle group weakness and atrophy may be prevented by electrical stimulation (71).

Finally, a muscle that is immobilized in a certain position becomes contracted, and, as muscle is replaced by fibrous tissue, normal length and function can be difficult, if not impossible, to restore.

VI. GENITOURINARY SYSTEM

Urinary complications due to immobility include development of renal calculi and urinary tract infections. In the supine position, both renal blood flow and renal water elimination are increased, leading to an increase in sodium and potassium excretion (71). Hypercalciuria is frequently found (72–74), and, when combined with hyperphosphaturia and an altered ratio of citric acid to calcium, can lead to stone formation. Gravity assists in urinary drainage from the renal pelvis and ureters. When supine, urine stagnates and dissolved mineral precipitates, promoting stone formation. Bladder emptying may also be decreased when recumbent as a result of decreased intra-abdominal pressure, incomplete pelvic floor relaxation, restricted diaphragm movement, and loss of gravitational assistance. Enlargement of the prostate produces additional outflow obstruction when present. Incomplete bladder elimination results in conditions for stone formation (72).

Bladder stones, especially struvite and carbonate-apatite stones, are found in 15–30% of immobilized patients. Bladder stones foster bacterial growth and can decrease the efficiency of antibiotic treatment. Bladder stones may also irritate the bladder mucosa and lead to infection (52,75).

VII. GASTROINTESTINAL SYSTEM

A lack of physical activity can lead to loss of appetite, especially for protein-rich foods, atrophy of the intestinal mucosa and glands, and a slower rate of absorption. These factors may result in a nutritional hypoproteinemia: immobilization also causes increased adrenergic stimulation, which inhibits peristalsis and causes sphincter contraction (64). The slower peristalsis, along with the loss of plasma volume and dehydration, often results in constipation. Constipation may be further aggravated by use of a bedpan, as it requires a nonphysiological position (76). Narcotic medications slow peristalsis even further and should be avoided if at all possible for the immobilized patient.

VIII. METABOLIC AND ENDOCRINE SYSTEMS

Characteristically, metabolic changes of inactivity have an insidious onset and a delayed recovery period with return to activity. The most basic changes with reduced activity would be expected to alter the basal metabolic rate (BMR), caloric requirements (77), and dietary intake. In one study, the BMR declined 6.9% within 20–24 h and remained stable (66). The BMR usually returns to normal 3 weeks after the subject returns to active life (1).

When subjected to bed rest, most individuals lose weight, usually from a combination of factors, including the known diuresis, a decreased caloric need, and the shift from actively metabolizing lean body mass to body fat (78). The loss of body fat appears to be proportional to the decrease in metabolic rate, while the loss of lean body mass is independent of metabolic rate and results from the relative inactivity (66). Because of a loss of appetite, particularly for proteins, it is desirable to reduce the dietary content of carbohydrates and fat and to increase the intake of protein (79,58). In most immobilized individuals, 30–40 kcal per kilo of body weight per day will meet the dietary needs. Immune system functions may be deleteriously affected by the change in diet and the lack of appetite.

A. Water and Salt Metabolism

When supine, approximately 700 cc of blood shift from the lower to the upper parts of the body. This stimulates cardiopulmonary receptors and carotid and aortic baroreceptors, resulting in an increase of prostaglandin and natriuretic factor and inhibition of the sympathetic nervous system, the renin-angiotensin-aldosterone system, and antidiuretic hormone (70). These mechanisms combine to increase urinary sodium and water excretion and diuresis with resultant decrease in blood volume. The loss of blood volume by diuresis, which results in a negative water balance, is rhythmic and periodic. Although extracellular fluid is primarily lost during the first few days of bed rest, further loss comes from intracellular fluids. In addition, interstitial volume (extracellular minus plasma volume) increases (58,80).

B. Catecholamine Response

The vascular system responds to a decrease in circulating blood volume by a release of catecholamines which would be expected during bed rest. In contrast, Leach (81) found a significant decrease in urinary norepinephrine excretion with no change in epinephrine. The lack of increase in norepinephrine may also cause decreased orthostatic tolerance following bed rest (82).

C. Glucose Metabolism

Impaired glucose tolerance is regularly found with inactivity and the degree of abnormality is proportional to the degree of immobilization (83). A hyperinsulinemic response to a glucose load is apparent after only 2 days of bed rest and is more enhanced with increasing duration.

The excessive hyperinsulinemia is caused by higher secretion rates from the pancreas and not by diminished clearance from the circulation (84). Under conditions of inactivity, an insulin resistance develops, requiring greater amounts of insulin to maintain normal glucose levels (85). Although the precise mechanism for insulin resistance is unknown, it could result from a defect in insulin-sensitive tissues or the presence of circulating insulin antagonists. The usual insulin antagonists—growth hormone, catecholamine, cortisol, and free fatty acids—are probably not responsible because they do not increase significantly and may even decrease during prolonged immobilization (86,87).

Daily exercise decreases the hyperinsulinemic response to glucose load, but does not eliminate it. With return to activity, 7–14 days are required to restore plasma glucose to normal in nonexercising individuals, compared with 7 days in those who exercised during bed rest.

Last, an altered metabolic state may affect the rate at which drugs are absorbed, distributed, bound, metabolized, or excreted, which will, in turn, affect the availability and effectiveness of a medication (81,90–92).

IX. PSYCHOLOGICAL SYSTEM

Bed rest entails sensory deprivation, isolation, and confinement. The lack of stimulation may result in sleep disturbances, increased emotional lability and fatigue, neurological changes, and deterioration in motivation and cognitive performance (93–95). Perceptual impairment may be found even after 7 days of immobilization (96).

Circadian rhythmicity deteriorates also and there is a shift from 24- or 12-h bimodal rhythmic patterns, which may result from a combination of immobilization, neuropsychological dysfunction, and reduced effectiveness of environmental synchronizers. Both light and dark cycles (97) and social interaction are involved in the synchronization or circadian rhythms and, when impaired, can decrease performance, sleep quality, and psychological well being (98). The degree of circadian dysrhythmia is also dependent upon individual characteristics including structure, interactions, environmental stressors, and the duration of immobilization (99). Restlessness, anxiety, decreased pain tolerance, irritability, hostility, insomnia, and depression may occur and may affect the ability of the patient to return to normal activity. These deleterious psychological effects may be countered by instituting a program of sensory stimulation.

Similarly, it is necessary to provide intellectual challenges to these patients and to make them perform specific tasks (e.g., arithmetic, comment on news) in order to preserve intellectual function at their premorbid level (88).

X. INTEGUMENTARY SYSTEM

One of the major hazards of immobilization is the breakdown of the skin and underlying tissues. The extent and duration of immobilization are crucial factors in the development of impaired tissue integrity (100). Tissue breakdown occurs from either pressure, shear, or a combination of the two. Skin breakdown is a result of interference with capillary blood flow and the resultant inability to provide nutrients and remove waste products.

Pressure is highest on the skin overlying bony prominences, especially the sacrum, ischial tuberosities, greater trochanters, heels, occiput, and elbows. Pressure sore formation is dependent on both the magnitude of the pressure and also the duration of the pressure. Other factors, including edema, malnutrition, loss of sensation, anemia, soiling of the skin with urine and feces, and excessive perspiration, contribute significantly to the formation of pressure sores (101). Prevention positioning and frequent turning with monitoring of other risk factors are the keys to protecting vulnerable skin areas against pressure sores. Once impaired tissue integrity has occurred, healing may be difficult and prolonged and may require surgical intervention (102,103).

XI. SUMMARY

Thus we see that for human beings, *movement* is like voting in a democracy: both a privilege and an obligation. The lack of movement, whether because of iatrogenic immobilization of a fracture or torn ligament or because of prolonged bed rest, has been shown by many researchers, over the past four decades, to result in profound physiological and biochemical changes in practically all organs and systems of the body (66,52,104–106). Conversely, regular range of motion and therapeutic exercise have been shown not only to prevent the complications of immobility, but also to promote general good health and fitness, improve quality of life, and greatly decrease risk factors for many chronic diseases, such as hypertension (107,108), diabetes (109), osteoporosis (110), and coronary heart disease (111).

REFERENCES

1. Browse NL. Physiology and Pathology of Bedrest. Springfield: Charles C Thomas, 1965: 1–221.
2. Steinberg FU. The Immobilized Patient, Functional Pathology and Management. New York: Plenum Press, 1980: 1–156.
3. Miller MG. Iatrogenic and neurogenic effects of prolonged immobilization of the ill aged. J Am Geriatr Soc 1975; 23(8): 360–369.
4. Taylor HL. The effects of rest in bed and of exercise on cardiovascular function. Circulation 1968; 38(6): 1016–1017.
5. Turner AH. The circulatory minute volume of healthy young women in reclining, sitting, and standing positions. Am J Physiol 1927; 80: 601–630.
6. Vernikos-Danellis J, Winget CM, Leach CS, Rambaut PC. Circadian endocrine and metabolic effects of prolonged bedrest: two 56-day bedrest studies NASA Technical bulletin, No Tm V-3051, US National Aeronautics and Space Administration, 1974: 1–45.
7. Gazenko OG, Shumakov VI, Kakurin LI, et al. Central circulation and metabolism of the healthy man during postural exposures and arm exercise in the head-down position, Aviat Space Environ Med 1980; 51(2): 113–120.
8. Hagan RD, Diaz FJ, Horvath S. J Appl Physiol 1978; 45(3): 414–417.
9. Padfield PL, Morton JJ. In Robertson JLS, ed. Handbook of Hypertension, Vol. 1. Amsterdam: Elsevier, 1983: 348–364.
10. Convertino VA, Hung J, Goldwater D, De Busk RF. Circulation 1982; 65: 134–140.
11. Gauer OH, Henry JP, Behn C. Ann Rev Physiol, 1970; 32: 547–595.
12. Goetz KL, Bond GC, Bloxham DD. J Appl Physiol 1975; 55: 157–205.
13. Greenleaf JE, Silverstein L, Bliss J, Langenheem V, Rossow H, Chao C. Physiological Responses to Prolonged Bed Rest: A Compendium of Research (1974–1988). NASA TM-81324 US National Aeronautics and Space Administration, Washington, DC, 1982.
14. Burkovskaya TY, Illyukhin AV, Jobachek VI, Zhidowv VV. Space Biol and Aerosp Med 1980; 14(S): 75–80.
15. Morse JT, Staley RW, Juhos LT, Van Beaumont W. Fluid and electrolyte shifts during bed rest without isometric and isotonic exercises. J Appl Physiol 1977; 42: 59–66.
16. Books GA, Fahey TD. Exercise Physiology. New York: John Wiley & Sons, 1884.
17. Vogt FB. Effects of intermittent leg cuff inflation and intermittent exercise on the tilt table response after ten days' bed recumbency. Aerosp Med 1966; 37: 943–946.
18. Sandler H, Popp RL, Harrison DC. (1985). Aviat Space Environ Med 1985; 56: 489.

19. Sandler H, Winter DL. Physiological Responses of Women to simulated weightlessness: A Review of the Significant Findings of the First Female Bed Rest Study. NASA SP-430, 1978: 1–87.

20. Saltin B, Blomqvist G, Mitchell JH, et al. Response to exercise after bed rest and after training, Circulation 1968 (Suppl VII): 1–78.

21. Taylor HL, Henschel A, Porozek J, Keys A. Effects of bed rest on cardiovascular function and work performance. J Apply Psychol 1949; 2: 223–229.

22. Todd J. Deep venous thrombosis in acute spinal cord injury: a comparison of 1251 fibrinogen ligament scanning, impedance plethysmography and venography. Paraplegia 1976; 1450.

23. Kovalenko YA, Gurovsky NN. In Sandler H, Vernikos J (eds.), Inactivity: Physiological Effects. Orlando: Academic Press Inc., 1986: 77–97.

24. Fiorentini C, Polese A, Olivari MT, Guazzi MD. Cardiac performance in hypertension re-evaluated through a combined haemodynamic ultrasonic method. Br Heart J 1980; 43(3): 334–350.

25. Gibbs NM. Venous thrombosis of the lower limbs with particular reference to bedrest. Br J Surg 1957; 191: 209–235.

26. Micheli LJ. Thromboembolic complications of cast immobilization for injuries of the lower extremities. Clin Orthoped 1975; 108: 191–195.

27. Enneking WF, Horowitz M. The intra-articular effects of immobilization on the human knee. J Bone Joint Surg [Am] 1972; 54: 973.

28. Wright HP, Osborn SB, Hayden M. Venous velocity in bedridden medical patients. Lancet 1952; 2: 699.

29. Memmer MK. Acute orthostatic hypotension. Heart Lung 1988; 17: 134–143.

30. McCally M, Piemme TE, Murray RH. Tilt table responses of human subjects following application of lower body negative pressure. Aerosp Med 1966; 37: 1247.

31. Melada GA, Goldman JH, Luestscher JA, Zager PG. Hemodynamics renal function, plasma renin, and aldosterone in man after 5 to 14 days of bedrest. Aviat Space Environ Med 1975; 46(9): 1049–1055.

32. Sandler H, Vernikos J, et al. Effects of inactivity on muscle. In Sandler H, Vernikos J., eds.), Inactivity: Physiological effects. New York: Academic Press, 1986: 77–97.

33. Convertino VA, Alson L, Goldwater D, Sandler H. Aerosp Med Assoc Reprints 1979: 47–48.

34. Hung J, Goldwater D, Convertino V, McKillop J, et al. Am J Cardiol 1981; 47: 477.

35. Sandler H, Webb P, Ammes JF, et al. Aviat Space Environ Med 1983; 54(3): 191–201.

36. Hamrin E. Anatomical and functional changes in joints and muscles during long-term bed rest. Nord Med 1970; 85: 293–298.

37. Saltin B, Rowell LB. Functional adaptation to physical activity and inactivity. Fed Proc 1980; 39(5): 1506–1513.

38. Takayama H, Tomiyama M, Managawa A, et al. The effect of physical exercise and prolonged bed rest on carbohydrate, lipid and amino acid metabolism. Jpn J Clin Pathol 1974, 22 (Suppl): 126–136.
39. Svanberg L. Influence of posture on lung volumes ventilation and circulation in normals. Scand J Clin Lab Invest 1957; 9: 25.
40. Stremel RW, Convertino VA, Greenleaf JE, Bernauer EM. Response to maximal exercise after bed rest. Fed Proc 1974; 33: 327.
41. Stremel RW, Convertino VA, Bernauer EM, Greenleaf JE. Cardiorespiratory deconditioning with static and dynamic leg exercise during bedrest. J Appl Physiol 1976; 41: 905–909.
42. Stegemann J, Framing HD, Schiefeling M. Influence of a six hour immersion in thermoindifferent water on circulatory control and work capacity in trained and untrained subjects. Pflugers Arch Eur Physiol 1969; 312(4): 129–138.
43. Stegemann J, Meier U, Skipka W, Hartlieb W, Hemmer B, Tibes U. Effects of a multi-hour immersion with intermittent exercise on urinary excretion and tilt table tolerance in athletes and non-athletes. Aviat Space Environ Med 1975; 46(1): 26–29.
44. Stegemann J, Busert A, Brock D. Influence of fitness on the blood pressure control system in man. Aerosp Med 1974, 45(1): 45–48.
45. Puchelle E, Zahm JM, Bertrand A. Influence of age on bronchial mucociliary transport. Scand J Resp Dis 1979; 60(6): 307–313.
46. Arnaud SB, Schnuder VS, Morey-Holton E. In Sandler H, Vernikos J, eds), Inactivity: Physiological Effects. Orlando, Academic Press, Inc., 1986: pp. 49–75.
47. Lerman S, Canterburg JM, Reiss E. Parathyroid hormone and the hypercalcemia of immobilization. J Clin Endocrinol Metab 1977; 45(3): 425–488.
48. Prockop DJ, Juva K. Synthesis of hydroxyproline in vitro by the hydroxylation of proline in a precursor of collagen. Proc Natl Acad Sci USA 1965; 53: 661–668.
49. Muller EA. Influence of training and of inactivity on muscle strength. Arch Phys Med Rehabil 1970; 51: 449–463.
50. Uhthoff HK, Tarvorski ZFG. Bone loss in response to long-term immobilization. JBJS (Br) 1978; 60: 420–429.
51. Giannetta CL, Castleberry HB. Influence of bed rest and hypercapnia upon urinary mineral excretion in man. Aerosp Med 1974; 45: 750–754.
52. Kottke FJ. The effects of limitation of activity upon the human body. JAMA 1966; 196: 117–122.
53. Halar EM, Bell KR. Contracture and other deleterious effects of immobility. In DeLisa Joel A, ed., Rehabilitation Medicine Philadelphia: Lippincott, 1988: 448–462.
54. Greenleaf JE, Van Beaumont W, Convertino VA, Starr JE. Aviat Space Environ Med 1983; 54: 696–700.

55. Rose GA. Immobilization osteoporosis. Study of extent, severity and treatment with bendrofluazide. Br J Surg 1966; 53: 769.
56. Moore-Ede MC, Burr RG. Circadian rhythm of urinary calcium excretion during immobilization. Aerosp Med 1973; 44: 495–498.
57. Giannetta CL, Castleberry HB. Influence of bed rest and hypercapnia upon urinary mineral excretion in man. Aerosp Med 1974; 45: 750–754.
58. Greenleaf JE, Bernauer EM, Young HL. Fluid and electrolyte shifts during bed rest with isometric and isotonic exercise. J Appl Physiol 1977; 42: 59–66.
59. Eichelberger L, Roma M, Moulder PV. Effects of immobilization on the histochemical characterization of skeletal muscle. J Appl Physiol 1958; 12: 42.
60. Heath HJ III, Earl JM, Schaff M, et al. Serum ionized calcium during bed rest in fracture patients and normal men. Metabolism 1972; 21: 633–640.
61. Rosen FJ, Woolin DA, Finberg L. Immobilization hypercalcemia after single limb fracture in children and adolescents. Am J Dis Child 1978; 132: 560–564.
62. Hyman LR, Boner G, Thomas JC, Segar WC. Immobilization hypercalcemia. Am J Dis Child 1972; 124: 723–727.
63. Henke JA, Thompson NW, Kaufer H. Immobilization hypercalcemia crisis. Arch Surg 1975; 110(3): 321–323.
64. Ivy AC, Grossman MI. Gastrointestinal function in convalescence. In symposium on physiological aspects of convalescence and rehabilitation. Fed Proc 1944; 3: 236–239.
65. Partridge REH, Duthie TTR. Controlled trial of the effect of complete immobilization of the joints in RA. Am Rheum Dis 1963; 22: 91.
66. Deitrick JE, Whedon GD, Shorr E. Effects of immobilization upon various metabolic and physiologic functions of normal men. Am J Med 1948; 4: 3–32.
67. Johnson PC, Driscoll RD, LeBlank A. D. In "Biomedical results from Skylab." NASA SP-377 US National Aeronautics and Space Administration. Washington, DC, 1977: 235–241.
68. Pestronk A, Drachmann B, Griffin JW. Effect of muscle disuse on acetylcholine receptors. Nature 1976; 260:352–353.
69. Eldrige L, Liebhold M, Steinback JH. Alterations in cat skeletal neuromuscular junctions following prolonged inactivity. J Physiol 1981; 313: 529–545.
70. Taylor HL, Erickson L, Henschel A. The effect of bed rest in the blood volume of normal young men. Am J Physiol 1945; 144: 227–232.
71. Greenleaf JE, Young HL, Bernauer EM. Effects of Isometric and Isotonic exercise on Body Water Compartments during 14 days bed rest. Aerosp Med Assoc Rep, Washington, DC, 1973.
72. Carlson HE, Ockerblad NF. Stones of recumbency. S Med J 1940; 33: 582.

73. Issekutz B, Blizzard JJ, Birkhead NC, et al. Effect of prolonged bed rest on urinary calcium output. J Appl Physiol 1966; 21: 1013–1020.
74. Sedkutz B Jr, Blizzard JJ, Birkhead NC, Rodahl K. Effect of prolonged bed rest on urinary calcium output. J Appl Physiol 1966; 21: 1013–1020.
75. Leadbetter WF, Engster HE. Problems of renal lithiasis in convalescent patients. J Urol 1957; 53: 269.
76. Deitrick JE, Whedon GD, Shorr E. Effects of immobilization upon various metabolic and physiological functions of normal man. Am J Med 1948; 4: 3–36.
77. Lecocq FR. "The effect of bedrest on glucose regulation in man," NASA SP-269. US National Aeronautics and Space Administration, Washington, DC, 1971; 268.
78. Piemme TE. Effects of 2 weeks of bed rest on carbohydrate metabolism, hypogravity and hypodynamic environments, NASA Special publication No. 269, US National Aeronautics and Space Administration, Washington DC, 1971.
79. Pace N, Kodama AM, Price, DC, et al. Life Sci Space Res 1976; 14: 269–274.
80. Melada GA, Goldman RH, Luestscher JA, Zager PG. Hemodynamics, renal function, plasma renin, and aldosterone in man after 5 to 14 days of bed rest. Aviat Space Environ Med 1975; 46: 1049–1055.
81. Leach CS, Hulley SB, Raumbaut PC, Dietlein LF. The effect of bed rest on adrenal function. Space Life Sci 1973; 4: 415–423.
82. Chobanian AV, Lillie RD, Tercyak A, Blevins P. The metabolic and hemodynamic effects of prolonged bedrest in normal subjects. Circulation 1974; 49(3): 551–559.
83. Whedon GD. New research in energy metabolism. J Am Diet Assoc 1959; 35(7): 682–686.
84. Wirth A, Diehm C, Mayer H, et al. Plasma C-peptide and insulin in trained and untrained subjects. J Appl Physiol 1981; 50(1): 71–77.
85. Duckworth WC, Jallipalli P, Solomon SS. Arch Phys Med Rehabil 1983; 64(3): 107–110.
86. Cardus D, Valbona C, Spencer WA. The effect of bed rest on various parameters of physiological function: VI The effect of the performance of periodic Flack maneuvers on preventing cardiovascular deconditioning of bedrest, publication No. NASA-CR-176, US National Aeronautics and Space Administration, 1965.
87. Lipman RL, Schnure JJ, Bradley EM, Lecocq FR. Impairment of peripheral glucose utilization in normal subjects by prolonged bed rest. J Lab Clin Med 1970; 76: 221–230.
88. Zubek JP, Boyer L, Milstein S, Shepard JM. Behavioral and physiological changes during prolonged immobilization plus perceptual deprivation. J Abnorm Psychol 1969; 74: 230.

89. Graham DH. Anesthesiology 1980; 52(1): 74–75.
90. Kates RE, Harapat SR, Keefe DL, Goldwater D, Harrison DC. Influence of prolonged recumbancy on drug disposition. Clin Pharmacol Ther 1980; 28(5): 624–628.
91. Vernikos-Danellis J, Leach CS, Winget CM, Changes in glucose, insulin and growth hormone levels associated with bedrest. Aviat Space Eniron Med 1976; 47(6): 583–587.
92. Levy G. Effect of bed rest on distribution and elimination of drugs. J Pharm Sci 1967; 56: 928–929.
93. Corrodi H, Fuxe K, Kokfelt T. The effects of stress on the activity of the central monoamine neuron. Life Sci 1968; 7: 107–112.
94. Downs FS. Bedrest and sensory disturbances. Am J Nurs 1971; 74: 434–438.
95. Smith MJ. Changes in judgement of duration with different patterns of auditory information for individuals confined to bed. Nurs Res 1975; 24: 93–98.
96. Banks R, Cappon D. Effects of reduced sensory input on time perception. Percept Motor Skills 1962; 14: 74.
97. Wever RA, Polasek J, Wildgruber CM. Bright light affects human circadian rhythms. Pflugers Arch 1983; 396(1): 85–87.
98. Kamas NA, Fedderson WE. "Behavioral, Psychiatric, and Sociological Problems of long-duration Space Missions" NASA Technical bulletin, TM X-58067, US National Aeronautics and Space Administration, Washington, DC, 1971.
99. Ryback RS, Lewis OF, Lessard CS. Psychobiologic effects of prolonged bed rest (weightlessness) in young healthy volunteers (Study II). Aerosp Med 1971; 42: 529–535.
100. Kosiak M Etiology and pathology of ischemic ulcers. Arch Phys Med Rehab 1959; 40: 62–69.
101. Williams A. A study of factors contributing to skin breakdown. Nurs Res 1972; 21: 238–243.
102. DeLisa JA, Mikulic MA. Pressure ulcers: What to do if preventive management fails. Postgrad Med 1985; 77: 209–220.
103. Bach CA. Studies of pressure on skin under ischial tuberosities and thighs during sitting. Arch Phys Med Rehab 50: 207.
104. Long CL, Bonilla LE. Metabolic effects of inactivity and injury. In Downey JA (ed.), Physiological Basis of Rehabilitation Medicine. Philadelphia: Saunders, 1971.
105. Spencer WA, Vallbona C, Carter RE. Physiologic concepts of immobilization. Arch Phys Med Rehabil 1965; 46: 89–100.
106. Browse NL. The Physiology and Pathology of Bed Rest. Springfield, IL: Charles C Thomas, 1965.
107. Blair SN, Goodyear NN, Gibbons LW, et al. Physical fitness and incidence of hypertension in healthy normotensive men and women. JAMA 1984; 252(4): 487–490.

108. Paffenbarger RS Jr, Wing AL, Hyde RT, et al. Physical activity and incidence of hypertension in college alumni. Am J Epidemiol 1983; 117(3): 245–257.
109. Helmrich SP, Ragland DR, Leung RW, et al. Physical activity and reduced occurrence of non-insulin-dependent diabetes mellitus. N Engl J Med 1991; 325: 14.
110. Pocock NA, Eisman JA, Yeates MG, et al. Physical fitness is a major determinent of femoral neck and lumbar spine bone mineral density. J Clin Invest 1986; 78(3): 618–621.
111. Powell KE, Thompson PD, Caspersen CJ, et al. Physical activity and the incidence of coronary heart disease. Annu Rev Pub Health 1987; 8: 253–287.

13

Rehabilitation Management of Mobility Impairment

WENDY S. KELLNER

Hospital for Special Care, New Britain, Connecticut

I. MOBILITY

Mobility for a disabled person involves movement from one location to another or a change in bodily position in the same location. Walking is functional if it is self-serving and can be done safely. It is, however, only one form of mobility.

Bed mobility involves several movements, including sit to supine, side to side, supine to sit, and weight shifting within the bed. Transfers require movement from bed to chair, within the bathroom, and in and out of a car. Wheelchair mobility is needed for those individuals who cannot ambulate or sustain ambulation.

Identifying mobility goals should be accomplished after a careful history and physical examination by the physician. Whenever possible, the patient should be an active participant in the goal-setting process. In situations where the patient is incapable of participating, as a result of cognitive dysfunction or in the case of a young child, the family should be involved.

In order to monitor functional changes in mobility, several validated and reliable scales of mobility function have been designed. A thorough discussion of each scale is beyond the scope of this chapter, but the reader is referred to the excellent review article by Applegate et al., (1) summarizing scales such as the Barthel index, the Performance test of ADL, and the Kenny self-care scale. All of these scales require administration and observation by an interviewer and help quantify changes in mobility.

When mobility impairment is a result of an uncomplicated problem such as a simple ankle fracture, prescription of the most appropriate assistive device and of the therapy needed to restore function is fairly straightforward. However, when the etiology of the impairment is more complicated or multisystemic, referral to a rehabilitation team may be indicated.

II. THE REHABILITATION TEAM

A *physiatrist* is a physician specializing in Physical Medicine and Rehabilitation. The physiatrist functions as team leader, prescribing the appropriate therapies and assuring a coordinated, multidisciplinary effort.

The physical therapist (PT) is primarily involved in large muscle group activities, including gait training, transfers, trunk and lower extremity strengthening, and endurance activities and balance.

The PT is also a contributor in the process of evaluation for lower extremity orthotics or prosthetics, and in wheelchair prescription. When ambulation is not a feasible goal, the physical therapist is responsible for teaching wheelchair mobility and management, as well as transfers. They also have specialized training in the application of various modalities, including superficial heat, ultrasound, icing, and other forms of cryotherapy. Many of those are used successfully in the treatment of contractures, that is, shortening of muscle or tightness of joint capsules that may preclude ambulation in an otherwise potentially ambulatory patient.

The occupational therapist (OT) works on upper extremity function and activities of daily living (ADL), including bathing, dressing, bed mobility, and home management. The OT is also involved in perceptual motor evaluation. There can be significant impact on all forms of mobility if visual-spatial dysfunction or neglect is present, and these problems must be identified and treatment initiated. As part of ADL training, the OT instructs patients about safe transfers in the bathroom, e.g., tub and toilet. If mobility is severely impaired, a commode chair may be used. Occupational therapists are trained in the assessment of the home, work place, etc., for any modifications needed to improve accessibility. Recommendations may range from rearranging furniture or picking up scatter rugs to major renovations in the case of individuals who are wheelchair dependent or severely impaired. The addition of a ramp outside a house or widening selected doorways may open previously impossible opportunities to an individual. Finally, the OT may be asked to do a predriving evaluation if patient has had a neurological event such as a stroke or traumatic brain injury. This battery of tests examines the patient's depth perception, visual field, reaction time, and glare recovery, among other things. It provides valuable information to both the therapist and the patient regarding the prospect of resuming driving.

The therapeutic recreation specialist (TRS) has an important role in the restoration of mobility. The TR provides patients with extensive education in community-based activities. Their sessions may involve planning a visit to a restaurant or store, investigating transportation for the disabled, anticipating and negotiating architectural barriers, and dispelling "attitudinal barriers" the patients themselves may harbor toward their own disability. More will be discussed about this in Sec. IX.

Other members of the rehabilitation team called upon to participate in maximizing mobility may include a prosthetist, orthotist, rehabilitation engineer, and nurse. A psychologist or psychiatrist is often involved, to assist with adjustment to changes in lifestyle and independence, and a social worker may become involved to facilitate adjustment and to provide additional information to the patient and family regarding available community resources and services.

III. LOWER EXTREMITY ORTHOTICS

A. Weight-Bearing Modifications

Lower extremity orthotics can be utilized for a variety of functions. In some patients, it is necessary to decrease or, if possible, eliminate weight bearing throughout all or part of a lower limb. Many femoral fractures are being treated successfully with an ischial weight-bearing orthosis or cast brace (Fig. 1). These orthoses are designed to transmit forces from

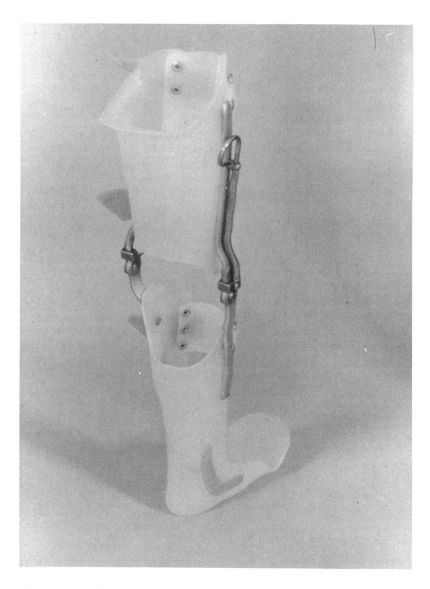

Figure 1   Ischial weight-bearing brace.

the ischium to the brace, then to the ground. Because only approximately 40% of the total force is transmitted through the ischial seat (1), and the rest through the soft mass of the thigh to the brace's skeletal structure, this orthosis does not provide total protection of the hip joint. Lehmann et al. determined the weight-bearing efficiency of the ischial weight-bearing orthosis, looking at design and training (2).

1. With a locked knee and a Patten or rocker bottom, 100% of the weight is transmitted through the orthosis.
2. With the knee locked and the ankle fixed and with patient training to decrease push-off, 86% of body weight is transmitted through the orthosis.
3. With a locked knee, fixed ankle but without patient training, 50% of body weight is borne by the orthosis.

A patellar–tendon-bearing orthosis (PTB) or a total contact PTB-like cast has been successfully used for several years in fracture rehabilitation (Fig. 2). While many believe the orthosis is accurately named pattelar—tendon bearing, other investigators believe that a total contact cast molded over the entire leg provides the real weight-bearing relief. (3) In the construction of these orthoses, patellar tendon indentation and high condylar flares are provided, to maximize rotational stability. Weight-bearing forces in this brace are transmitted from the ground, to the proximal tibia, bypassing the fracture site.

According to Davis et al. (4), short-term use of the PTB orthosis is indicated in the following conditions:

1. Os calcis fracture healing.
2. Postoperative ankle fusions.
3. Painful heel conditions, refractory to conservative management, when surgery is not indicated.

Long-term use of the orthosis is recommended in the following conditions:

1. Delayed or non-union of fractures.
2. Avascular necrosis of the talar body.
3. Degenerative arthritis of the ankle.
4. Os calcis osteomyelitis.
5. Sciatic nerve injury with insensate distal limb.
6. Diabetic skin ulceration.
7. Chronic conditions of the foot not correctable with surgery.

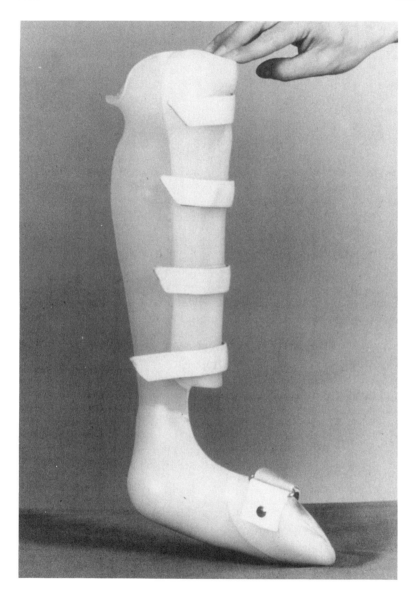

Figure 2   Patellar tendon-bearing brace.

B. Wound Healing

Diabetic plantar ulcers often complicate ambulation and historically have been very difficult to treat. While many therapeutic modalities have been employed, they do not treat the underlying cause of the ulcers. (5) According to Kosiac and others, (6) the primary cause of diabetic foot ulcers is excessive pressure on an insensate foot. Even in the presence of aggressive wound-healing techniques, a plantar sore will persist until the cause of the excessive pressure is removed. A case report by Mueller and Diamond (7) described a diabetic patient with a plantar ulcer under the second and third metatarsal heads. The ulcer remained refractory to traditional treatments but healed in 85 days, after the patient was placed in a total contact below knee cast with a walking heel. Weight-bearing instructions were one-third his usual amount. To provide long-term protection after healing, the patient was provided with a custom-molded ankle foot orthosis (AFO) and bilateral rocker bottom shoes (in an effort to disperse weight bearing over the entire plantar surface). Other studies have demonstrated similar results with total contact casting. (8) Diabetic food disease is discussed further in Chapter 9.

C. Joint Alignment

Lower extremity orthoses may also be used to maintain or correct joint alignment. One of the most common sites of joint dysfunction and progressive malalignment in the lower extremities is at the knee. Arthritis often causes weakening of the medial collateral ligament with progressive valgus deformity. To counteract this deformity, a corrective force needs to be applied medially at the knee, with two countering forces laterally, one above and one below the knee joint.

Another common alignment problem at the knee is genu recurvatum or back knee. This may be seen in situations where muscle imbalance is present, or where the patient stabilizes the knee by maintaining an extension moment. This extension force is checked by the posterior joint capsule, which is weak and over time will yield, producing hyperextension. Genu recurvatum may also occur in individuals with contracture of the gastrocnemius and soleus. In this case, treatment should be directed at the cause of the extension, i.e., stretching or motor point blocks, for example. Otherwise, the recurvatum can be managed with an AFO set in some dorsiflexion at the ankle to create a knee flexion moment at heel strike. In more severe cases, a knee–ankle–foot orthosis

(KAFO) stabilizing the knee in a few degrees of flexion will be needed. A knee cage has been used in some individuals, fabricated with a stop to prevent hyperextension. (9) The same knee orthoses have some limited benefit in treating genu valgus as well.

D. Compensation for Weakness

Perhaps the most frequent use of orthoses is in those patients with lower extremity weakness resulting from upper or lower motor neuron disease, or muscle pathology.

The AFO is the most commonly used orthosis. Indications for prescription of this brace include mediolateral instability at the ankle, toe drag, or foot drop, decreased push-off, and, in some instances, weakness about the knee.

There are two types of the most commonly used AFOs. The first is the metal double upright brace (Fig. 3). The ankle joint in the double upright AFO determines the amount of dorsiflexion and plantar flexion. A free ankle offers no restriction to plantar flexion or dorsiflexion. A single axis ankle may be equipped with a plantar flexion stop to restrict plantar flexion at a predetermined angle. Finally, a dual-channeled ankle joint can be adjusted to restrict plantar flexion and dorsiflexion. A plantar flexion stop is a substitute for weak foot dorsiflexors. The dorsiflexion stop, when used with a metal sole plate in the shoe, helps simulate push-off as the body moves forward in stance. In this respect, it can compensate for weak gastrocnemius and soleus muscles.

Additionally, the amount of dorsiflexion and plantar flexion permitted at the ankle has a definite effect on knee movement and stability. An AFO set in 5 degrees of plantar flexion holds the knee center back, resulting in a knee extension moment. In a patient with weakness of the knee extensors, setting the brace in a few degrees of plantar flexion may produce greater knee stability. However, one must be careful to avoid excessive knee locking as this may produce genu recurvatum. Also, there will be less toe clearance during swing phase when the brace is set in plantar flexion and this too must be considered before constructing the AFO. Setting the orthosis in 5 degrees of dorsiflexion will increase toe clearance during the swign phase of ambulation. However, this creates a significant knee-bending moment at heel strike, potentially destabilizing a weak knee joint. Thus, there is a trade-off between toe clearance and knee stability and AFO prescriptions must take this into account.

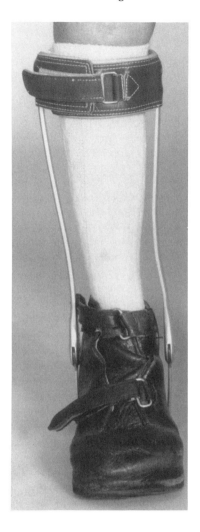

Figure 3 Double upright ankle foot orthosis.

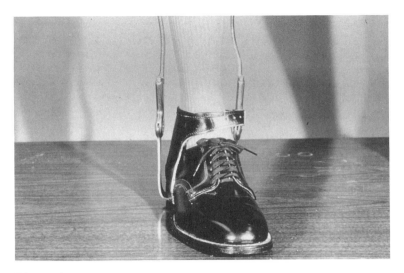

Figure 4   T-strap.

A double upright metal AFO generally provides good mediolateral support to the ankle. In some patients with significant spasticity,
however, the standard components of the brace may be overridden by
the tendency of the foot toward varus. In these situations, a T-strap (Fig.
4) can be added to the brace, attached to the lateral aspect of the shoe,
encircling the medial upright of the AFO. When buckled tightly, the
strap has the effect of pulling the foot toward the medial, i.e., immov-
able bar, decreasing the varus. A medial T-strap can similarly be used to
correct excessive ankle valgus.

The second major category of AFO is the molded plastic AFO.
This brace is molded over a positive mold taken from a cast of the leg
and foot. The orthosis can provide minimal or extensive mediolateral
support depending on the trim lines at the level of the ankle. This AFO
can virtually encase the malleoli in plastic, with maximum mediolateral
control (Fig. 5), or can be constructed with very narrow trim lines, well
behind the malleoli, offering little or no mediolateral support (Fig. 6).
The full trim line, or solid ankle AFO is also comparable to a double
upright brace with a plantar flexion and dorsiflexion stop, allowing no
movement at the ankle. As with the metal AFO, dorsiflexion and

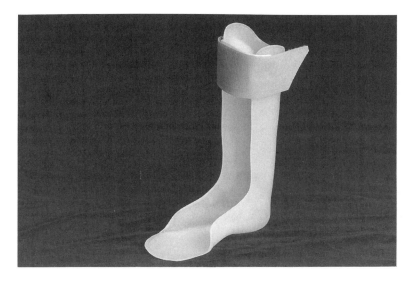

Figure 5 Solid ankle ankle-foot orthosis.

plantar flexion can be controlled, here, by positioning the foot at the desired angle during casting. Knee stability is determined by the amount of plantar flexion or dorsiflexion built into the ankle portion of the brace. While the plastic AFO has the advantage of being transferable from one pair of shoes to another, unlike the metal brace, it is critically important that the heel and sole heights of all shoes used match those of the shoes used for casting. The lighter weight and improved comesis of the plastic AFOs has made them the first choice of many patients. The major advantages of the double upright brace are that (1) it can be used in patients with fluctuating lower extremity edema; and (2) it can be used in patients with open areas on the skin of their legs.

A third AFO, less often prescribed, is the Veteran's Administration Prosthetics Center (VAPC) shoe clasp orthosis. This brace is clasped onto the counter of a shoe. It provides moderate toe pick-up and no mediolateral stability. It has no effect on knee stability.

The knee–ankle–foot orthosis (Fig.7) is also used to compensate for either upper or lower motor neuron weakness. This brace is indicated for patients who have weakness not only of the foot and ankle but

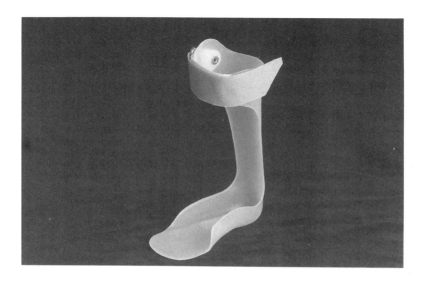

Figure 6   Narrow trim line ankle-foot orthosis.

also significant weakness or instability of the knee. KAFOs are often prescribed for individuals who have had a stroke, for those with a variety of neuromuscular diseases, and, in many instances, for spinal cord injury. Knee stabilization is usually excellent and may be further improved by the addition of a knee cap strap to the brace.

E. Electrophysiological Bracing

Electrophysiological bracing by direct muscle stimulation continues to be an area of research and exploration. The locations for use of electrical stimulation range from specific, even single nerve selection, to significantly larger areas involving multiple nerves. In a study investigating peroneal nerve stimulation in hemiplegic patients, stimulators were designed to stimulate muscle that effect dorsiflexion of the ankle, facilitating the swing phase of ambulation. (10) The circuit was closed when the affected heel was lifted off the floor and was deactivated when the same heel returned to the floor at heel strike. Later studies sought to refine the indications for this application of electrical stimulation and assess results. (11) The current applied was often not well tolerated by patients and the

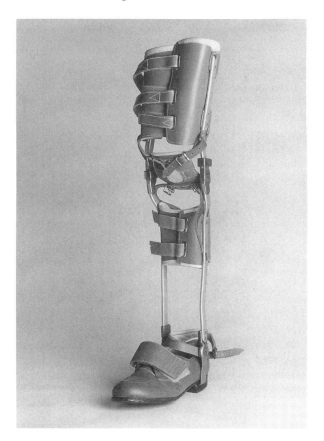

Figure 7 Knee-ankle-foot orthosis.

stimulators were difficult to apply. Nonetheless, it was believed that there was benefit to gait training with the assist of the functional stimulation, with some carryover noted even without the stimulator. (11)

More recently, investigators have looked at the use of implantable stimulators, individually used or as part of a multichannel system. (12) Bracing for paraplegic patients, long a challenge because of the weight of the orthotics and the energy expenditure needed, is one area of exploration. Multiple stimulators, either surface electrodes or implantable, are needed to activate muscles needed for ambulation.

IV. SHOES

A. Shoes and Mobility

Among those with impaired mobility, shoes are often attached to lower extremity orthoses. In order to fulfill this function, the shoes, as well as the brace or braces, must be thoughtfully prescribed. The sole of the shoe should be constructed of leather, as rubber or Neoprene will not hold the orthotic rigidly in place. It is important that the shoes used have a good quality steel shank or are amenable to modification by the orthotist or shoe specialist. There is a tendency for a shoe to distort in the region of the longitudinal arch when an orthosis is attached. This distortion may precipitate pain or discomfort in many joints of the foot, resulting in a worsening of the individual's gait pattern as he or she flexes the knee to relieve stress at the brace and shoe.

B. Longitudinal Arch Support—Medial

Medial depression of the longitudinal arch is commonly seen in pes planus. Here, the navicular becomes prominent and the forefoot pronates. There are several shoe modifications that can be considered. A steel shank can be used, either alone, or in conjunction with a cookie. The cookie is a rigid leather support in the shape of the longitudinal arch. It can be removable, thus allowing it to be used in any shoe or it can be cemented in place.

A scaphoid or navicular pad is similar to a cookie and also provides medial arch support. However, it is made of compressable rubber and is used for those patients who cannot tolerate the cookie. Placement within the shoe is the same as with the cookie.

The University of California Biomedical Lab (UCBL) (13) is a newer modification that provides medial support along the sole but, more important, supports the calcaneus in the proper position (Fig. 8). This insert must be custom made and can be transferred between different pairs of shoes.

Medial wedging of the shoe may be prescribed if there is a greater need for shifting the body weight laterally than for support of the medial arch. (14) Wedging may be applied to the medial heel, sole, or along the entire length of the medial aspect of the shoe. Heel wedges shift weight in the region of the talocalcaneal and talonavicular joints. Sole wedges are used for changes in weight shifting in the tarsal and metatarsal areas. The full foot, or heel and sole wedge, is often used in valgus or medial arch depression and may be used in conjunction with an arch support.

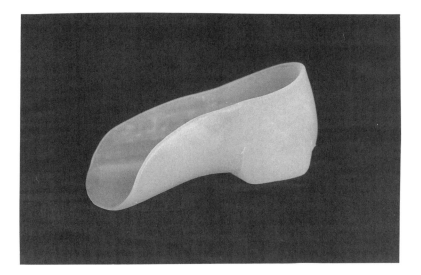

Figure 8   University of California Biomechanical Laboratory insert.

C. Longitudinal Arch Support—Lateral

The need for lateral longitudinal arch support arises in conditions including lateral pes planus, varus, and ankylosis. In all three, support and medial weight shift may be helpful. In these cases, wedging the lateral heel and sole may be of some help but often is ineffective in varus deformities, unless the deformity is nonrigid. Flaring the heel and/or sole may also offer some correction. In severe or very painful cases of varus or valgus, a T-strap may be used in conjunction with a brace as described in the orthotic section.

D. Metatarsal Support

Difficulty with adequate support or protection of the anterior metatarsal arch is responsible for many disabilities of the foot. Metatarsalgia pes cavus, fractures, plantar warts, and some deformities of the great toe are among the many deformities that can cause foot pain and gait dysfunction. Callus formation, which occurs as a result of pressure intolerance, further increases pain. There are several supports that may be prescribed to alleviate discomfort at the metatarsal heads and improve

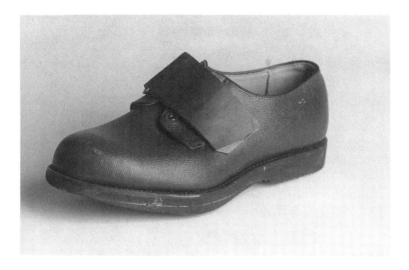

Figure 9   Rocker bottom shoe.

weight bearing by distributing weight over a more diffuse area. Chapter 9 reviews this area further.

Inside the shoe, a metatarsal pad may be used. This elevates the inner sole behind the metatarsal heads, off-weighting the painful areas.

A metatarsal bar is an external support that can be used alone or in conjunction with an insert. It is attached to the sole of the shoe in such a position that after heel strike, and roll over, the weight is borne behind the metatarsal heads not over them. Another external modification is the rocker bar or bottom (Fig. 9). The rocker bottom shoe overlay extends further over the toe than the metatarsal bar and, in addition to unweighting the metatarsal heads, reduces mid and hindfoot weight-bearing forces during push-off.

V. PROSTHETICS

A discussion of the process of prosthetic evaluation, prescription, and training is beyond the scope of this chapter. Several excellent texts and articles have been written and the reader is referred to them for additional information. (15)

VI. ASSISTIVE DEVICES FOR WALKING

Walking aids or assistive devices are often prescribed in order to improve balance, increase support, provide protection, and reduce lower extremity pain. The greater an individual's disability, the more extensive the assist needed. The most appropriate aid, as well as the safest gait pattern should be determined by a physician and/or a physical therapist.

A. Canes

Canes provide a minimal amount of support (Fig. 10). Up to a quarter of the patient's weight can be supported by a cane. (15) The tip of the cane, plus the patient's two feet create a tripod of support. The cane is generally held in the hand of the contralateral side, in cases of unilateral lower extremity involvement. The advantages of a straight cane are that they are inexpensive, and fit easily on stairs. The major disadvantage is the small base of support.

Canes are also available with a quadriped base of support (Fig. 11). The bases are available in several sizes. These aids increase an individual's base of support and thus provide more stability than a single point cane. They are often, however, difficult to use on stairs and some of the wider based quadriped canes will not fit on a standard-depth step.

B. Hemiwalker

A hemiwalker is also an assistive device with four feet. (Fig. 12) It combines features of a walker and a quadriped cane. In progressive gait training, it is often a transition between the parallel bars or walker and a quadriped cane. Its base of support is wider than a quadriped cane, and it is usually collapsible, making it easier to transport. The hemiwalker is particularly helpful with hemiplegic patients.

C. Walkers

Walkers provide the greatest amount of stability in balance during ambulation. They come in many models and sizes and are generally adjustable and can often be folded. A walker is frequently used early in gait training when balance and confidence are decreased. The main disadvantages are a slow, cumbersome gait; difficult maneuvering, particularly in close quarters such as the bathroom; the need to use both upper extremities; and great difficulty on stairs. A standard walker (Fig. 13) requires that the patient have sufficient standing balance and upper extremity

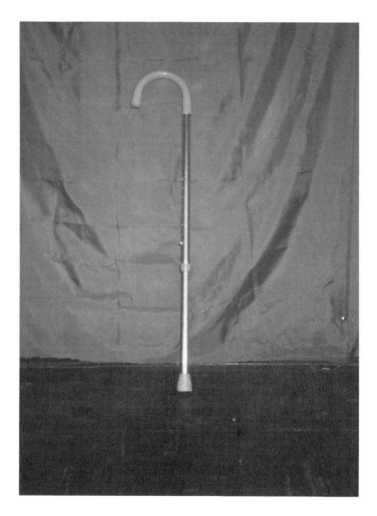

Figure 10 Straight cane.

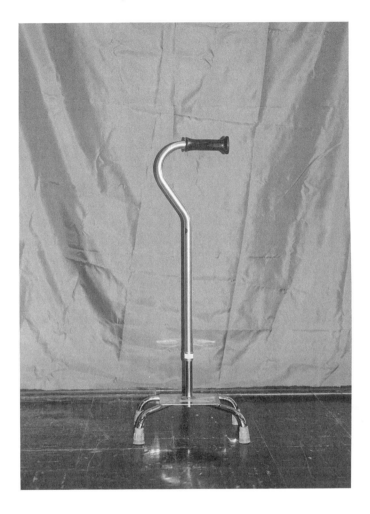

Figure 11 Quadriped cane.

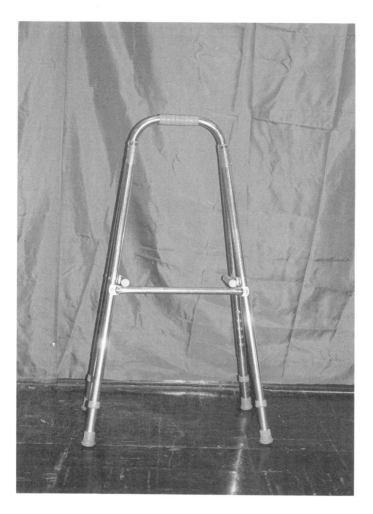

Figure 12 Hemiwalker.

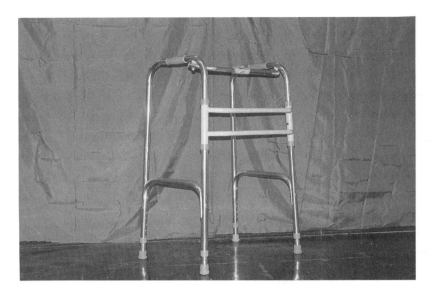

Figure 13 Walker.

strength to coordinate a forward movement by lifting the walker off the floor in order to advance it.

A rolling walker, or rollator (Fig. 14) has wheels on the front legs. The walker is advanced by lifting the back two legs and rolling the walker forward. This type of walker may be helpful for patients with upper extremity weakness or significant problems with balance, where lifting the entire walker is difficult. Problems have been noted, however, with diminished stabilization of the wheels.

D. Crutches

Crutches provide more support than canes. The standard axillary crutch requires good-to-normal upper extremity strength (Fig. 15). Many are adjustable. Standard axillary crutches are made of wood. The "ortho-crutch" is a single bar aluminum crutch, considered lighter than the wood. Axillary crutches can transfer 80% of body weight (16). Advantages of axillary crutches include good lateral stability, low cost, and ease of fit on stairs. The major disadvantage is the tendency of the

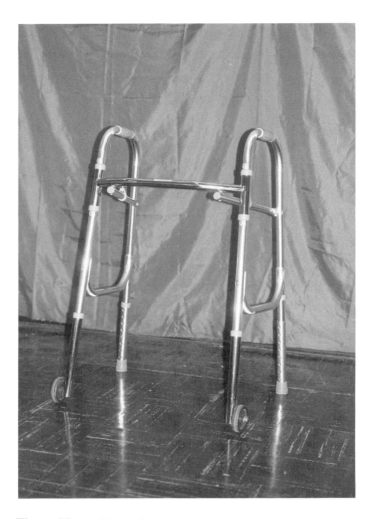

Figure 14   Rolling walker.

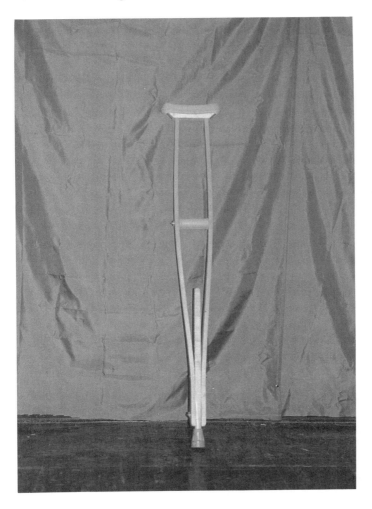

Figure 15 Axillary crutch.

patient to lean against the axillary piece, especially on stairs. Radial nerve compression or "crutch palsy" may occur.

Individuals with weak elbow extensors may have less difficulty with some of the upper arm crutches. The most commonly prescribed is the triceps crutch or Canadian. It has two cuffs, one above and one below the elbow. This type of crutch can transfer 40–50% of body weight (16). Patients using this type of walking aid can release the grip, without dropping the crutch. These crutches do require better control than do axillary crutches.

Loftstrand crutches have a forearm cuff to increase stabilization (17) during weight bearing (Fig. 16). They do not provide support above the elbow, as with the triceps crutches, but are otherwise comparable. Both nonaxillary crutch types are more expensive than their wooden axillary counterparts.

The platform crutch provides a horizontal platform or trough on which to rest the forearm, and a vertical hand grip (Fig. 17). Weight is distributed all along the forearm and wrists, instead of solely at the wrist and fingers. This crutch is especially useful for arthritic patients who

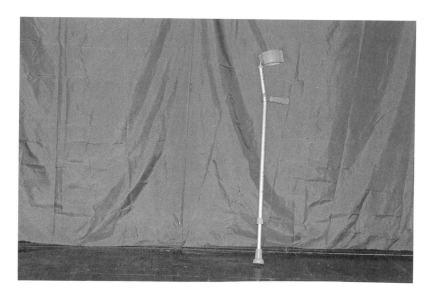

Figure 16 Forearm crutch.

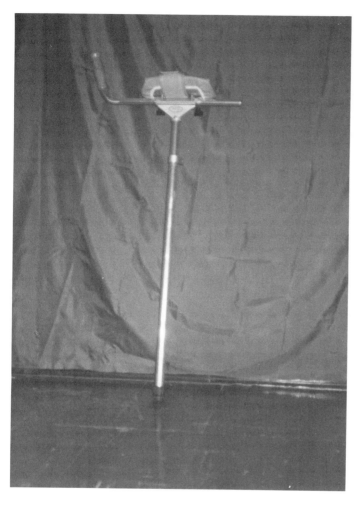

Figure 17 Platform crutch.

have a painful wrist or hand. Weakness of the fingers, flexion contracture of the elbow, or above the elbow amputation are also indications for prescription. Other attempts to provide adequate support during ambulation without exacerbating painful wrist and finger arthritis have been documented. Lofkvist et al. have constructed custom-molded handles on canes and crutches to allow their arthritic patients to sustain their level of mobility without significant negative effects on the upper extremity. (18) Their results have been encouraging, with most patients expressing great satisfaction and pain relief.

E. Fitting

Proper fitting of an assistive device is critical to its use. Cane length is determined by measuring from the top of the greater trochanter to the floor. (19) The elbow will be flexed approximately 30 degrees. A walker is fitted by positioning it 10–12 in. in front of the patient. The height should be adjusted until elbows are flexed approximately 20 degrees. The initial measurement for axillary crutches is often done with the patient supine. Measurement is taken from the anterior axillary fold to the bottom of the shoe heel. If the patient is barefoot, 1–2 in. should be added. The hand bar should be placed so that the elbow is in 30 degrees of flexion.

F. Gait Training and Patterns

In order for assistive devices to work properly, supporting and balancing the body, strength, and mobility of the upper extremities must be optimized. This strengthening program can and should be started even before the patient is ambulatory. The most important muscle groups of the shoulder girdle and upper extremity are the shoulder depressors (latissimus dorsi, lower trapezius, and pectoralis major), to stabilize the upper extremity and prevent hiking of the shoulder on weight bearing; elbow extensors (triceps and anconeus) to stabilize this joint during weight bearing by preventing flexion; wrist extensors (extensor carpi radialis and ulnaris) to hold the wrist in proper position to bear weight on the hand piece (19).

Determining the most appropriate assistive device depends on several things: trunk control, balance, upper body status, and weight bearing. Crutch walking can be divided into swing gaits and point gaits. The swing gaits are either swing-to or swing-through. Swing-to ambulation involves placing the crutches ahead first, then swinging the body to them. The swing-through gait requires more energy and necessitates the patient swinging his body beyond the level of the crutches.

A two-point gait sequence is opposite arm and leg moving simulta-neously. This is a stable gait and is effective for individuals with ataxia. The three-point gait involves moving both crutches or canes and the weaker, painful, lower extremity together, then the sound leg. This minimizes weight bearing on the affected leg and thus is preferred when that limb must be nonweight bearing. A four-point gait sequence is right crutch or cane, left foot, left side, right foot. Three points of support are always in contact with the floor making this a very stable, albeit slow, gait pattern. When only one cane is used, it should be contralateral to the affected extremity. The cane and affected limb are advanced first, making this either two- or three-point.

VII. WHEELCHAIR AND MOBILITY

A. Evaluation and Prescription

A wheelchair is a means of locomotion. It should be prescribed for those individuals who should not or cannot walk. It should also be available for those who may be capable of limited ambulation but lack the endur-ance or strength for sustained walking.

There are many different commercially available wheelchairs and a careful evaluation of the patient's needs and abilities should be com-pleted prior to prescription. The weight of the chair is often an impor-tant issue, either for the individual who propels it, or the caregiver who lifts it into a car. The lightest chair weighs approximately 24 pounds while a standard wheelchair is about 46 pounds. A motorized wheelchair can weigh 200 pounds.

B. Standard Wheelchair

The most commonly used wheelchair is the rearwheel drive chair (Fig. 18). This can be used by an individual with fair to fair-plus upper extrem-ity strength, on level surfaces. Insufficient hand grip strength can be compensated for by a hand rim projection and this type of wheelchair can also be motorized.

C. Amputee Wheelchair

Specialized amputee wheelchairs are also available (Fig. 19). These are constructed with the rear axle and rear (large) wheels set off posteriorly. This safety feature decreases the risk of tipping posteriorly when an

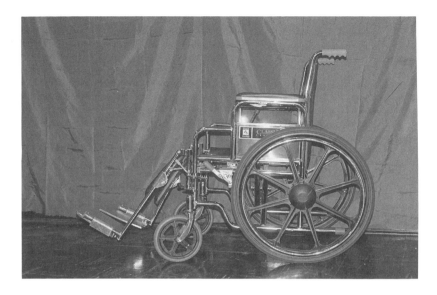

Figure 18   Standard wheelchair.

amputee leans backward while propelling the chair. It may also be advisable for patients with a strong upper body but with atrophic lower limbs. Tipping may also occur when propelling the wheelchair up an incline. When a patient without legs is using a standard wheelchair instead of an amputee chair, it is recommended that a sandbag of 10–15 pounds be positioned on the foot rests. (17)

D. One-Arm Drive Wheelchair

A one-arm drive wheelchair provides opportunity for independent wheelchair propulsion for those patients with absence or paralysis of an upper limb. In this chair, both wheels are driven by two hand rims mounted on the same side of the chair. This type of wheelchair is successfully used by many hemiplegic patients. However, a significant number of stroke patients can be taught to propel a standard wheelchair by coordinating propulsion by the unaffected foot with that of the unaffected arm. The one-arm drive chair is more expensive and heavier than a standard chair and may be more difficult to learn to use.

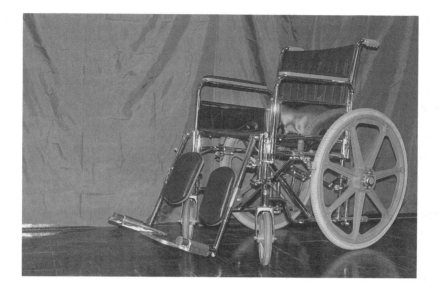

Figure 19 Amputee wheelchair.

E. Recliner

A reclining wheelchair is helpful for those individuals who cannot tolerate a seated position for long periods (Fig. 20). It is also used for quadriplegic patients whose sitting balance is not secure enough for them to be completely vertical. Recliners can be adjusted from near horizontal to upright. Although the reclining position does take some pressure off the buttocks and ischia, there is an increased shearing force acting on the posterior sacrum and sacral pressure is increased directly.

F. Motorized Chair

Motorized wheelchairs are indicated for those individuals with insufficient energy to propel a manual wheelchair or with significant paralysis (Fig. 21). This type of chair is generally operated by a joy stick or tiller, requiring only minimal movement from the user. More severely disabled patients can operate the chairs through breath control (sip and puff) or through the use of their voice.

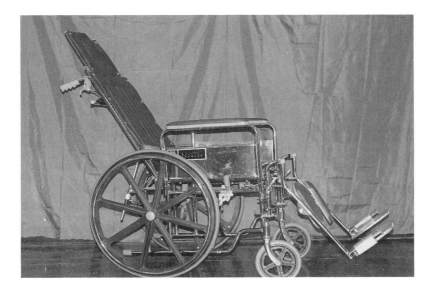

Figure 20   Recliner wheelchair.

These chairs rely on an electric battery for their power. The battery is usually 12 V. A fully charged battery provides power for 8 miles. Recharging can take place overnight.

The three-wheeled motorized chairs or scooters require better trunk and hand control. The central steering column makes transfers difficult, even if the seat swivels. It also makes it harder in some cases to come to a table. These scooters are often used for outdoor mobility only, as in patients with significant cardiac or pulmonary disease.

G. Wheelchair System

The components of a wheelchair system need to be evaluated carefully. A firm seat provides a surface for symmetric weight bearing. Lateral pads may help stabilize the trunk, preventing scoliosis. Head and neck supports provide proper positioning to patients with poor head control.

Arm rests give support to upper extremities, helping maintain trunk balance and offer support in sitting down or coming to stand. Removable arm rests can facilitate transfers, either those done by the patient or by caregivers. Desk arms are cut away at the front corners so

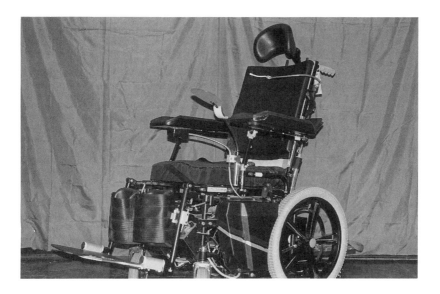

Figure 21   Motorized wheelchair.

that the wheelchair can roll further under a table. They are often removable, so that they can be reversed, positioning the existing parts of the arm rest at the wheelchair front. This provides support needed for push-off in transfers, or in coming to stand.

Foot plates or foot rests are often a part of wheelchair equipment. They can be shortened or lengthened according to the patient's leg length or seating position. Shortening foot rest length will often shift the patient's weight posteriorly, increasing weight over the ischia. Longer foot rests increase weight distribution over distal thighs. The user of swing-away or detachable foot rests facilitate movement onto and off the chair. Elevating foot rests are indicated in the treatment of lower extremity edema, either unilateral or bilateral. These leg rests require a calf piece to support the leg and prevent undue stress on the knee. Individuals with long leg casts or knee extension contractures should also be given wheelchairs with leg rests that can be raised. In many cases, it is advantageous to remove the foot rests, in order to permit propulsion to be done by the lower limbs. Some cardiac and pulmonary patients find this less fatiguing than propulsion by upper extremities.

VIII. ENERGY EXPENDITURE AND MOBILITY

The human body appears to have developed biomechanically to minimize energy expenditure. Our center of gravity has minimal displacement vertically or laterally. The forces influencing energy utilized in gait have been carefully investigated.

A. Normal Gait

Saunders et al. (20) described the six determinants of normal gait that act to minimize energy expenditure. Vertical displacement is smoothed by pelvic rotation, pelvic tilt, and knee flexion. Pelvic rotation elevates the end of the arc, and pelvic tilt and knee flexion lower the apex. The fourth determinant of gait, lateral displacement of the pelvis, reduces excess horizontal or lateral movement. The final two determinants are foot and ankle mechanisms. These help smooth the point of intersection of arcs of translation of the center of gravity. The end result is a sinusoidal pathway during gait.

In ambulation, energy expenditure is analyzed in terms of kilocalories per meter (kcal/m). Several studies have researched the energy expenditure during walking by normal subjects. At 80 m/min, Macdonald (20) found energy expenditures to be lowest—0.0083 kcal/m/kg body weight (BW) for men and 0.0076 kcal/m/kg BW for women. Other researchers have calculated the most energy-efficient speeds of ambulation to vary from the mid 70 m/min to 83 m/min (22–24).

B. Amputee Gait

In the amputee population, speeds of ambulation and energy expenditure change. Ralston (25) examined two below-knee (BK) amputees. At 48.8 m/min, their energy expenditure per unit time was similar to or less than that of normals walking at 73.2 m/min. He found their energy expenditure (kcal/unit distance) to be within the normal range. He determined that although the energy expenditure per step is higher in the amputee subjects, their energy expenditure per minute is similar to normal subjects when they can choose their most comfortable walking rate.

Gonzales et al. (26) studied BK amputee subjects walking at various speeds. Although they are comfortable at walking speeds slower than that of normal subjects (64.4 m/min versus 83.1 m/min), their energy expenditure was the same (0.062 kcal/min/kg versus 0.063 kcal/min/kg). He also noted that bilateral amputees walked 21% slower and expended 41% more energy per unit distance than normals.

C. Hemiplegia

In hemiplegia, changes also occur in gait and energy expenditure. Corcoran et al. (27) studied hemiplegic patients ambulating with plastic short leg braces, metal short leg braces, or without any brace. They found that oxygen consumption at various speeds without the braces in the hemiplegic subject was 64% higher than in normals. A metal brace reduced this to 54% above normal and plastic to 51% above normal. Significantly, the choice of metal or plastic made no statistical difference in oxygen consumption, walking speed, or stair climbing. Comfortable walking speeds without braces were 46% slower than in normal subjects. This improved to 39% when either type of brace was used.

D. Paraplegia

Paraplegic ambulation requires significant increases in energy. Clinkingbeard et al. (28) studied paraplegics at the thoracic and lumbar levels. Thoracic paraplegics ambulated at the average of 4.75 m/min and consumed 0.0076 kcal/m/k. They consumed nine times the energy per meter expended by normal subjects walking at their comfortable speed. The paraplegics with lesions in the lumbar region walked an average of 20.0 m/min and consumed 0.0024 kcal/m/kg, which was three times the energy expenditure of a normal subject at comfortable walking speed.

E. Wheelchair Mobility

A comparison of walking and wheelchair energetics in paraplegic patients was performed by Cerny et al. (29) in California. All subjects required bilateral KAFOs to walk. Level of injury was lower thoracic to upper lumbar. The investigators found that walking was significantly more inefficient than wheelchair propulsion, even for those paraplegic subjects who customarily used KAFOs for locomotion. The average velocity for the ambulators was less than half that for normal subjects, and the rate of oxygen uptake increased 50%. The oxygen uptake was increased to six times the value in normal subjects. When wheelchair propulsion was compared to normal walking, however, wheelchair propulsion was found to be an efficient mode of locomotion. Velocity was only 10% higher than normal subjects. Data showed that the energy cost of wheelchair propulsion approximated that of normal walking.

Other studies have also looked at wheelchair locomotion and support the findings of Cerny et al. Hildebrandt's group (30) studied individuals who had been wheelchair dependent for at least 2 years. At speeds ranging from 16.6–50 m/min, the net energy expenditure for wheelchair propulsion was found to be less than that used in walking at corresponding speeds. A linear relationship was noted between speed of propulsion and energy expenditure. Heart rate was significantly higher during wheelchair locomotion at all speeds, a result, perhaps, of increased heart rate with increased upper extremity work.

F. Crutch Walking

The increased energy expenditure associated with crutch walking varies, according to the type of crutches being used. Axillary crutch ambulation has been found to require no significant increase in energy expenditure over prosthetic ambulation in an above-knee amputee. (31) In contrast, the forearm crutch user walked about 33% slower than the AK prosthetic user and utilized approximately 40% more kcal/unit distance. (32) In a study using normal adults, McBeath et al. (33) found that both types of crutches, axillary and forearm, required about equal amounts of energy per minute for a swing-to gait.

IX. COMMUNITY MOBILITY

A. Architectural Barriers

For most travelers, the major factor limiting travel is cost. Yet for many individuals with impaired mobility, the opportunity for community mobility and travel may be limited as a result of architectural and transportation barriers. Architectural barriers can include curbs, stairs, and narrow doorways. The opportunity to return to work may be denied to an individual simply because the bathroom cannot accommodate a wheelchair or walker. The OT, TR Specialist, or PT, alone or in combination, can visit the worksite and evaluate its accessibility. Similar evaluations can be done for school or for the home.

Certain basic requirements will greatly facilitate mobility within a space as well as entry and exit from it. Doors should be 80 cm or more in width. Door knobs should be no higher than 90 cm from the floor.

Ramps are often used to alleviate the barriers imposed by stairs or curbs. The standard ramp gradient is 2.5 cm of rise per 30 cm of length (1 in. per foot). Newer studies (34) have demonstrated, however, that in certain cases ramp gradients of 1:10 or even 1:8 can be used, shortening the amount of ramp length required and perhaps facilitating installation.

B. Transportation Barriers

The obstacles imposed by architectural barriers, however significant, can often be overcome, particularly with the technology we possess. The issue of transportation barriers, however, has only recently begun to be addressed. Most people do not realize how insurmountable such seemingly minor obstacles as steps into a bus, curbs, or subway turnstiles can be. While modifications have begun and most towns offer some accessible transportation, the needs of those with impaired mobility are not being met.

The recently passed Americans with Disabilities Act (ADA), has mandated equal accessibility to the disabled in the workplace and on public transportation. More buses with lifts will be required as well as improved access to trains and airplanes. The ADA is being phased in over a period of years and so, for many, the struggle for community reintregation is not over.

C. Driving

Partly as a result of the difficulties utilizing public transportation, many individuals with special mobility needs will opt for driving. The number of disabled drivers varies. If it is defined as individuals in wheelchairs, the the number is small. However, if the definition is broadened to include other mobility impairments such as loss of a limb or arthritis, then the number of drivers increases and is a significant percentage of the total driving population. (35)

Many modifications are available to assist disabled drivers. Individuals with a missing or nonfunctional left leg may be unable to use the dimmer switch or parking brake. This can be compensated for with a hand-operated switch. Drivers with a missing or nonfunctional right leg may require a left foot accelerator. A bilateral lower extremity amputee or a paraplegic can be taught to use a hand-operated accelerator and brake. Here, too, a hand-operated dimmer switch and a parking brake may be needed.

An individual who has had a stroke may need a spinner knob mounted on the steering wheel to facilitate turning. Extensions may be needed to permit use of controls on the involved side.

A low-level quadriplegic—one who can transfer into a car—can use hand controls, a parking brake extension, a specialized steering system, a grab bar or strap for transfers, and specialized restraints.

A high-level quadriplegic will probably require a modified van in which to drive from the wheelchair. These vans have special lifts, raised roofs, and more elaborately constructed hand controls. Some controls can be controlled by head movement.

REFERENCES

1. Applegate WB, Blass JP, Williams TF. Instruments for the functional assessment of older patients. New Eng J Med 1990;332:1207–1214.
2. Nickel VL Mooney V. The application of lower extremity orthotics to weight bearing relief. Final narrative report. Rancho Los Amigos Hospital, Downy, California.
3. Lehmann JF, Warren CG, deLauter BJ, et al. Biomechanical evaluation of axial loading in ischial weight-bearing braces of various desings. Arch Phys Med Rehab 1970;51:331–337.
4. Sarmineto A, Sinclair WF. Application of prosthetics-orthotics principles to treatment of fractures. Artificial Limbs, 1967;11:28–32.
5. Davis FJ, Fry LR, Lippert FC, et al. The patellar tendon bearing brace: Report of 16 patients. J Trauma 1974;14:216–221.
6. Kosiak M. Decubitus ulcers. In: Krusen FH. Handbook of Physical Medicine and Rehabilitation, 2nd ed. Philadelphia, PA: W.B. Saunders Co., 1971:643–648.
7. Brand PW. The diabetic foot. In: Ellenberg M, Rifkin H, eds. Diabetes Mellitus: Theory and Practce, 3rd ed. New Hyde Park, New York: Medical Examination Publishing Co., Inc., 1983: 829–849.
8. Mueller MJ, Diamond JE. Biomechanical treatment approach to diabetic plantar ulcers: A case report. Phys Ther 1917–1920;1988.
9. Walker SC, Helm PA, Pullium G. Total contact casting and chronic diabetic neuropathic foot ulcerations: Healing rates by wound location. Arch Phys Med Rehab 1987;67:217–221.
10. Moebermon M. Crutches and cane exercises and use. In: E. Licht, ed. Therapeutic Exercise, Chapter 15, New Haven: Yale University Press, 1958:228–255.
11. Kamenetz HL. Wheelchairs and other indoor vehicles for the disabled. In: Redford JB. Orthotics Etcetera, 3rd ed. Baltimore: Williams and Wilkins, 1986:464–517.

12. Liberson WT, Holmquest MJ, Scot D, and Dow M. Functional electrotherapy. Stimulation of the peroneal nerve synchronized with swing phase of the gait of hemiplegic patients. Arch Phys Med 1961;42:101–105.
13. Lehmann JF. Lower limb orthotics. In: Redford JB. Orthotics Ectetera, 3rd ed. Baltimore: Williams and Wilkins, 1986:278–351.
14. Inman VT. UC-BL dual axis ankle control system and UC-BL shoe insert. Bull Prosthet Res 1969:10–11.
15. Zamosky I, Redford JB. In: Redford JB. Orthotics Etcetera, 3rd ed. Baltimore: Williams and Wilkins, 1986:388–452.
16. New York University Postgraduate Medical School. Lower Limb Prosthetics and Orthotics, rev ed. New York University, 1982.
17. Lofkvist VB, Braatstrom M, Geborek P, Lidgren L. Individually adapted lightweight walking aids with moulded handles for patients with severely deforming chronic arthritis. Scand Rheumatol 1988;17:167–173.
18. Okamoto GA, Gait disorders. In: Okamoto GA, Physical Medicine and Rehabilitation. Philadelphia: W.B. Saunders Company, 1984:6–12.
19. Jebsen R. Use and abuse of ambulation aids. JAMA 1967;199:63–68.
20. Takebe K, Kukulka C, Mysore GN, Milner M, et al. Peroneal nerve stimulator in rehabilitation of hemiplegic patients. Arch Phys Med 1975; 56:237–239.
21. Vauken E, Jeglic AG. Application of an implantable stimulator in the rehabilitation of paraplegic patients. Int Surg 1976;61:335–339.
22. Saunders JB, Inman VT, Eberhard HD. Major determinants in norman and pathological gait. J Bone Joint Surg (Am) 1953;35:543–558.
23. McDonald I. Statistical studies of recorded energy expenditure of man. Nutrit Abstr Rev 1961;31:739–762.
24. Ralston HJ. Energy-speed relation and optimal speed during level walking. Int Z Angew Physiol Einscert Arbeits Physiol 1958;17:277–283.
25. Corcoran PJ, Brengelmann GL. Oxygen uptake in normal and handicapped subjects, in relation to speed of walking beside velocity-controlled cart. Arch Phys Med Rehab 1970;51:78–87.
26. Waters RL, Perry J, Antonelli D, Hislop H. Energy cost of walking of amputees: influence of level of amputation. J Bone Joint Surg (Am) 1976;58:42–46.
27. Ralston HJ. Dynamics of the human body during locomotion: The efficiency of walking in normal and amputee subjects. Biomechanics Laboratory, University of California, San Francisco (Berkeley). Final Report, SRS Grang RD 2849-M, August 1971.
28. Gonzalez EG, Corcoran PJ, Reyes RL. Energy expenditure in below-knee amputees: correlation with stump length. Arch Phys Med Rehab 1974;55: 111–119.
29. Corcoran PJ, Jebsen RH, Breglemann GL, Simms BC. Effects of plastic and metal leg braces on speed and energy cost of hemiparetic ambulation in the traumatic paraplegic. Arch Phys Med Rehab 1970;51:69–77.

30. Clinkingbeeard JR, Gersten JW, Moehn D. Energy cost of ambulation in the traumatic paraplegic. Am J Phys Med 1964;43:157–165.
31. Cerny K, Waters R, Hislop H, Perry J. Walking and wheelchair energetics in persons with paraplegia. Phys Therapy 1980;60:1133–1139.
32. Hildebrandt G, Voight ED, Bahn D, Berendes B, et al. Energy costs of propelling wheelchair at various speeds: Cardiac response and steering accuracy. Arch Phys Med Rehab 1970;51:131–136.
33. Erdman WJ II, Hettinger T, Saez P. Comparative work stress for above-knee amputees using artificial legs or crutches. Am J Phys Med 1960;39: 225–232.
34. Inman VT, Barnes GH, Levy SW, Loon HE, et al. Medical problems of amputees. California Med 1961;94:132–138.
35. McBeath AA, Bahrke M, Balke B. Efficiency of assisted ambulation determined by oxygen consumption requirement. J Bone Joint Surg (Am) 1974;56:994–1000.
36. Sweeny GM, Harrison RA, Clarke AK. Portable ramps for wheelchair use–an appraisal. Int Disabil Stud 1989;11:68–70.
37. Vehicles and Adaptive Aides—A Buyer's Guide. Les Communications MVM Inc., Montreal, 1986.

14

The Impact of Physical Activity and Physical Fitness on Functional Capacity in Older Adults

LINDA S. PESCATELLO

New Britain General Hospital, New Britain, Connecticut

JAMES OAT JUDGE

University of Connecticut Health Center, Farmington, Connecticut

> All parts of the body which have a function, if used in moderation and exercised in labours in which each is accustomed, become thereby healthy, well-developed and age more slowly, but if unused and left idle they become liable to disease, defective in growth, and age quickly.
>
> Hippocrates (1)

I. INTRODUCTION

In 1900 the average life expectancy from birth was 47 years of age. By 1985 it was 75 years, and by 2050 it has been projected to be 80 years.

The older population, defined as individuals 60 years of age and older, has grown at a rate twice that of the entire United States population. In 1980, Americans 60 years of age and older for the first time surpassed two other age segments of the population, children less than 10 years of age and teenagers (2).

If these current trends continue, the most rapidly growing portion of the population will be the group most susceptible to disability and degenerative disease, persons aged 85 and older. Several futurists have proposed that the aging of our population will lead to an increased amount of time older persons will be afflicted with chronic disease, a greater period of dependence, and substantial increases in the demands for health care (3–5). Despite the social and economic hardships that potentially would occur as a result of these projections, medical care of the older person has typically disregarded the importance of functional living (6).

Aging has been defined as a decreased ability to adapt to stress, resulting from a decline in structure and function of the organ systems (7). The onset and rate of deterioration in these systems varies considerably from person to person. Furthermore, a decrement in one system may lead to dysfunction in another. For instance, maximum aerobic capacity ($\dot{V}O_2$ max) decreases with age (8,9). However, physical inactivity increases with age (10). Thus, the reported age-related decline in $\dot{V}O_2$ max may be due more to a decrease in physical activity than to decrements in determinants of cardiovascular function such as heart rate (HR), stroke volume (SV), and cardiac output ($\dot{Q}$). This example illustrates the difficulty in separating the alterations that occur with aging per se from those that have been associated with age such as disuse, depression, poor nutrition, and disease.

As seen in Table 1, the similarities between changes in structure and function that occur with age, and those that result from lack of physical activity are striking. Older persons are often limited in their activities because of generalized weakness, poor endurance, abnormal gait, and/or recurrent falls. Therefore, as Hippocrates suggested, an active lifestyle may attenuate the aging process by extending active life expectancy, the expected duration of functional wellbeing (11,12).

II. PHYSICAL ACTIVITY, PHYSICAL FITNESS, EXERCISE AND HEALTH

Individuals who are physically active, as well as those who are physically fit, have been found to have more positive cardiovascular risk factor

Table 1 Similar Physiological Alterations Associated with Age and Disuse

Characteristic	Aging	Disuse[a]
Body composition		
Lean body mass	↓ [b]	↓
Fat mass	↑ [c]	↑ , ↓
Bone mass	↓	↓
Cardiovascular function		
Exercise capacity ($\dot{V}O_2$ max)	↓	↓
Cardiac output (resting, maximal)	↓ , -[d]	↓
Stroke volume, resting	↓ ,−	↓
Stroke volume, maximal	↓ , ↑	↓
Heart rate, resting	↑ ,−	↓ ,−
Heart rate, maximal	↓	↑
Baroreceptor function	↓	↓
A - $\bar{V}O_2$ difference	↓ ,−	↓ ,−
Musculoskeletal system		
Muscle fiber number and size (type II> type I)	↓	↓
Muscle strength	↓	↓
Capillary density	↓	↓
Muscle oxidative capacity	↓	↓
Intramuscular fat and connective tissue	↑	↑
Metabolic/hematologic systems		
Basal metabolic rate	↓	↓
Exercise-induced hyperthermia	↑	↑
Glucose tolerance	↓	↓
Insulin sensitivity	↓	↓
Calcium balance	↓	↓
Cholesterol levels (low-density liproprotein)	↑	↑ ,−

[a] Disuse data were taken from studies of hypokinesia, immobilization, bed rest, or weightlessness.
[b] ↓ Decreased.
[c] ↑ Increased.
[d] No change in a majority of studies to date.
Source: Reprinted from *Topics in Geriatric Rehabilitation*, Vol. 5, No. 2, p. 64 with permission of Aspen Publishers, Inc., (c) 1990.

profiles compared to their sendentary counterparts. An active lifestyle has been shown to result in such health-related benefits as reduced incidence of osteoporosis (13), lower blood pressure (14, 15), more favorable blood lipid profiles (16,17), enhanced glucose tolerance and insulin sensitivity (18–20), greater muscle mass (21,22), controlled body weight (23–25) and improved psychosocial functioning (26). In addition, recent epidemiological evidence has found low levels of physical activity and physical fitness to be associated with an increased incidence of coronary heart disease (27) and all-cause mortality, especially in persons 60 years of age and older (28).

For an older person to function independently, a combination of cardiorespiratory endurance, muscle fitness, agility, and balance is needed. For instance, independence in shopping for food and household requires the cardiovascular fitness to walk up to a quarter mile, adequate balance to reach and carry items, and the muscle strength and agility to remove the bag contents (and oneself) from the bus or car. Independence in stair climbing and descending requires balance, strength, and cardio-vascular fitness as well.

In order to understand the impact of physical activity and physical fitness on functional capacity in older adults, it is necessary to define and distinguish between these commonly misued terms. *Physical activity* is bodily movement produced by the skeletal muscles that results in energy expenditure ranging from low to high. Physical activity is a behavior for which there is no standard measurement (29). Methods utilized to determine levels of physical activity include continual monitoring of physiological responses to movement with mechanical or electrical devices, and questionnaires designed to calculate self-reported weekly energy expenditure.

Exercise is a subset of physical activity. It is physical activity that is planned, structured, repetitive, and designed to improve or maintain physical fitness (29). Exercise-type activities are often associated with organized sports.

Physical fitness is classically defined as the ability to perform prolonged work and is measured by $\dot{V}O_2$ max. It is a set of characteristics that a person has or strives to achieve (29). Physical fitness is divided into two components: (1) skill-related, which includes agility, balance, coordination, speed, power, and reaction time; and (2) health-related, including cardiorespiratory endurance, body composition and muscle fitness, consisting of muscular strength, muscular endurance, and flexibility. The health-related components of physical fitness pertain to an ability to perform daily activities with vigor and demonstration of capacities associated with a low risk of developing premature degenerative disease (30,31). Because of their greater influence on function in older persons, our discussion will focus on the health-related component of physical fitness, namely, cardiorespiratory endurance and muscular fitness.

III. AGE-RELATED DECLINE IN $\dot{V}O_2$ MAX

The relationship between cardiovascular function and $\dot{V}O_2$ max is described by the Fick equation (32):

$$\dot{V}O_2 \text{ max} = \dot{Q} \text{ max} \times (a - \bar{V}O_2 \text{ diff}) \text{ max},$$

where $\dot{Q}$ max = maximal cardiac output and $(a - \bar{V}O_2 \text{ diff})$ max = maximal arteriovenous O_2 difference, or the ability of the muscles to extract O_2 from the blood.

There is general consensus in the literature that cardiorespiratory endurance, as measured by $\dot{V}O_2$ max, progressively declines with age (8,9,33–35). Beginning at 25 years of age, cross-sectional studies show a linear rate of decline in $\dot{V}O_2$ max of 0.40 to 0.50 ml/kg/min/yr, or approximately a 9% per decade decrease in sendentary men. Longitudinal studies generally report two times the age-related decline in $\dot{V}O_2$ max that cross-sectional studies have found (8). This range of variability has been attributed to limitations inherent in studies on exercise and aging such as: difficulty in isolating the true effects of aging from those of inactivity, problems in attaining a true $\dot{V}O_2$ max, and finding study volunteers who are representative of the older population (8,9,36,37). In addition, ambiguity also ensues from viewing populations from two different reference points, namely, cross sectionally at one point in time, or longitudinally over time.

Based upon an age-related decline or 0.45 ml/kg/min/yr, a sedentary 25-year-old man with a $\dot{V}O_2$ max of 45 ml/kg/min would be predicted to have a $\dot{V}O_2$ max of 18 ml/kg/min at 85 years of age. An old person with this low physical work capacity would find doing such activities of daily living as food shopping, general house cleaning, showering, and walking to be near maximal efforts, and probably would avoid them and/or be unable to perform them. Such a person would no longer be able to function independently, solely as a result of this sedentary lifestyle.

A. The Influence of Physical Training

The age-related decline in $\dot{V}O_2$ max can be attenuated when physical training is maintained. Heath and co-workers (33) matched young endurance athletes ($\bar{X}=22$ yr) with older endurance athletes ($\bar{X}=59$ yr) in a cross-sectional design. They found $\dot{V}O_2$ max to be lower in the master compared to the young athletes, 58.7 vs. 69.0 ml/kg/min, respectively. This decrease in $\dot{V}O_2$ max of 5% per decade in master athletes was half that reported in sedentary persons of comparable age. Because O_2 pulse ($\dot{V}O_2$ max/HR) was similar in both groups, these authors concluded that the decline in $\dot{V}O_2$ max was primarily due to the reduction in HR max that occurs with the aging process.

Rivera et al. (35) compared unmatched old ($\bar{X}=66$ yr) and young ($\bar{X}=32$ yr) distance runners, and found $\dot{V}O_2$ max to be reduced in the young runners from 70.4 to 45.0 ml/kg/min in the older runners. They attributed this decrement in $\dot{V}O_2$ max of 11% per decade to reduced training and decreases in HR max and SV in the old compared to young runners. Thus, it appears that younger athletes who reduce their activity levels will experience reductions in their physical work capacity as they age. Even though the relative amount of the age-related decrease in $\dot{V}O_2$ max is similar to sedentary persons, the absolute decline is less since their initial $\dot{V}O_2$ max was comparatively higher. Based upon a 0.45 ml/kg/min/yr linear decrease in $\dot{V}O_2$ max, a 25-year-old endurance athlete with a VO_2 max of 60 ml/kg/min at 25 would be estimated to have a VO_2 max of 33 ml/kg/min at 85 if training was reduced. A functional capacity of this value would enable this person to engage comfortably in self-care activities, contrasted to the sendentary individual described earlier.

Pollock and co-authors (34) studied 24 men between 50 and 82 years over a 10-year period. The subjects were divided into two groups: a competitive group who maintained their training level, and a post-competitive group who decreased their level of training. Over the 10-year period, $\dot{V}O_2$ max was reduced from 53.3 to 49.3 ml/kg/min for both groups combined. However, the $\dot{V}O_2$ max of the competitive groups decreased only 2% over this time period, from 54.2 to 53.3 ml/kg/min; whereas the $\dot{V}O_2$ max of the postcompetitive group declined 13% from 52.5 to 45.9 ml/kg/min. In summary, the age-related decline in $\dot{V}O_2$ max is attenuated in older men who maintain their level of physical training whether studied cross-sectionally or longitudinally.

With all the appropriate training stimulus, aerobic capacity can be improved at all ages. Even though the cardiovascular adaptations to physical training are relatively similar in older and younger individuals, the conditioning takes longer to occur and the absolute changes are less in older adults (38,39). Seals and co-workers (40) studied the effects of 6 months of low-intensity exercise (50% $\dot{V}O_2$ max) followed by 6 months of high-intensity exercise (85% $\dot{V}O_2$ max) in 11 men and women 60 years of age and older. $\dot{V}O_2$ max increased from 25.4 to 32.9 ml/kg/min, with the major portion of the increase occurring during the high-intensity exercise program. Since $\dot{Q}$ max was unchanged, the authors attributed the elevation in $\dot{V}O_2$ max to an increase in the a $- \bar{V}O_2$ diff. Interestingly, they reported orthopedic injuries to be more common and of greater severity during the high- rather than the low-intensity program.

More recently, Belman and Gaesser (41) examined the effects of training at exercise intensities below and above the threshold of lactate production in 17 older subjects from 65 to 75 years of age. Study volunteers were divided into a low-training intensity group (50% $\dot{V}O_2$ max), and a high-training intensity group (80% $\dot{V}O_2$ max) for 8 weeks. The increases in $\dot{V}O_2$ max were significantly different in pre- as compared to post-training, but they were not different between the groups, 25.4 to 27.2 ml/kg/min for the low-intensity group, and 24.3 to 26.1 ml/kg/min for the high-intensity group.

B. The Effects of Physical Activity and Physical Fitness

Despite the proported benefits of an active lifestyle, the amount of physical activity and physical fitness necessary to result in favorable health outcomes remains to be defined in older persons. Blair and co-workers (28) recently reported that the major reduction in all-cause death rates occurred between the low and moderately fit groups. Minimal additional benefit was conferred to the high fit individuals. In fact, the American College of Sports Medicine's Position Stand on the recommended quantity and quality of exercise for developing and maintaining cardiorespiratory and muscular fitness in healthy adults recently stated (42):

> . . . the quantity and quality of exercise needed to attain health-related benefits may differ from what is recommended for fitness benefits. It is now clear that lower levels of physical activity than recommended by this position statement may reduce the risk for certain chronic degenerative

diseases and yet may not be of sufficient quantity or quality to improve $\dot{V}O_2$ max.

Older adults are more predisposed to musculoskeletal and cardiovascular injury when exercising vigorously compared to younger persons (43). Therefore, the effect of increasing levels of physical activity on health outcomes and active life expectancy may be of greater magnitude than on physical fitness in this population.

In order to test this hypothesis, we studied the cross-sectional association of physical activity, as assessed from weekly energy expenditure by the Yale Physical Activity Survey, and physical fitness, as measured by estimated $\dot{V}O_2$ max to measures of resting cardiovascular function in 11 women and 14 men from 60 to 84 years of age (44). The Yale Physical Activity Survey contains five categories of common groups of activities pertinent to older persons. These categories include work, yard work, caretaking, transportation, and recreational activity (45). Resting diastolic blood pressure (DBP) and mean arterial pressure (MAP) were inversely related to weekly energy expenditure, whereas resting systolic blood pressure and HR were not. With a weekly energy expenditure of at least 6099 kcal/week, resting DBP was less for each increasing level of caloric expenditure. Similarly, for subjects reporting an weekly energy expenditure of greater or equal to 6099 kcal/week, resting MAP was lower compared to subjects who recalled expending less than this amount. In contrast, resting blood pressure did not show a significant association with $\dot{V}O_2$ max.

Our findings in older adults are consistent with reports in middle-aged populations that resting blood pressure is inversely related to weekly energy expenditure in healthy, active persons of middle age. A possible explanation for our observation of a stronger association of physical activity than physical fitness with resting blood pressure in older adults is that the movement pattern of active, older individuals is constant in nature and of low intensity (46). Active, older persons may expend enough kilocalories per week to result in lower resting blood pressure, but the intensity of their activities may not be of sufficient magnitude to significantly improve their $\dot{V}O_2$ max.

Our results (44), as well as those of Belman and Gaesser's (41), suggest that exercise programs for a majority of the older population should be conducted at low-to-moderate exercise intensities. Older adults should be primarily encouraged to move and increase their activity levels. An ideal activity that meets these criteria for older adults is walking. Regular walking is a weight bearing, yet low impact, activity that can be conducted at low-to-moderate exercise intensities. Furthermore, it results in sustained caloric expenditure. Further investigation is needed to quantify the dose of exercise that maximizes the health-related benefits of physical activity while minimizing the health-related risks in these individuals.

IV. AGE-RELATED ALTERATIONS IN MUSCULAR FITNESS

A. The Interrelationships of Cardiovascular and Muscle Fitness to Functional Status

Muscle mass, muscle strength, aerobic capacity, and functional status are inextricably related in older persons. Fleg and Lakatta (47) have shown parallel declines in muscle mass and aerobic capacity in longitudinal studies of healthy aging men. When they corrected $\dot{V}O_2$ max for lean body mass, much of the age-related decline in $\dot{V}O_2$ max disappeared. They concluded that much of the decrease in cardiovascular fitness in older persons when expressed as $\dot{V}O_2$ max in ml/kg, was due to reductions in muscle mass. Therefore, a loss of muscle mass, whether by disease or disuse, will result in a loss of cardiovascular fitness.

The hypothesis that aerobic fitness is dependent on muscle mass is further supported by two recent intervention studies. Frontera and co-authors (48,49) trained thigh muscles of 12 older men from 60 to 72 years using an intense resistance training program. Maximum weight lifted increased from 20 to 40 kg, isokinetic strength at different speeds increased from 8 to 18%, and cross-sectional area of thigh muscle increased 11% on Computerized Axial Tomography Scan. The thigh muscles had increased capillary density per muscle fiber, and increased capillary density per muscle fiber, and increased oxidative enzyme activity. Following the weight training program, there was an 11% improvement in $\dot{V}O_2$ max measured during leg cycle ergometry from 36.8 to 40.5 ml/kg fat free mass/min, but no change in $\dot{V}O_2$ max during arm ergometry. Since the study volunteers did not participate in an aerobic training program, these results support the hypothesis that the improvement in leg oxygen consumption was due to peripheral adaptations to resistance training.

An exercise program designed to improve aerobic capacity has been shown to enhance muscle strength in older persons which further illustrates the interrelatedness of cardiovascular endurance and muscle mass in this population. A long-term program of aerobic training and low-resistance exercise in older women (X=72 yr) improved $\dot{V}O_2$ max from 19.8 to 23.0 ml/kg/min and isokinetic strength 6.5% This program also increased muscle cross-sectional area (50). Another aerobic training intervention in older men improved cardiovascular fitness 38% and improved maximal isokinetic work performed in 30 s 12% (51).

B. Age-Related Decreases in Muscle Strength

As with $\dot{V}O_2$ max, muscle mass and muscle strength decline with advancing age, resulting in profound changes in body composition. In women over 60 years, body mass is stable or declines only slightly, but muscle mass is lost at a rate of about 0.5 kg annually. This results in an increase in percent body fat of approximately 1% annually in women and 0.5% in men who are over 60 years (52,53).

There is a preferential loss of type II or fast twitch fibers with increasing age, and diminished cross-sectional area of individual fibers. As the cross-sectional area of a muscle is the best predictor of force generation, the loss in cross-sectional area is responsible for much of the age-associated loss in strength. In longitudinal and cross-sectional data analyses, Kallman et al. (54) found an accelerated loss of upper extremity strength after age 70. When grip strength was compared with strength predicted by cross-sectional area of the forearm muscles, there was a decrease in force generation per cross-sectional area of muscle with increasing age.

Using a more quantitative measure of muscle area, Klitgard and co-authors (55) tested the strength/cross sectional area ratio of older men with different levels of physical activity. They compared healthy, sendentary older men with runners and weight lifters. As expected, weight lifters had substantially greater muscle mass than either the runners or sendentary men. However, runners and weight lifters were able to generate greater force/cm^2 of muscle than the sedentary men. These results imply that the pattern of usual activity may be a determinant of muscle strength in older persons. Furthermore, increasing levels of usual physical activity were associated with continued functional independence and lower rates of hip fractures in cohort studies of older persons (56, 57).

C. Functional Outcomes from Losses in Muscle Mass

A decreased muscle mass/total body mass ratio may be partially responsible for the loss of functional independence in older individuals. As this ratio declines, climbing stairs or getting up from a couch requires a greater activation of the remaining muscle. Activities that formerly required only 30% of maximal strength may now require 50 to 60% of maximal strength. Few people enjoy performing activities that involve muscle contractions at a high percentage of maximum strength. Thus, certain activities may become too demanding or unpleasant to perform regularly or repeatedly. Less stimulus to the muscle leads to further muscle weakness and functional impairment.

As discussed in Chapter 8, gait velocity is highly related to functional status. Thus, interventions that are successful in maintaining a normal pattern of gait will likely have profound effects on functional independence. If the pattern of gait is normal, walking at a normal pace does not require substantial muscle activation. However, there is probably a threshold of muscle strength below which the pattern of gait will be impaired. In a community sample, Bassey et al. (58) found moderate relationships (Pearson $r=.42$ for men, $r=.36$ for women, $p<.001$) of plantar flexor (calf) strength and gait velocity. In a small sample of nursing home patients who all had slow gait speeds, Fiatarone and co-workers (59) found a strong relationship between lower extremity strength to gait speed. Buchner and DeLatuer (60) also suggested a curvilinear effect of muscle strength on stride length in a larger study of community-dwelling older persons. In ambulatory life-care community residents over age 74, we found a substantial loss of gait velocity and stride length (corrected for height), when knee extension strength was below 48 N m (61). A thirteen week training program of lower leg resistance training and balance exercises increased usual gait velocity 8% (3-13%) from 1.04 ± 0.07 m s^{-1} to $1.12\pm$p$=0.06$ m s^{-1}, $p=.006$. This increase in gait was suprising in that the exercise program did not train walking, but trained the components necessary for adequate gait balance and strength.

Skeptics may argue that the loss in strength and function is due primarily to disease, and that disease causes limitations in activity which then lead to loss in cardiovascular fitness, muscular strength, and muscle mass. Prospective studies are addressing these issues. The relationship of muscle strength and gait is being assessed prospectively in the FICSIT (Frailty and Injuries: Cooperative Studies of Intervention Techniques) trials, which are testing exercise and behavioral interventions in persons over 75 years (62). These studies will determine whether interventions that improve muscle strength or balance will improve gait measures and functional status in older persons with multiple diseases.

V. CONCLUSIONS

Older persons ($\geq$ 60 yr) are often limited in their activities of daily living because of generalized muscle weakness, poor cardiorespiratory endurance, abnormal gait, and/or recurrent falls. Unfortunately, cardiorespiratory endurance, as measured by $\dot{V}O_2$ max, and muscle mass and muscle strength decline with advancing age. Maintenance of cardiovascular fitness and muscle strength through formal or home-based exercise programs may be a critical component of independent function in older individuals.

With the appropriate training stimulus, aerobic capacity and muscle strength can be enhanced at any age. Recent evidence indicates the major health benefits result from participation in physical activity done at low-to-moderate intensity that is performed on a frequent basis. In addition, the pattern of usual activity may also be a determinant of muscle strength, and thus continued functional independence in older persons. Since an active lifestyle may attenuate the aging process in certain older individuals by extending active life expectancy, health clinicians should encourage movement and increased activity in this population.

REFERENCES

1. Wallace AG. Fitness, health and longevity: A question of cause and effect. Inside Track 1986; 2(5): 3.
2. Dyckwall K, and Flower J. Age wave: challenges and opportunities for an aging America, New York: St. Martin's Press, 1989.
3. Manton KG. Changing concepts of morbidity and mortality in the elderly population. Milbank Mem Fund Q 1982; 60: 183.
4. Manton KG, and Soldo BJ. Dynamics of health changes in the oldest old: New perspectives and evidence. Milbank Mem Fund Q 1985; 63: 206.
5. Schneider EL, Brody JA. Aging, natural death and the compression of morbidity: Another view. N Engl J Med 1983;309(14): 854.
6. Katz S, Branch LG, Branson MH, Papsidero JA, Becka JC, Greer DS. Active life expectancy. N Engl J Med 1983;309: 1218.
7. Kennedy RA. Physiology of aging. A synopsis. Chicago: Year Book Medical Publishers, Inc., 1984.
8. Buskirk ER, Hodgson JL. Age and aerobic power: the rate of change in men and women. Fed Proc 1987; 46: 1824.
9. Hagberg JM. Effect of training on the decline of $\dot{V}O_2$ max with aging. Fed Proc 1987;46: 1830.
10. Blair SN, Brill, PA, Kohl III, HW. Physical activity patterns in older individuals. In American Academy of Physical Education Papers (No. 22),

Physical activity and aging. Champaign, IL: Human Kinetics Books 1988: 120–139.

11. Bortz WM. Disuse and aging. JAMA 1982;248: 1203.

12. Fiatarone MA, Evans WJ. Exercise in the oldest old. Top Geriatr Rehab 1990;5(2): 63.

13. Dalsky GP. The role of exercise in the prevention of osteoporosis. Comp Ther 1989;15: 30.

14. Tipton CM. Exercise, training, and hypertension. In Terjung RL, ed. Exercise and Sport Science Reviews. Lexington, MA: Collamore Press, 1984: 245.

15. Tipton CM. Exercise, training and hypertension. In Holloszy JO. ed. Exercise and Sport Science Reviews. Lexington, MA: Collamore Press, 1991: 447.

16. Cook TC, Laporte RE, Washburn RA, Traven ND, Slemenda CW, Metz KF. Chronic low level physical activity as a determinant of high density lipoprotein cholesterol and subfractions. Med Sci Sports Exerc 1986; 18(6): 653.

17. Dannenberg AL, Keller JB, Wilson PWF. Leisure-time physical activity in the Framingham Offspring Study. Am J Epidemiol 1989;129: 76.

18. Helmrich SP, Ragland DR, Leung RW, Paffenbarger RS. Physical activity and reduced occurrence of non-insulin dependent diabetes mellitus. N Engl J Med 1991;325: 147.

19. Seals DR, Hagberg JM, Allen WK. Glucose tolerance in young and older athletes and sedentary men. J Appl Physiol 1984;56: 1521.

20. Sherman WM, Albright A. Exercise and type I Diabetes, Sports Science Exchange. Chicago, IL: Gatorade Sports Science Institute, 1990:3(25).

21. Ballor DL, Katch VL, Becque MD, Marks CR. Resistance weight training during caloric restriction enhances lean body weight maintenance. J Clin Nutr 1988;47: 19.

22. Saris WHM, Van Dale D. Effects of exercise during VLCD diet on metabolic rate, body composition and aerobic power. Pooled data of four studies. Intern J Obesity 1989;13(Suppl 2): 169.

23. Lennon D, Nagle F, Stratman F, Shirago E, Dennis S. Diet and exercise training effects on resting metabolic rate. Intern J Obes 1985;9: 39.

24. Molè PA, Stern JS, Schultz CL, Bernaver EM, Holcomb BJ. Exercise reverses depressed metabolic rate produced by severe caloric restriction. Med Sci Sports Exerc 21(1): 29.

25. Poehlman ET, Melby CL, and Goran MI. The impact of exercise and diet restriction on daily energy expenditure. Sports Med 1991;11: 78.

26. Morgan WP, Goldston, SE. Exercise and mental health. Hagerstown, MD, Hemisphere Publishing Co., 1987.

27. Leon AS, Connett J, Jacobs DR, Rauramaa R. Leisure-time physical activity levels and risk of coronary heart disease and death. The Multiple Risk Factor Intervention Trial. JAMA 1987;258: 2388–2395.

28. Blair SN, Kohl III HW, Paffenbarger RS, Clark DG, Cooper, KH, Gib-

bons, LW. Physical fitness and all-cause mortality. A prospective study of healthy men and women. JAMA 1989;262: 2395.

29. Caspersen CJ, Powell KE, Christenson GM. Physical activity, exercise and physical fitness: definitions and distinctions for health-related research. Public Health Rep 1985;100(2): 126.

30. American College of Sports Medicine. Guidelines for exercise testing and prescription, 4th ed.. Philadelphia: Lea and Febiger, 1991.

31. Pate RR. The evolving definition of physical fitness. Quest 1988;40: 174.

32. Astrand P, Rodahl K. Textbook of work physiology. Physiological bases of exercise. New York: McGraw-Hill, 1986.

33. Heath GW, Hagberg JM, Ehsani AA, Holloszy JO. A physiological comparison of young and old endurance athletes. J Appl Physiol 1981;51(3): 634.

34. Pollock ML, Foster C, Knapp D, Rod JL, Schmidt DH. Effect of age and training on aerobic capacity and body composition of master athletes. J Appl Physiol 1987;62(2): 725.

35. Rivera AM, Pels AE, Sady SP, Sady MD, Cullinane EM, Thompson PD. Physiological factors associated with the lower maximal consumption of master runners J Appl Physiol 1989;66: 949.

36. Gerstenblith G, Renlund DG, Lakatta EG. Cardiovascular response to exercise in younger and older men. Fed Proc 1987;46: 1834.

37. Shephard RJ. The aging of cardiovascular function. In American Academy of Physical Education. Physical activity and aging. Champaign, IL: Human Kinetics Books, 1988:175–185.

38. Ehsani AA. Cardiovascular adaptations to exercise training in the elderly. Fed Proc 1987;46: 1840.

39. Pollock ML, Wilmore JH. Exercise in health and disease. Evaluation and prescription in prevention and rehabilitation, 2nd ed. Philadelphia: W.B. Saunders Co., 1990.

40. Seals DR, Hagberg JM, Hurley BF, Ehsani AA, Holloszy JO. Endurance training in older men and women. I. Cardiovascular responses to exercise. J Appl Physiol 1984;57:1024–1029.

41. Belman MJ, Gaesser GA. Exercise training below and above the lactate threshold in the elderly. Med Sci Sports Exerc 1991;23(5): 562.

42. American College of Sports Medicine. The recommended quantity and quality of exercise for developing and maintaining cardiorespiratory and musclar fitness in healthy adults. Med Sci Sports Exerc 1990;22: 265.

43. Shephard RJ. Can we identify those for whom exercise is hazardous? Sports Med 1984;1: 75.

44. Pescatello LS, DiPietro L, Fargo AE, Caspersen CJ, Ostfeld AM, Nadel ER. The impact of physical activity and physical fitness on health outcomes in older adults. J Aging Phys Activ 2:2.

45. DiPietro L, Caspersen CJ, Ostfeld AM, Nadel ER. The comparison of two surveys for assessing physical activity in older adults. Med Sci Sports Exerc 25:628.

46. Folsom AR, Caspersen CJ, Taylor HJ. Leisure time activity and its relationship to coronary risk factors in a population based sample. Am J Epidemiol 1985;121(4): 570.
47. Fleg JL, Lakatta EG. Role of muscle loss in the age-associated reduction in ˙VO₂ max. J Appl Physiol 1988;65: 1147.
48. Frontera WR, Meredith CN, O'Reilly KP, Evans WJ. Strength training and determinants of V̇O₂ max in older men. J Appl Physiol 1990;68: 329.
49. Frontera WR, Meredith CN, O'Reilly KP, Knuttgen HG, Evans WJ. Strength conditioning in older men: skeletal muscle hypertrophy and improved function. J Appl Physiol 1988;64: 1038.
50. Cress ME, Thomas DP, Johnson J, Kasch FW, Cassens RG, Smith EL, Agre JC. Effects of training on V̇O₂ max, thigh strength, and muscle morphology in septuagenarian women. Med Sci Sports Exerc 1991; 23(6): 752.
51. Jones NL, McCartney N. Influence of muscle power on aerobic performance and the effects of training. Acta Med Scand 1986;711(Suppl.): 115.
52. Aloia JF, McGowan DM, Vaswani AN, Ross P, Cohn SH. Relationship of menopause to skeletal and muscle mass. Am J Clin Nutr 1991;53: 1378.
53. Flynn MA, Nolph GB, Baker AS, Martin WM, Krause G. Total body potassium in aging humans: a longitudinal study. Am J Clin Nutr 1989;50: 713.
54. Kallman DA, Plato CC, Tobin JD. The role of muscle loss in the age-related decline of grip strength: cross-sectional and longitudinal perspectives. J Gerontol 1990;45(3): M82.
55. Klitgaard H, Mantoni M, Schiaffino S, Ausoni S, Forza L, Laurent-Winter C, Schnohr P, Saltin B. Function, morphology and protein expression of aging skeletal muscle: a cross-sectional study of elderly men with different training backgrounds. Acta Physiol Scand 1990;140: 41.
56. Farmer ME, Harris T, Madans JH, Wallace RB, Cornoni-Huntley J, White LR. Anthropometric indicators and hip fracture. J Am Geriatr Soc 1989; 37: 9.
57. Harris T, Kovar MG, Suzman R, Kleinman JC, Feldman JJ. Longitudinal study of physical ability in the oldest-old. Am J Publ Health 1989;79: 698.
58. Bassey EJ, Bendall MJ, Pearson M. Muscle strength in the triceps surae and objectively measured customary walks activity in men and women over 65 years of age. Clin Sci Lond 1988;74: 85.
59. Fiatarone MA, Marks EC, Ryan ND, Meredith CN, Lipsitz LA, Evans W. High intensity strength training in non-agenarians: effects on skeletal muscle. JAMA 1990;263: 3029.
60. Buchner D, DeLateur B. The importance of skeletal muscle strength to physical function in older adults. Ann Behav Med (in press).
61. Judge JO, Underwood M, Gennosa T. Exercise improves gait velocity in older persons. Arch Phys Med Rehabil (in press).
62. Ory M, Schechtman K, Miller, JP, Fiatarone M, Province M, Arfken C, Morgan D, Weiss S. Frailty and injuries in later life: The FICSIT trails. J Am Geriatr Soc (in press).

Index

[Arthritis]
  seronegative, in foot and ankle,
    214
Assistive devices,
  for fall prevention, 260
  for walking, 303–312
Ataxia, 123, 129, 234–238
Avoidance strategies, 67

Balance, 81, 85–86, 247
Basal ganglia,
  anatomy, 131
  locomotion, role in, 61, 68, 133
Base of support, 107
Benzodiazepines, 234
Binswanger's disease, 84, 162
Bracing (*see* Orthotics)

Cane, 303
Center of gravity, 105
Cerebellar system,
  anatomy, 118–122
  anterior lobe syndrome, 123, 127
  Friedreich's disease, 128
  gait, 85
  role in gait control, 123
  vestibulocerebellar dysfunction,
    127
Chloroquine, 230
Chorea, 140
  differential diagnosis, 144
  see also specific diseases
Clofibrate, 231
Clozapine, 234
Cognitive maps, 72
Computerized gait analysis (*see*
    Gait, clinical analysis of)

Core locomotor pattern, 55, 57–60
Corns and calluses, 200
Cortico-basal degeneration, 83,
    135
Crutches, 307–312
  axillary, 307
  Canadian, 310
  energy expenditure, 320
  forearm, 310
  gait patterns, 312–313
  platform, 310

Diabetic foot disease, 194, 195,
    218–219
  orthotic in, 293
Disequilibrium, 85
Diuretics, 229–230, 231
Dopamine, 134
Driving, 321–322
Drugs (*see* Medications)
Dystonia, 84, 143–149
  classification, 146
  see also specific diseases

Elderly (*see* Older adults)
Electronystagmography (ENG), 98
Electrophysiological bracing, 298–
    300
Equilibrium, 62, 65, 80
Essential tremor, 149
Exercise, 328, 331
  for fall prevention, 259
  health benefits of, 331–333
  walking, 333
Extrapyramidal motor system (*see*
    Basal ganglia)

About the Editor

BARNEY S. SPIVACK is Director of the Geriatrics Subsection of the Department of Medicine and an Attending Physician at Norwalk Hospital, Connecticut, and an Assistant Clinical Professor in the Department of Internal Medicine at Yale University School of Medicine, New Haven, Connecticut. The author or coauthor of numerous professional publications, Dr. Spivack is a Fellow of the American College of Physicians and the American College of Rheumatology, and a member of the American Geriatrics Society, among others. He received the B.A. degree (1974) in English from Brooklyn College of the City University of New York, New York, and the M.D. degree (1978) from Mount Sinai School of Medicine of the City University of New York, New York.